Placenta and Trophoblast

METHODS IN MOLECULAR MEDICINE™

John M. Walker, SERIES EDITOR

METHODS IN MOLECULAR MEDICINE™

Placenta and Trophoblast

Methods and Protocols

Volume 2

Edited by

Michael J. Soares

Institute of Maternal–Fetal Biology
Division of Cancer and Developmental Biology
Department of Pathology and Laboratory Medicine
University of Kansas Medical Center, Kansas City, KS

Joan S. Hunt

University Distinguished Professor, Vice Chancellor for Research
Department of Anatomy and Cell Biology
University of Kansas Medical Center, Kansas City, KS

HUMANA PRESS ✳ TOTOWA, NEW JERSEY

Library of Congress Cataloging in Publication Data
Placenta and trophoblast: methods and protocols / edited by Michael J. Soares and Joan S. Hunt.
       p. ; cm. — (Methods in molecular medicine ; 121-122)
    Includes bibliographical references and index.
    ISBN 1-58829-404-8 (alk. paper) — ISBN 1-58829-608-3 (alk. paper)
    1. Placenta. 2. Molecular biology.
    [DNLM: 1. Placenta. 2. Molecular Biology. WQ 212 P6974 2005] I.
    Soares, Michael J. II. Hunt, Joan S. III. Series.
    QP281.P5435 2005
    612.6'3—dc22   2005006428

Preface

The aim of the two-volume set of *Placenta and Trophoblast: Methods and Protocols* is to offer contemporary approaches for studying the biology of the placenta. The chapters contained herein also address critical features of the female organ within which the embryo is housed, the uterus, and some aspects of the embryo–fetus itself, particularly those of common experimental animal models. In keeping with the organization used effectively in other volumes in this series, each chapter has a brief introduction followed by a list of required items, protocols, and notes designed to help the reader perform the experiments without difficulty. In both volumes, sources of supplies are given and illustrations highlight particular techniques as well as expected outcomes. A key aspect of these volumes is that the contributors are at the forefronts of their disciplines, thus ensuring the accuracy and usefulness of the chapters.

Placenta research has progressed rapidly over the past several decades by taking advantage of the technical advances made in other fields. For example, the reader will note that many techniques, such as reverse transcriptase polymerase chain reaction, northern and western blotting, microarray analyses and *in situ* hybridization experiments, are routinely used for dissecting a wide range of experimental questions. Protein analysis and functional experiments on tissues and cells that comprise the maternal–fetal interface benefit from studies in endocrinology, immunology, and developmental biology. These volumes also present new ideas on investigating gene imprinting and gene transfer via viral vectors.

In developing these volumes we encountered the problem of how to organize the contents so as to be reader-friendly. Our decision was to subdivide in large part by the chronology of pregnancy so that in vivo aspects of implantation come first, followed by in vitro systems of investigation, then protocols for phenotypic analyses of placentas of several species. Special techniques mentioned above conclude Volume I. Volume II continues with protocols for studying trophoblast invasion, followed by dissection of how invading trophoblast cells might be received by uterine immune cells. Returning to the placenta itself, methods for researching trophoblast endocrine and transport functions are followed by a final series of chapters on how placentas adapt to disease. In this latter group, two chapters offer help to investigators interested in animal models of human placental disorders and two address working with the oxygen switches that program gene expression in early pregnancy, a concept entirely unexplored less than a decade ago. The reader is referred to the Introductions in each of the two volumes for a more detailed description of the contents.

This project would not have been possible without the contributions of many individuals. We wish to express our gratitude to the contributing authors for their time, effort, creativity, and their willingness to share their knowledge and expertise. Our deep appreciation and gratefulness also goes to Stacy Mc-Clure for her dedicated efforts in maintaining the organization of the manuscripts and the correspondence between the editors and the authors. During this process the publisher has provided us with helpful guidance and instruction essential for the completion of this effort.

Finally, we hope that these volumes are useful and provide a valuable resource for both trainees and established scientists striving to advance our understanding of this unique, entirely essential organ of reproduction.

Michael J. Soares
Joan S. Hunt

Contents

vii

Contributors

VIKKI M. ABRAHAMS • *Reproductive Immunology Unit, Department of Obstetrics and Gynecology, Yale University School of Medicine, New Haven, CT*

RUPASRI AIN • *Institute of Maternal-Fetal Biology, Division of Cancer & Developmental Biology, Department of Pathology & Laboratory Medicine, University of Kansas Medical Center, Kansas City, KS*

ADAM R. ALT • *Institute of Maternal-Fetal Biology, Division of Cancer & Developmental Biology, Department of Pathology & Laboratory Medicine, University of Kansas Medical Center, Kansas City, KS*

JOHN APLIN • *Academic Unit of Obstetrics and Gynaecology, Division of Human Development, Medical School, University of Manchester, Manchester, United Kingdom*

KENNETH L. AUDUS • *Department of Pharmaceutical Chemistry, School of Pharmacy, University of Kansas, Lawrence, KS*

ELIZABETH BALL • *Departments of Obstetrics and Gynaecology, Royal Victoria Infirmary, University of Newcastle upon Tyne, Newcastle upon Tyne, United Kingdom*

CHARLES BALZLI • *Department of Physiology and Biophysics, University of Mississippi Medical Center, Jackson, MS*

ELLEN M. BARBER • *Center for Study of Reproductive Biology and Women's Health, Department of Developmental and Molecular Biology, Albert Einstein College of Medicine of Yeshiva University, Bronx, NY*

FULLER W. BAZER • *Center for Animal Biotechnology and Genomics, Department of Animal Science, Texas A&M University, College Station, TX*

WILLIAM BENNETT • *Department of Obstetrics and Gynecology, University of Mississippi Medical Center, Jackson, MS*

CLAUDIA J. BODE • *Department of Pharmaceutical Chemistry, School of Pharmacy, University of Kansas, Lawrence, KS*

GENNADIY I. BONDARENKO • *National Primate Research Center, University of Wisconsin-Madison, Madison, WI*

EDITH BREBURDA • *National Primate Research Center, University of Wisconsin-Madison, Madison, WI*

JUDITH N. BULMER • *Department of Pathology, Royal Victoria Infirmary, University of Newcastle upon Tyne, Newcastle upon Tyne, United Kingdom*

GRAHAM J. BURTON • *Department of Anatomy, University of Cambridge, Cambridge, United Kingdom*

JUDITH E. CARTWRIGHT • *Department of Basic Medical Sciences, Biochemistry and Immunology, St. George's Hospital Medical School, London, United Kingdom*

DERRICK CHANDLER • *Department of Physiology and Biophysics, University of Mississippi Medical Center, Jackson, MS*

CHIWEN CHANG • *Department of Pathology, University of Cambridge, Cambridge, United Kingdom*

D. STEPHEN CHARNOCK-JONES • *Department of Obstetrics and Gynaecology, University of Cambridge, Cambridge, United Kingdom*

THOMAS J. COOK • *Department of Pharmaceutics, Ernest Mario School of Pharmacy, Rutgers, The State University of New Jersey, Piscataway, NJ*

KATHY COCKRELL • *Department of Physiology and Biophysics, University of Mississippi Medical Center, Jackson, MS*

B. ANNE CROY • *Department of Anatomy and Cell Biology, Queen's University, Kingston, Ontario, Canada*

SVETLANA V. DAMBAEVA • *National Primate Research Center, University of Wisconsin-Madison, Madison, WI*

MAUREEN DURNING • *National Primate Research Center, University of Wisconsin-Madison, Madison, WI*

ASGERALLY T. FAZLEABAS • *Department of Obstetrics & Gynecology, Center for Women's Health & Reproduction, University of Illinois, Chicago, IL*

YOU-JUN FEI • *Department of Biochemistry and Molecular Biology, Medical College of Georgia, Augusta, GA*

VADIVEL GANAPATHY • *Department of Biochemistry and Molecular Biology, Medical College of Georgia, Augusta, GA*

LUCY GARDNER • *Department of Pathology, University of Cambridge, Cambridge, United Kingdom*

ARIEH GERTLER • *Institute of Biochemistry, Food Science and Nutrition, Faculty of Agriculture, The Hebrew University of Jerusalem, Jerusalem, Israel*

JOCELYN D. GLAZIER • *Academic Unit of Child Health, Human Development and Reproductive Healthcare Academic Group, University of Manchester, St. Mary's Hospital, Manchester, United Kingdom*

THADDEUS G. GOLOS • *National Primate Research Center and Department of Obstetrics and Gynecology, University of Wisconsin-Madison, Madison, WI*

NORBERTO C. GONZALEZ • *Department of Molecular and Integrative Physiology, University of Kansas Medical Center, Kansas City, KS*

JOEY P. GRANGER • *Department of Physiology and Biophysics, University of Mississippi Medical Center, Jackson, MS*

JONATHAN A. GREEN • *Department of Animal Science, University of Missouri-Columbia, Columbia, MO*

SUSAN L. GREENWOOD • *Academic Unit of Child Health, Human Development and Reproductive Healthcare Academic Group, University of Manchester, St. Mary's Hospital, Manchester, United Kingdom*

INDIRA GULERIA • *Transplantation Research Center and Center for Neurologic Diseases, Children's Hospital at Harvard University, Boston, MA*

MYRIAM HANSSENS • *Department of Obstetrics and Gynaecology, University Hospital Gasthuisberg, Katholieke Universiteit Leuven, Leuven, Belgium*

WILLIAM W. HAY, JR. • *Perinatal Research Center, Department of Pediatrics, University of Colorado School of Medicine, Aurora, CO*

JENNIFER K. HO-CHEN • *Institute of Maternal-Fetal Biology, Department of Molecular and Integrative Physiology, University of Kansas Medical Center, Kansas City, KS*

JOAN S. HUNT • *Department of Anatomy and Cell Biology, University of Kansas Medical Center, Kansas City, KS*

ERIC JAUNIAUX • *Academic Department of Obstetrics and Gynaecology, Royal Free and University College, London, United Kingdom*

HONG JIN • *Department of Pharmaceutical Chemistry, School of Pharmacy, The University of Kansas, Lawrence, KS*

S. ANANTH KARUMANCHI • *Department of Medicine, Obstetrics and Gynecology, Harvard Medical School and Beth Israel Deaconess Medical Center, Boston, MA*

GREGORY T. KNIPP • *Department of Pharmaceutics, Ernest Mario School of Pharmacy, Rutgers, The State University of New Jersey, Piscataway, NJ*

B. BABBETTE D. LAMARCA • *Department of Physiology and Biophysics, University of Mississippi Medical Center, Jackson, MS*

DAUDI K. LANGAT • *Department of Anatomy and Cell Biology, University of Kansas Medical Center, Kansas City, KS*

DANIEL I. H. LINZER • *Department of Biochemistry, Molecular Biology, and Cell Biology, Northwestern University, Evanston, IL*

RAMSEY H. MCINTIRE • *Department of Anatomy and Cell Biology, University of Kansas Medical Center, Kansas City, KS*

ASHLEY MOFFETT • *Department of Pathology, University of Cambridge, Cambridge, United Kingdom*

GIL MOR • *Reproductive Immunology Unit, Department of Obstetrics and Gynecology, Yale University School of Medicine, New Haven, CT*

PEDRO J. MORALES • *Department of Anatomy & Cell Biology, University of Kansas Medical Center, Kansas City, KS*

HEINER MÜLLER • *Department of Obstetrics and Gynecology, University of Rostock, Rostock, Germany*

JACQUIE NORTHFIELD • *Department of Pathology, University of Cambridge, Cambridge, United Kingdom*

JOSEPH ORLY • *Department of Biological Chemistry, The Alexander Silberman Institute of Life Sciences, The Hebrew University of Jerusalem, Jerusalem, Israel*

JUDITH L. PACE • *Department of Molecular and Integrative Physiology, University of Kansas Medical Center, Kansas City, KS*

MARGARET G. PETROFF • *Department of Anatomy and Cell Biology, University of Kansas Medical Center, Kansas City, KS*

TERESA A. PHILLIPS • *Department of Internal Medicine, University of Kansas Medical Center, Kansas City, KS*

ROBERT PIJNENBORG • *Department of Obstetrics and Gynaecology, University Hospital Gasthuisberg, Katholieke Universiteit Leuven, Leuven, Belgium*

JEFFREY W. POLLARD • *Department of Developmental and Molecular Biology, Center for Study of Reproductive Biology and Women's Health, Albert Einstein College of Medicine of Yeshiva University, Bronx, NY*

PUTTUR D. PRASAD • *Department of Obstetrics and Gynecology, Medical College of Georgia, Augusta, GA*

TIMOTHY R. H. REGNAULT • *Perinatal Research Center, Department of Pediatrics, University of Colorado School of Medicine, Aurora, CO*

R. MICHAEL ROBERTS • *Life Sciences Center, University of Missouri-Columbia, Columbia, MO*

STEPHEN C. ROBSON • *Department of Obstetrics and Gynaecology, Royal Victoria Infirmary, University of Newcastle upon Tyne, Newcastle upon Tyne, United Kingdom*

ERIK RYTTING • *Department of Pharmaceutical Chemistry, School of Pharmacy, The University of Kansas, Lawrence, KS*

MONA SEDEEK • *Department of Physiology and Biophysics, University of Mississippi Medical Center, Jackson, MS*

NOA SHER • *Department of Biological Chemistry, The Alexander Silberman Institute of Life Sciences, The Hebrew University of Jerusalem, Jerusalem, Israel*

COLIN P. SIBLEY • *Academic Unit of Child Health, Human Development and Reproductive Healthcare Academic Group, University of Manchester, St. Mary's Hospital, Manchester, United Kingdom*

PETER S. SILVERSTEIN • *Department of Pharmaceutical Chemistry, School of Pharmacy, University of Kansas, Lawrence, KS*

IGOR I. SLUKVIN • *National Primate Research Center and Department of Obstetrics and Gynecology, University of Wisconsin-Madison, Madison, WI*

MICHAEL J. SOARES • *Institute of Maternal-Fetal Biology, Division of Cancer & Developmental Biology, Department of Pathology & Laboratory Medicine, University of Kansas Medical Center, Kansas City, KS*

THOMAS E. SPENCER • *Center for Animal Biotechnology and Genomics, Department of Animal Science, Texas A&M University, College Station, TX*

ISAAC E. STILLMAN • *Department of Pathology, Harvard Medical School and Beth Israel Deaconess Medical Center, Boston, MA*

SHAWN L. STRASZEWSKI-CHAVEZ • *Reproductive Immunology Unit, Department of Obstetrics and Gynecology, Yale University School of Medicine, New Haven, CT*

ANITA TRUNDLEY • *Department of Pathology, University of Cambridge, Cambridge, United Kingdom*

LISBETH VERCRUYSSE • *Department of Obstetrics and Gynaecology, University Hospital Gasthuisberg, Katholieke Universiteit Leuven, Leuven, Belgium*

MARK WAREING • *Maternal and Fetal Health Research Centre, Academic Unit of Obstetrics and Gynaecology and Reproductive Health Care, St. Mary's Hospital, Manchester, United Kingdom*

JOHN G. WOOD • *Department of Molecular and Investigative Physiology, University of Kansas Medical Center, Kansas City, KS*

XUEMEI XIE • *Department of Environmental Biology, University of Guelph, Guelph Ontario, Canada*

YAN XU • *Department of Pharmaceutics, Ernest Mario School of Pharmacy, Rutgers, The State University of New Jersey, Piscataway, NJ*

AMBER M. YOUNG • *Department of Pharmaceutical Chemistry, School of Pharmacy, University of Kansas, Lawrence, KS*

ANA C. ZENCLUSSEN • *Reproductive Immunology Group, Institute of Medical Immunology, Charite, Medical University of Berlin, Berlin, Germany*

BEIYAN ZHOU • *Department of Biochemistry, Molecular Biology, and Cell Biology, Northwestern University, Evanston, IL*

Contents of Volume 1

Companion CD-ROM

This book is accompanied by a CD-ROM that contains all the color illustrations.

I

INTRODUCTION

1

Placenta and Trophoblast: Methods and Protocols: Overview II

Michael J. Soares and Joan S. Hunt

1. Introduction

The placenta has multiple functions that are vital to the success of pregnancy. Trophoblast cells are specialized constituents of the placenta that are responsible in large part for these unique functions. In some species, trophoblast cells acquire invasive properties. These cells penetrate the uterus where they interact with and modify uterine vasculature. In other instances, trophoblast cells acquire the capacity to fuse with themselves or with maternal cells, or undergo the peculiar process of endoreduplication, where DNA replication continues independent of karyokinesis and cytokinesis *(1,2)*. The placentas of all species contain a population of trophoblast cells, which possess a barrier function. These cells regulate molecular and cellular transit between maternal and fetal compartments *(3)*. Trophoblast cells have also acquired the ability to modulate maternal and fetal physiology via production and secretion of regulatory factors and through cell–cell interactions. The outcome is reprogramming of metabolic and immune activities, which has a positive impact on maternal and fetal health and ensures the success of pregnancy.

In this volume, methods for studying placental function are presented. Parts II (Analysis of Trophoblast Cell Invasion) and III (Analysis of Uteroplacental Immune Cells and Their Functions) focus exclusively on biological events associated with hemochorial placentation.

Chapters in part II describe investigative protocols for studying the invasive character of trophoblast cells, and chapters in part III deal with protocols for learning more about how encounters between trophoblast cells and uterine

From: *Methods in Molecular Medicine, Vol. 122: Placenta and Trophoblast: Methods and Protocols, Vol. 2*
Edited by: M. J. Soares and J. S. Hunt © Humana Press Inc., Totowa, NJ

immune cells influence the course of pregnancy. Chapters in part IV (Analysis of Trophoblast Cells and Placental Function: Transport and Endocrinology) address methods for investigating the movement of molecules across the placenta and the production and action of hormones produced by the placenta. The final section of this volume, part V (Analysis of Trophoblast Cell and Placental Adaptations to Disease), describes specific in vivo model systems for studying pathologies of the placenta and functional adaptations in this critical organ during disease.

2. Analysis of Trophoblast Invasion

A hallmark of hemochorial placentation is the movement of trophoblast cells into the uterine parenchyma. Trophoblast cells home in large part to the uterine spiral arteries. These blood vessels are modified, allowing maternal blood to directly bathe trophoblast cells and facilitating nutrient and waste exchange. Invasive trophoblast cells represent a specialized trophoblast lineage. The course of their development and functions are poorly understood, as are the regulatory factors in the uteroplacental milieu that guide their journey. Abnormalities in trophoblast invasion are a prominent feature of diseases of pregnancy, including preeclampsia and anemias *(4)*. This important link to human pathology has resulted in considerable efforts directed toward studying mechanisms regulating invasive trophoblast cells. The early work has been dominated by the development of strategies for studying human trophoblast and will represent the subject material for the chapters in this section. Chapter 2 presents a critical examination of research used for analyzing invasive trophoblast cells developing *in situ*. In vitro protocols for studying trophoblast invasion are described in Chapters 3 and 4. These chapters include experimental procedures for investigating trophoblast cell interactions with extracellular matrices and blood vessels.

3. Analysis of Uteroplacental Immune Cells and Their Functions

As trophoblast cells enter the uterine environment they are likely to encounter cells of the maternal immune system that reside in the uterine stroma or migrate into the decidua as a consequence of high levels of chemoattractant molecules that are a feature of the uterus during pregnancy. The main decidual immune cells in species with hemochorial placentation are natural killer (NK) cells and cells of the mononuclear phagocyte lineage, which are comprised of macrophages and dendritic cells. Part III describes methods for isolating and studying the functions of these two types of leukocytes, which are critical components of the uterine natural immune system, and their interactions with trophoblast cells. Chapter 5 presents an in vivo experimental system for studying

NK cell trafficking within the murine uterus that features utilization of genetically modified mice. The protocols describe analyses of NK cell migration in mice where proteins believed to be central to regulation of the NK cells are altered. Protocols for the isolation and characterization of cells situated at the maternal-fetal interface from the rhesus monkey and human are presented in Chapters 6 to 8. The techniques rely on the use of specific antibodies for isolating uteroplacental cells and characterizing the resulting populations. In Chapters 8 and 9, methods for investigating macrophages and macrophage-trophoblast interactions are addressed. The final two chapters in this section present strategies for studying trophoblast major histocompatibility complex (MHC) antigens, which differ dramatically from MHC antigens expressed by other types of cells. In Chapter 10, methods for investigating baboon placental MHC antigens are described, and in Chapter 11, research strategies for investigating the immunobiology of the soluble isoforms of the human histocompatibility antigen, human leukocyte antigen (HLA)-G, are described in detail.

4. Analysis of Placenta Function: Transport and Endocrinology

Among the major functions of the placenta are (1) regulation of the flow of nutrients and wastes between maternal and fetal compartments, and (2) modification of maternal and fetal environments by secreting hormones, cytokines, and growth factors as well as other proteins that modify the activities of these ligands. These functions are mainly achieved by trophoblast cells, although some are accomplished by placental stromal cells which include fibroblasts, macrophages, and endothelial cells. In some species, transport and endocrine functions are segregated to distinct subpopulations of trophoblast cells, whereas in other species, multifunctional trophoblast cells accomplish both tasks. In part IV of this volume, protocols are given for investigations of both transport and endocrine functions of the placenta.

In the first six chapters (Chapters 12 through 17), in vivo and in vitro methods are described to analyze transport across the placental barrier. Experimental procedures for the in vivo analysis of placental transport across the sheep placenta that are adaptable to other animal models are presented in Chapter 12. Protocols for blood vessel cannulation and mathematical models are provided for accurate assessment of the hemodynamic and transport properties of the maternal–fetal interface. Chapters 13 through 17 include methods for dissecting transport systems and transporters at cellular and biochemical levels. For example, Chapter 13 describes procedures for establishing and characterizing cell culture systems that have been designed to investigate transcellular transport in trophoblast cells. These methods can be used to evaluate transport and efflux mechanisms for a range of endogenous substances and xenobiotics. In vitro protocols specifically targeted for studying placental amino acid transport are presented in Chapters 14 and 15, and procedures for investigating placental fatty acid trafficking are provided in Chapter 16. The transport section concludes with protocols for the analysis of specific transporter proteins (Chapter 17). Strategies are presented for the expression of transporter proteins and their biochemical and biological characterization.

The remaining chapters in part IV (Chapters 18 through 23) present a range of techniques for analyzing the biosynthesis and actions of hormones and cytokines produced by the placenta. Chapter 18 introduces protocols for studying the biosynthesis of steroid hormones by rodent trophoblast cells, with a special emphasis on the enzymes responsible their production. The following chapter (Chapter 19) provides detailed procedures for establishing an enzyme-linked immunoassay that specifically detects one of the major secretory products of bovine trophoblast binucleate cells, pregnancy-associated glycoprotein. This assay provides an effective means of monitoring the function of trophoblast binucleate cells both in vitro and in vivo.

Chapters 20 through 23 focus on investigating the biological actions of placental hormones/cytokines. Experimentally valuable tags can be introduced into protein hormones using recombinant DNA techniques. The tagged proteins can be used to identify cellular targets for the protein hormones (Chapter 20). Efficient procedures for generating recombinant protein hormones are described in Chapters 21 and 22. These protocols allow for the production of biologically active hormones that can be used to investigate the physiology of pregnancy. Finally, Chapters 22 and 23 include methods for investigating specific biological processes. Techniques for analyzing placental hormone regulation of hematopoiesis are presented (Chapter 22), as are procedures for examining the action of trophoblast-derived interferons (Chapter 23). Each of the protocols described in this section should be adaptable for the analysis of other hormones, cytokines, or growth factors produced by the placenta.

5. Analysis of Placenta Adaptation to Disease

In part V of this volume, the focus is on techniques for investigating placenta dysfunction and adaptation to disease. Chapters 24 through 26 describe experimental procedures for establishing and characterizing rodent models suitable for studies on pregnancy-associated vascular dysfunction. Each of these models reproduces some of the features of the clinical disorder called preeclampsia. A mechanical strategy for restricting uterine perfusion is described in Chapter 24. The surgical manipulation affects maternal cardiovascular function and the flow of nutrients to the developing fetus, resulting in intrauterine growth restriction. In Chapter 25, a preeclampsia-like disease is established by treating rats with adenoviruses overexpressing a soluble version of the Flt1 receptor. Dysregulation of growth factor networks controlling blood vessel development is effectively produced, and the result is a pregnancy-associated disease typified by increased maternal blood pressure, renal disease, and intrauterine growth restriction. In Chapter 26, an immunological approach is used to create a mouse model of preeclampsia. The technique relies on increased inflammation leading to many if not all of the symptoms and signs of preeclampsia.

Many diseases of pregnancy, including preeclampsia, impact nutrient flow to the placenta and fetus. One of the essential nutrients is oxygen. Chapter 27 presents in vitro methods for studying the effects of oxygen on trophoblast cell development. This chapter describes protocols for studying trophoblast cell adaptive responses to restricted oxygen and following exposure to oxidative stress. In Chapter 28, a simple procedure is outlined for exposing pregnant rodents to hypoxia. Either rats or mice are easily placed into a hypobaric chamber, which simulates high altitude and creates a hypoxic atmosphere. Adaptive responses can be investigated in the uteroplacental compartment or elsewhere in maternal and fetal tissues.

The final chapter in this section (Chapter 29) presents an effective strategy for investigating uteroplacental development and immune responses following introduction of a bacterial pathogen. *Listeria monocytogenes* is used as a tool to elucidate mechanisms utilized by the pregnant mouse to restrict bacterial infection. Techniques are included for creating the infection and for evaluating trophoblast and immune cell responses.

References

1. Wooding, F. B. P. and Flint, A. P. F. (1994) Placentation, in *Marshall's Physiology of Reproduction, Fourth Edition, Vol. 3* (Lamming, G. E., ed.). Chapman & Hall, London: pp. 233–460.
2. Rossant, J. and Cross, J. C. (2002) Extraembryonic lineages, in *Mouse Development* (Rossant, J. and Tam, P.P.L., eds.). Academic, San Diego: pp. 155–190.
3. Audus, K. L., Soares, M. J., and Hunt, J. S. (2002) Characteristics of the fetal/maternal interface with potential usefulness in the development of future immunological and pharmacological strategies. *J. Pharmacol. Exp. Ther.* **301,** 402–409.
4. Kaufmann, P., Black, S., and Huppertz, B. (2003) Endovascular trophoblast invasion: implications for the pathogenesis of intrauterine growth retardation and preeclampsia. *Biol. Reprod.* **69,** 1–7.

II

Analysis of Trophoblast Invasion

2

In Vivo Analysis of Trophoblast Cell Invasion in the Human

Robert Pijnenborg, Elizabeth Ball, Judith N. Bulmer, Myriam Hanssens, Stephen C. Robson, and Lisbeth Vercruysse

Summary

In vivo analysis of trophoblast cell invasion is highly dependent on histological techniques, which are amply described in standard textbooks. The emphasis of this chapter therefore lies on material collection and interpretation of tissue sections, rather than on histological techniques *per se*. Proper identification of vascular structures on placental bed histological sections is important, the more because invading trophoblastic cells induce significant structural changes in uterine blood vessels, which may be disturbed in complicated pregnancies. Guidelines for distinguishing several vascular structures are provided, and different approaches for qualitative and quantitative assessment of spiral artery changes are discussed. The purpose of such studies is not only to obtain a better insight into mechanisms of trophoblast invasion and associated maternal tissue changes, but also to understand placental bed defects in various pregnancy complications.

Key Words: Placental bed; placental bed biopsies; human; extravillous trophoblast; trophoblast invasion; trophoblast quantitation; histological methods; immunohistochemistry; spiral arteries; uteroplacental blood flow; vascular smooth muscle; cytokeratin; elastica; preeclampsia; complicated pregnancies.

1. Introduction

Studies on trophoblast invasion in the human were initially inspired by pioneering studies of maternal placental blood flow, which revealed impaired flow in hypertensive patients *(1)*. Because vascular lesions in underlying maternal arteries were suspected to be the cause of this impaired flow, biopsies were collected from the placental bed for histological evaluation of the uterine vasculature. This first collection event was followed by a learning period of several years, necessary for understanding the nature of the unfamiliar "physiologically changed" vascular structures, which were hypothesized to result from the action of invading trophoblast *(2)* (**Fig. 1**). An important find-

From: *Methods in Molecular Medicine, Vol. 122: Placenta and Trophoblast: Methods and Protocols, Vol. 2*
Edited by: M. J. Soares and J. S. Hunt © Humana Press Inc., Totowa, NJ

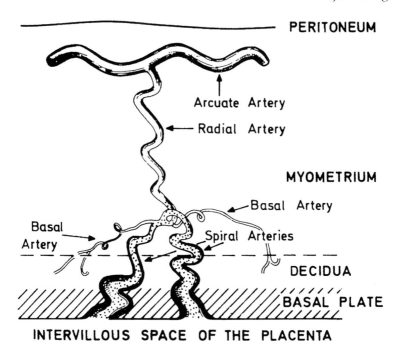

Fig. 1. Diagram showing uteroplacental arterial blood supply in human pregnancy. Intraluminal stippling indicates the extent of physiological change in spiral arteries. Reproduced from **ref. 2**, with permission.

ing was the significant restriction of the extent of physiological change in preeclamptic women *(3)*, which was assumed to be due to limited trophoblast invasion *(4)*. These results were so striking at that time that placental bed changes in preeclamptic as compared with normal pregnancies were considered a straightforward, black-and-white process. In later years, however, realization of the complexity of preeclampsia, the findings of placental bed defects in other pregnancy complications *(5)*, and the problems of clinical classification *(6)* resulted in the more subtle view that defects in the placental bed show a spectrum of pathological changes partly related to the severity of the disease *(7,8)*. This newer concept also implies that a good evaluation of placental bed changes critically depends on the extent to which the biopsy material is representative, as well as on a good methodology.

It is obvious that complete pregnant uteri provide the best study material for evaluating trophoblast invasion. Only in such material can topographical differences in density and extent of invasion be assessed throughout the placental bed. In this way, marked variation has been described in the patterns of interstitial and endovascular trophoblast invasion and in the associated modifications of the spiral arteries from the center to the margins of the placental bed *(9,10)*. Such an approach is not routinely feasible in a clinical context, however. Most of the time, we have only small tissue samples available for study, and it is really a bold leap to extrapolate from the findings in small tissue fragments to the whole placental bed. The task is particularly challenging for the study of biopsies from complicated pregnancies, in which invasion may be irregular and vasculopathies may occur focally.

The only comprehensive review on the methodology of placental bed research was published nearly 20 yr ago by Robertson and colleagues *(11)*. Over the years, there have been changes, technically as well as conceptually, in our understanding of tissue dynamics, as well as in clinical practice. In this review, our aim was to combine the experience of two centers in order to provide a series of useful guidelines for studies on the placental bed.

2. Materials

2.1. Delivered Placentas

Early observations on the decidua were usually limited to tissue fragments attached to the maternal surface, i.e., the basal plate of a delivered placenta. The basal plate is defined as "the trophoblastic layer of the placenta that is attached to the endometrium," in other words "the placental floor" *(12)*. The term "placental bed," on the other hand, was deliberately chosen to emphasize that it includes "not only basal decidua but also underlying myometrium containing the origins of the uteroplacental (spiral) arteries" *(11)*. It is not necessary to point out that maternal tissue sticking to the basal plate of a delivered placenta is highly incomplete and does not even represent the whole thickness of the decidua. Nevertheless, papers are still published on the "placental bed" which, after scrutinizing the illustrations, can be suspected to be based on basal plate material only. Although such decidual fragments may indeed contain invaded spiral arteries, it should be clear that such material has only limited value for evaluating the depth of trophoblast invasion into spiral arteries which, according to Brosens and colleagues *(3)*, extends into the inner myometrium during normal pregnancy, but is restricted to the decidua in preeclampsia. On the other hand, Khong and colleagues *(13)* showed that in preeclampsia, not only are physiological changes restricted to the decidual segments of spiral arteries, but also fewer arteries are invaded. In that case, estimating the percentage of decidual spiral arteries with physiological change may be relevant, and it was therefore recommended to perform *"en face"* sectioning of flatly embedded basal plates in order to maximize the number of decidual spiral arteries examined *(14)*. Also, atherotic lesions may be detected in such material, and it should be added here that this lesion was actually first described in spiral artery segments clinging to delivered placentas *(15)*. Nevertheless, basal plate biopsies do not allow evaluation of the depth of the lesion, which may be relevant, since Robertson and colleagues *(11)* hinted that the myometrial spread of atherosis may indicate a more severe disease. Moreover, even in normal pregnancies, the basal plate may undergo involution with lipid deposition, especially near term *(16)*, so that information gathered from such material may be misleading.

2.2. Hysterectomy Specimens

Pregnant hysterectomy specimens, of course, provide the ideal material for study. In processing such specimens, it is recommended to prepare tissue sections comprising the complete placenta and underlying placental bed, which, of course, requires the special skill of sectioning large tissue blocks. Only in such complete preparations can one properly evaluate the distribution of changes throughout the depth of the uterine wall and from the central to the lateral parts of the placental bed. Furthermore, this approach also allows us to study changes in placental areas in association with the underlying spiral arteries.

Nowadays, hysterectomies of pregnant uteri are performed only in very exceptional situations, and collections of such material are therefore very rare and precious. Two famous historical collections are the J. D. Boyd collection (forming the basis of Boyd and Hamilton's famous papers on early placental development) *(17,18)* and the Bristol collection brought together by H. G. Dixon *(9,10,19,20)*.

Only very occasionally have complete hysterectomy specimens been obtained from complicated pregnancies. Brosens and Renaer *(21)* obtained a complete pregnant uterus from a preeclamptic woman, and were able to demonstrate that acute atherosis in spiral arteries is directly associated with overlying placental infarcts. Kadyrov and colleagues *(22)* reported on a series of hysterectomies from four normal, five preeclamptic, and six anemic women, in which they observed, respectively, restricted and increased depth of interstitial trophoblast invasion. It is not clear whether the whole placental bed was examined or whether their observations were limited to random parts; such information is important regarding the variability of trophoblast invasion from lateral to central areas.

2.3. Placental Bed Biopsies

The very first placental bed biopsy was taken at caesarean section by Dixon and Robertson *(23)*, who also introduced the term "placental bed" to emphasize that deep tissue layers were included, comprising not only decidua but also part of the inner myometrium.

2.3.1. Placental Bed Biopsies at Caesarean Section

Caesarean section biopsies may be taken under direct vision. After peeling off the placenta from the uterine wall, a fragment of decidua and underlying myometrium of approx 1.5 cm in diameter can be removed using a scalpel and/ or a pair of scissors. The biopsies should be taken from the central zone of the placental bed, which can be manually located before removing the placenta *(11)*. Some clinicians prefer to insert a needle through the uterine wall as a guide for determining the center of the placental bed *(7)*. As to the depth of the biopsy, it is unnecessary to go deeper than a few millimeters within the myometrium, because interstitial trophoblastic cell counting on complete hysterectomy sections revealed a greatly diminished volume density at 3 mm beneath the decidual–myometrial junction *(9)*. At the time of biopsy taking, besides a "random" tissue sample in the central zone, also additional biopsies may be collected in areas with suspected vascular lesions *(11)*, although we must realize that this introduces a sampling bias.

Obtaining adequate placental bed biopsies following this method depends greatly on the experience of the surgeon. Hanssens and colleagues *(24)* showed that after restarting the practice of placental bed collecting at the University Hospital in Leuven, the proportion of adequate biopsies, containing trophoblast and at least one spiral artery, showed, interestingly, first a drop from 1987 (54%) to 1988 (25%), followed by a steady rise to 75% in 1991. It is noteworthy that, in 1988, more gynecologists were involved in collecting biopsies who had less experience—and possibly less interest—in placental bed research. It was also found that the presence or absence of myometrial structures paralleled the size of the biopsy (**Table 1**). No complications related to the taking of placental bed biopsies have been reported. However, long-term evaluation with follow-up into the next pregnancies has not been performed.

2.3.2. Placental Bed Biopsies Under Ultrasound Guidance

2.3.2.1. Early Pregnancy

Khong and colleagues *(25)* first reported the use of ultrasound to guide placental bed sampling. Using curettage, they successfully obtained myometrial spiral arteries in a small group of women undergoing uterine evacuation for spontaneous miscarriage between 9 and 25 wk of pregnancy. Michel and colleagues *(26)* adapted the ultrasound-guided technique by using cervical biopsy forceps introduced through the cervix. Biopsies of the placental bed were collected from early normal and anembryonic pregnancies with the placenta still *in situ (27)*. The success rate of the technique was not reported, although examination of their published material suggests samples were mainly decidual.

Table 1
Adequacy of Placental Bed Biopsies Collected During Successive Years

	1987	1988	1989	1990	1991	1992
No. pregnancies	23	70	45	27	22	14
No. biopsies	24	157	90	48	45	25
Biopsy largest diameter						
<0.5 cm No. (%)	2 (8)	39 (25)	13 (15)	2 (4)	1 (2)	0 (0)
0.5–1 cm No. (%)	17 (71)	90 (57)	39 (44)	6 (13)	13 (29)	5 (20)
>1 cm No. (%)	5 (21)	28 (18)	37 (42)	40 (83)	31 (69)	20 (80)
no myometrium No. (%)	2 (8)	38 (24)	15 (17)	4 (8)	2 (4)	2 (8)
no trophoblast No. (%)	8 (33)	80 (51)	30 (33)	9 (19)	3 (7)	9 (36)
adequate + spir. artery	13 (54)	39 (25)	47 (52)	30 (63)	34 (75)	14 (56)

As presented in **ref. 23**.

Robson modified Michel's technique employing long, straight, laparoscopic biopsy forceps introduced through the cervix *(28)*. The movable jaw has a cutting edge and can be rotated through 360° to facilitate sampling posterior placentas (**Fig. 2**). In order to increase success, especially of obtaining myometrial spiral arteries, we perform biopsies after placental removal, having identified the site by prior ultrasound. The tip of the forceps is guided into the uterine wall adjacent to the placental site. The jaws are then opened and closed under ultrasound surveillance. Successful biopsy of the uterine wall has a characteristic tactile sensation and optimally yields samples of approx 5×5 mm (**Fig. 3**). We usually take four biopsies per patient.

Initial experience with this technique in 313 women undergoing termination of pregnancy under general anesthesia between 6 and 21 wk indicated successful biopsy of the placental bed, defined as the presence of interstitial trophoblast and more than one spiral artery in at least one biopsy, in 53% of cases with 32% having a myometrial spiral artery *(28)*. Slightly higher rates were obtained in 104 women with embryonic/fetal death prior to evacuation of retained products of conception (61% and 46%, respectively). In those with a successful biopsy, one-third had both a decidual and a myometrial spiral artery and one-third had more than one myometrial artery. Interestingly, there was a statistically significant correlation between gestational age and the proportion of cases with interstitial trophoblast (42% at <8 wk increasing to 92% at 18–21 wk).

Extensive experience with this technique in nearly 800 cases indicates that it is safe; total operative loss (blood and amniotic fluid) exceeds 500 g in 1% of cases, a rate comparable with nonbiopsied cases. We have encountered one uterine perforation in a woman of 13 wk gestation who had a difficult termina-

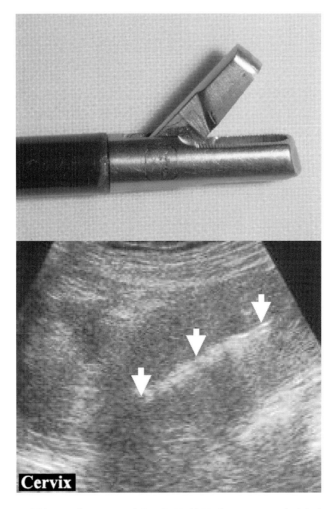

Fig. 2. Jaw of biopsy forceps (Richard Wolf Endoscopes, Wimbledon, UK). The transabdominal ultrasound scan after uterine evacuation shows the forceps (arrows) introduced through the cervix and positioned to take a fundal placental bed biopsy

tion after apparently straightforward biopsies. The fact that the perforation was on the opposite wall of the uterus to the site of the biopsies, which consisted of decidua and superficial myometrium, suggests that the perforation occurred at the time of the termination.

The great advantage of this biopsying technique is that it allows the study of placental bed samples throughout the period of placentation. Further, it affords the opportunity of studying placentation in a range of early pregnancy compli-

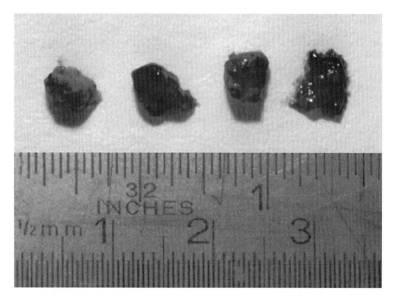

Fig. 3. Placental bed biopsy specimens, collected by the punch biopsy method under ultrasound guidance

cations, notably spontaneous miscarriage. Recent studies from our group have shown that trophoblast invasion and spiral artery transformation is deficient in late (>12 wk gestation) but not early spontaneous abortions *(29)*.

2.3.2.2. LATE PREGNANCY

Placental bed biopsies can also be obtained by punch biopsy at the time of caesarean section, a technique originally described by Gerretsen and colleagues *(30)*. Ultrasound guidance is not required and multiple biopsies (8 to 10) can be taken under direct vision, having identified the placental site prior to removal. Theoretical advantages of this method are that access to an anterior wall placental bed may be easier and, because biopsies are much smaller, morbidity may be less. Our experience with this technique (approx 150 cases) indicates that successful biopsy of the placental bed (as defined previously) occurs in 50% of cases, with more than one myometrial artery in 39% of cases *(28)*. This is a lower success rate than knife biopsy, at least when performed by an experienced operator, and caution must be exercised when interpreting multiple small biopsies, particularly in complicated pregnancies.

The method of transcervical placental bed biopsy under ultrasound guidance can also be used in late pregnancy. The placental site is carefully identified prior to the third stage of labor and then multiple biopsies are taken after placental expulsion. Because any intrauterine manipulation is uncomfortable, we have limited sampling to women with a functioning epidural block, inserted for labor analgesia. Limited experience suggests the success rate is comparable with early biopsy *(28)*. Obviously the advantage of this method is that cases delivering vaginally, e.g., fetal death, can be sampled.

3. Methods

3.1. Tissue Processing

3.1.1. Hysterectomy Specimens

3.1.1.1. FIXATION, PARAFFIN EMBEDDING, AND SECTIONING

Hysterectomy material offers technical and logistic problems for processing and sectioning, and proper fixation is a particular problem. As a first and necessary step, the amniotic fluid should be removed using a syringe and replaced by fixative. Large organs such as a pregnant uterus must remain immersed in fixative for a sufficiently long time in order to obtain satisfactory fixation. The use of an easily penetrating fixative such as buffered (para)formaldehyde is therefore necessary. In fact, whole uteri have been stored in fixative for several weeks and even months. However, if samples are to be used for immunohistochemistry, such long periods of storage in fixative should be avoided, and thinner tissue slices should be cut as soon as possible to allow a restricted fixation time. Experience with small biopsies has indicated that prolonged fixation of more than 24 h may result in antigen masking and elution of secreted material *(31)*, although recent methods of heat-mediated antigen retrieval may to some extent overcome this problem. Whole uteri should be cut in slices with a maximal thickness of 1 cm, covering the whole placental and placental bed area. The subsequent dehydration, clearing, and infiltration steps should be prolonged in order to obtain good penetration of the solvents. Sectioning such material may be difficult and, to allow easier cutting, it is recommended to pass the slices through two baths of cedar wood oil between the absolute alcohol and the toluene step. After transferring a slice to cedar wood oil, the tissue will initially float on top of the oil, but will gradually sink, becoming somewhat translucent. It should be transferred to toluene only after the tissue has reached the bottom of the receptacle, which can take several hours. The oil is cleared from the tissue in several baths of toluene.

Finally, cutting large sections is really a skill to be learned under the supervision of an experienced "master." A good and technically more realistic alternative for the cutting of large sections is the "labeled blocking method," in which the whole uterus with attached placenta is divided into successively labeled 1-cm thick slices, and every labeled slice is cut, perpendicular to the uterine lumen, into rigorously labeled blocks, allowing normal processing toward regularly sized paraffin sections. A complete picture of invasion and vascular remodeling in the whole placental bed can be reconstructed from the observations on the individual tissue blocks. The latter approach should be recommended whenever a precious whole pregnant uterus happens to be available, because it avoids application of technologies which are not routinely on hand in standard laboratory settings.

3.1.1.2. STAINING

Almost all published work on large hysterectomy sections was based on standard histological staining techniques, i.e., hematoxylin and eosin (H&E), periodic acid–Schiff (PAS), and the connective tissue methods such as Masson's trichrome and Van Gieson, which may be combined with an acid orcein staining for elastic fibers. Application of immunohistochemical staining to large tissue sections is not immediately obvious, and also for this reason the "labeled blocking method" for processing complete hysterectomy specimens is recommended.

Nevertheless, if it were possible, immunostaining of large tissue sections would be desirable and could be regarded as a "gold standard" for the definitive identification of cell types and their interrelationship. However, there are several technical and practical problems, which may be insurmountable. Prolonged fixation in formalin-based fixatives may irreversibly damage antigens. In this case, modern methods of antigen retrieval, particularly heat-mediated antigen retrieval by microwave or pressure cooking in citrate or Tris–ethylenediamine tetraacetic acid (EDTA) buffer, may allow some immunohistochemistry to be performed successfully. Even if antigens resist fixation or can be retrieved, the size of hysterectomy specimens implies that fixation is likely to be uneven throughout the tissue and results of immunohistochemical staining may be variable even within a single section. Moreover, heat pretreatment, particularly in EDTA buffer, may cause sections to lift and requires adhesion of sections to glass slides using substances such as 3-aminopropyl-triethoxysilane (APES); even if antigens were preserved after prolonged periods of storage at room temperature, any precut archival sections would be unlikely to have used this approach. A further practical problem is the volume of antibody required to stain a whole section, with consequent high cost. Although we have had some success in both single and double immunolabeling of archive sections from pregnant hysterectomy samples, the labeled blocking method described above is a more practical approach for immunohistochemical localization of different cell types in complete hysterectomy specimens. The pattern of trophoblast invasion and spiral artery transformation in the whole specimen may subsequently be reconstructed from the observations on the separate tissue blocks.

3.1.2. Placental Bed Biopsies

3.1.2.1. FIXATION, PARAFFIN EMBEDDING, AND SECTIONING

Because of their small size, more slowly penetrating fixatives may be used for biopsies, and indeed some antigenic epitopes may need an alternative fixation method. It was, for example, found that immunolocalization of renin was greatly improved using Bouin fixation instead of the more standard paraformaldehyde *(32)*. The processing of biopsies into paraffin blocks does not pose special problems. In order to reduce the painstaking step serial sectioning, it is recommended to divide the original 1-cm³ tissue blocks into 1- to 2-mm thick slices, perpendicular to the placenta insertion, while still in the fixative. These slices should be embedded flat on the cut side within the same paraffin block. This method allows a survey of the whole tissue sample, which is especially useful for the study of spiral artery sections.

Frozen tissue sections have also been used for some studies *(33–38)*. Although these are suboptimal for morphological assessment, the use of cryostat sections does allow localization of antigens which will not withstand fixation with formalin or other fixatives. However, as antigen retrieval methods improve, the requirement for frozen samples will be reduced. As well as less-satisfactory morphological preservation, there are other disadvantages of using frozen samples. First, placental bed tissues appear to be exquisitely sensitive to ice crystal artefact, probably because of the relatively high water content of decidualized endometrial stromal cells. Freezing must therefore be rapid, preferably in isopentane; this chemical has a rapid cooling curve and freezes tissues very rapidly, in contrast with freezing directly in liquid nitrogen, which may lead to formation of a gas bubble around the tissue and hence slow freezing. Handling after freezing is technically demanding; any warming of the sample, for example, while preparing for cryostat sectioning, may lead to disastrous loss of morphological preservation. Because of their very small size, punch biopsies of the placental bed are particularly at risk at this stage. Whereas paraffin sections are routinely sectioned at a thickness of 3–4 µm, frozen sections are generally no thinner and often thicker than 5 µm. Furthermore, the advantages of frozen sections in allowing detection of some antigens may be outweighed by the fact that other antibodies will perform less well on frozen tissues. There may be additional problems caused by leaching of cytoplasmic antigen out of cells, leading to poor localization. This can be a particular problem for detection of metalloproteinases *(39)*. Even some standard histochemical stains cannot be performed adequately on frozen sections; for example, we (JNB, EB) have been unable to demonstrate elastin using standard histochemical staining techniques in cryostat sections.

Frozen tissues can be successfully used for laser capture microdissection techniques. Using this approach, it is possible to sample specific areas of placental bed tissues, such as transformed and nontransformed spiral arteries, under direct vision and use these samples to gain quantitative data, either extracting RNA for real-time reverse-transcription (RT)-polymerase chain reaction (PCR) or extracting protein for analysis *(40)*. Because placental bed biopsies are precious samples which, particularly in pathological pregnancy, may not be readily available, it may be appropriate to prepare both frozen and fixed paraffin embedded samples wherever possible, in order to ensure that the appropriate tissue sample is available for a wide range of technical approaches.

3.1.2.2. STAINING

For many years, placental bed work was bedeviled by the virtual impossibility to distinguish with certainty the invading trophoblast from decidual cells, unless, of course, one wished to concentrate on the multinuclear giant cells. That was also the reason why Pijnenborg and colleagues *(9)* had restricted their quantitative work on interstitial trophoblast to the myometrium, where it was assumed that the trophoblast cells could reasonably well be distinguished from the spindle-shaped smooth muscle cells. Studying spiral arteries offers additional problems, because several different processes that are taking place more or less simultaneously must be considered . In the first place, during vascular remodeling, the medial smooth muscle cells themselves undergo regression or dedifferentiation. In addition, endovascular trophoblast makes its appearance and should be clearly distinguished from the maternal endothelium and vascular smooth muscle cells. For these reasons, the introduction of the epithelial cell marker cytokeratin was a major breakthrough in placental bed research *(41,42)*. Based on this technique, Meekins and colleagues *(43)* reported 39% "real" placental bed biopsies in a series of leftovers, previously dismissed on H&E-stained sections as being non-placental bed.

After its introduction, cytokeratin immunohistochemistry was enthusiastically applied, but in the investigators' eagerness, epithelium-lined remnants of glands were also sometimes interpreted as endovascular trophoblast-lined spiral arteries. A few years ago, some investigators became alarmed by the possible cross-reactivity of conventionally used cytokeratin antisera (such as MNF116) with myometrial smooth muscle *(44)*. For this reason, the more specific anti-cytokeratin 7 is now generally recommended for the identification of trophoblast. It is obviously true that this more specific antibody is absolutely required for studying isolated cells in vitro *(45)*. On the other hand, an experienced histologist usually has no problem in distinguishing real trophoblast cells from false-positive smooth muscle cells on histological sections after broad spectrum cytokeratin immunostaining. Apart from a difference in shape, the

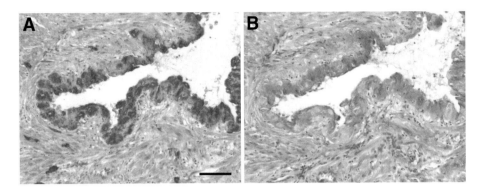

Fig. 4. Myometrial spiral artery with physiological change at 26 wk. (**A**) Cytokeratin immunostaining with hematoxylin and eosin counterstaining. A few scattered interstitial trophoblastic cells are present in the myometrial stroma; (**B**) periodic acid–Schiff staining to reveal the fibrinoid deposition which has replaced the original smooth muscle layer. (Bar = 100 μm.)

smooth muscle cells usually show different staining characteristics, lacking the typical filamentous appearance of the cytoskeleton. In our experience (RP, LV, MH, JNB), smooth muscle cross-reactivity in MNF116 or other broad-spectrum cytokeratin immunohistochemistry is biopsy-dependent, and is most pronounced in the outer myometrial layers, which are normally not included in a standard placental bed biopsy. On the other hand, scattered glandular epithelial cells are also positive for cytokeratin 7, and therefore this sometimes confusing cross-reactivity cannot be avoided even by the more specific antibody. It is also worth noting that in the third trimester the residual endometrial glands may be very distorted and lined by flattened epithelial cells, hindering their identification as glands and increasing the chance of confusion with trophoblast.

For a routine qualitative evaluation, we recommend the following staining methods:

1. Cytokeratin immunostaining, which may be counterstained lightly with H&E (**Figs. 4A** and **9A**) or, maybe even better, PAS for revealing the fibrinoid which is associated with the intramural (**Fig. 5**) and some of the perivascular trophoblast (**Fig. 6**) (*see* **Subheading 4.2.1.**). Amylase predigestion before applying PAS staining may be preferred in order to remove the sometimes distracting glycogen "blobs" from the section.
2. If not applied as counterstaining after cytokeratin, a PAS stain should be included, in order to detect physiologically changed spiral arteries "at a glance" during a rapid screening of the section (**Figs. 4B** and **9B**).

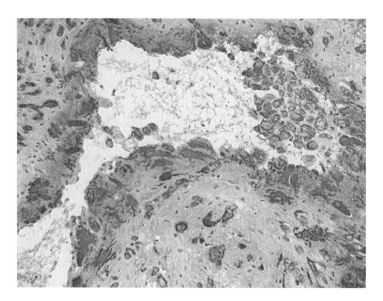

Fig. 5. Decidual spiral artery in a 15-wk punch biopsy, showing endovascular trophoblast becoming intramural. Cytokeratin immunostaining with periodic acid–Schiff
counterstaining to show fibrinoid deposition.

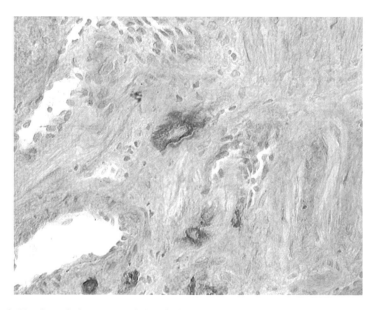

Fig. 6. Noninvaded myometrial spiral artery in a 19-wk punch biopsy, showing
perivascular trophoblast and associated fibrinoid. Cytokeratin immunostaining with
periodic acid–Schiff counterstaining.

3. A smooth muscle cell marker, either desmin or α-actin, is not only very helpful for evaluation of vessel wall disorganization, but also allows a clear outlining of decidua and myometrium, the latter tissue often being indistinct after H&E staining.
4. An elastica stain such as acid orcein is useful for evaluation of elastica break-down during physiological change of spiral arteries (**Fig. 9C**) *(46)*.

In addition, other antibodies reactive after paraffin-embedding are very useful, such as an endothelial cell marker (Von Willebrands factor, CD31, CD34, *Ulex europaeus* lectin), some leukocyte markers such as the macrophage markers CD68 and CD14, and the natural killer (NK) cell marker CD56, depending on the research program. Also, markers for cell proliferation (although extravillous trophoblast does not proliferate) or apoptosis may be of interest. Within the context of immunohistochemistry, it must be mentioned that biotin-linked techniques can cause prominent irrelevant staining in nuclei of endometrial glands, which cannot be blocked completely by applying avidin previous to the immunostaining. This means that enzyme-conjugated secondary antibodies should be used as a better detection alternative *(47)*.

For some purposes, staining of strictly parallel sections or, even better, double immunostaining is required, i.e., for the localization of different proteins in particular cell types *(48,49)* or for studies on cell interactions, which need multiple cell typing *(50)*. Double immunohistochemical labeling may be particularly useful for frozen sections, which are of necessity thicker and technically more demanding than paraffin sections, so that satisfactory parallel sections may be less easy to obtain. Various approaches may be used for double immunolabeling, and ample information is available on this matter either from the literature or from commercial suppliers. Whatever the approach, every cross reactivity between the detection systems for the two antigenic epitopes must be rigorously avoided, and the labeling pattern obtained for every epitope should be absolutely the same compared with a single-labeling experiment.

Double immunofluorescent labeling has been used in several studies *(33,51,52)*. In this technique, the two labeled antigens can be viewed either separately by the use of specific waveband filters or simultaneously by photographing the same field under the two filters and combining the images. However, immunofluorescence has the definite disadvantage that morphological features are often difficult to discern. Further drawbacks are the excessive background reactivity in paraffin sections and fading of the fluorescent signal upon storage at room temperature, making the preparations less permanent. In double immunohistochemistry, on the contrary, detailed morphological localization of the labeling is straightforward and preparations are permanent, albeit sometimes necessitating the use of an aqueous mountant according to the used chromogen. Because viewing of the two labels separately is not possible in this technique, the colors must be sufficiently different to allow clear distinction between the two types of single-labeled cells and double-labeled cells. For this purpose, a variety of enzyme conjugates can be used, making numerous color combinations possible. A constraint for all approaches may be the antigen retrieval pretreatments required for the two antibodies, which really must be the same in order for the technique to be successful. Undoubtedly, double immunohistochemical labeling is particularly successful if the two antigens are localized to different parts of the cell. Examples would include nuclear antigens such as Ki67 or steroid hormone receptors used in combination with membrane or cytoplasmic antigens such as human leukocyte antigen (HLA)-G or cytokeratin. Apart from different antigens, double labeling can of course also involve combinations with labeled lectins *(53)* or with the terminal deoxynucleotidyl transferase-mediated dUTP nick-end labeling (TUNEL) method *(54)*.

Because the definitive early studies of trophoblast invasion in pregnancy hysterectomy specimens preceded the development of immunohistochemistry, there is enormous scope for double immunohistochemical labeling to define accurately the relationships between different cell types in the placental bed at different stages of gestation.

3.2. Identification of Relevant Structures

3.2.1. General Strategy of Histological Evaluation

Because the purpose of this research is the interpretation of placental bed biopsies, a newcomer in the field should ideally have access to large hysterectomy preparations. The exercise of trying to recognize various structures and understanding their localization in such material will be extremely helpful for proper interpretation of biopsy specimens. Besides, only by studying such overview sections can the real extent and variability of trophoblast invasion be appreciated. Unfortunately, such specimens are rarely available for study.

Turning to biopsies, the first question is always whether the tissue sample is a "real" placental bed biopsy. The presence of trophoblast is the ultimate criterion and, therefore, application of cytokeratin immunohistochemistry is essential. At a first screening, one usually looks for the presence of interstitial trophoblast, which may occasionally be present in large numbers, but may also be very scarce. Studies on hysterectomy specimens have shown how the numbers of interstitial trophoblast decrease near the margins and in the center of the placental bed *(9)*. In the course of pregnancy, interstitial mononuclear trophoblastic cells fuse into multinuclear giant cells, and the presence of the latter provides an excellent indicator for a true placental bed biopsy, even when cytokeratin immunohistochemistry is not immediately available. When one sees small clusters of cytokeratin-positive mononuclear cells, it is advisable to check whether these are not part of tangentially cut endometrial glands.

Next, one must make sure that both decidua and myometrium are present. The presence of myometrium is essential for evaluating the depth of trophoblast invasion, especially in complicated pregnancies. Often, decidual tissue is very fragmentary, and the decidual–myometrial junction may be very irregular. α-Smooth muscle actin or desmin immunostaining is helpful for proper delineation of decidual and myometrial compartments. Remnants of endometrial glands are usually present in the decidua, even at term. The epithelial lining of the glands is often extremely flattened, and cytokeratin-immunostaining is required to distinguish residual glands from dilated capillaries or venules *(55)*. Glandular profiles may be numerous in a biopsy originating from the placental bed margin: based on observations on complete hysterectomy specimens it has been assumed that lateral expansion of the placenta pushes the glands aside, resulting in an accumulation of glandular profiles in these marginal areas *(56)*. Glandular structures may also be found in the inner myometrium, which is known as the phenomenon of adenomyosis.

3.2.2. Spiral Arteries

It is important to understand the basic anatomy of the vascular system in the uterus. The basic arterial supply has been described by Robertson and colleagues *(57)* as follows: "In the nonpregnant uterus the spiral arteries are the terminations of the radial arteries, the latter traversing the myometrium as offshoots of the arcuate system. Just internal to the myometrial–endometrial junction the radial artery gives off the spiral or coiled arteries, which are muscular arteries, 200–300 μm in diameter, with a well defined internal elastic lamina, which however, gradually disappears as the spiral artery penetrates into the endometrium. The radial arteries also give rise to smaller arteries, 100 μm or less in diameter, known as the straight arteries but which we prefer to call the basal arteries that ramify in the inner myometrium and terminate in the basal endometrium. They would appear to be much less hormone responsive than the spiral arteries, their function probably being nutritive only [to the uterus]..." The different arterial components can be recognized in the diagram of the placental bed, taken from Brosens *(2)* (**Fig. 1**).

3.2.2.1. Normal Pregnancy

During pregnancy, extensive modifications take place in the spiral arteries, which are invaded by trophoblast. Brosens and colleagues *(2)* coined the term "physiological changes" to emphasize the fact that they are not pathological. The development of these changes clearly is a multistep process *(58)*, occurring along both decidual and myometrial segments of these vessels. Physiological change may be complete, i.e., comprising the whole circumference of the

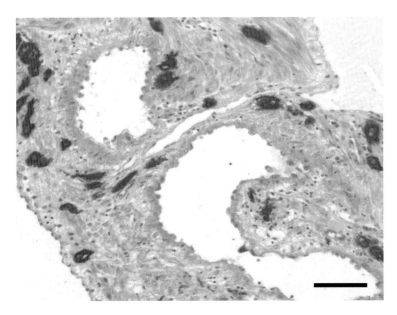

Fig. 7. Veins in the placental bed of a 26-wk pregnancy which have not undergone trophoblast invasion or physiological change. A few scattered interstitial trophoblastic cells are present. Cytokeratin immunostaining. (Bar = 100 μm.)

vessel, or partial, when the changes are restricted to a part of the arterial circumference (**Fig. 9**). It is claimed that also parts of the radial arteries may occasionally undergo trophoblast invasion and physiological changes *(3)*. Veins and basal arterioles on the other hand never undergo trophoblast invasion or associated vascular changes (**Figs. 7** and **8**).

Within first- and early second-trimester spiral artery cross sections, intraluminal trophoblast, which may be in the process of becoming embedded into the arterial wall (**Fig. 5**), can be readily found. Also, perivascular trophoblastic cells may be present, positioned at the adventitia of the vessel. The extent to which perivascular as well as endovascular trophoblast may contribute to the intramural trophoblast in the spiral artery wall requires further study. Histological and immunohistochemical studies of placental bed biopsies may provide some clues to this. Intramural trophoblast can often be identified within the wall of myometrial spiral arteries before endovascular trophoblast is detected, raising the possibility that at least a proportion of intramural trophoblast originates from interstitial (perivascular) trophoblast (JNB). Immunohistochemical studies also provide some support for a dual origin of intramural trophoblast from both endovascular and perivascular trophoblast. In contrast with other trophoblast populations within the placental bed, endovascular trophoblast

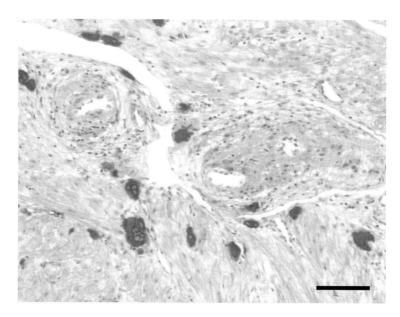

Fig. 8. Several sections through a basal artery of a normal pregnancy, taken at the same magnification as **Figs. 4, 7,** and **9–11**. A few multinuclear interstitial giant cells are present. Cytokeratin immunostaining. (Bar = 100 μm.)

expresses the adhesion molecule NCAM *(59)*. Intramural trophoblast in transformed spiral arteries in normal placental bed from the early second trimester onwards is both NCAM-positive and negative *(60)*, providing circumstantial evidence that the intramural trophoblast may originate from both NCAM-negative perivascular trophoblast and NCAM-positive endovascular trophoblast. However, even the most detailed histological and immunohistochemical studies cannot provide definitive evidence for the direction of cell movement in vivo. The development of in vitro models of spiral arteries may allow further clarification *(61)*, although in vitro studies may not be directly representative of the in vivo situation.

The origin and even the composition of the "fibrinoid," which is deposited in the spiral arteries as a part of the transformation process, is also uncertain. Fibrinoid reacts with antibodies to fibrinogen *(62,63)* and further components include complement factors and basement membrane components *(62–64)*. Based on ultrastructural observations, an origin from degenerating trophoblast, maternal serum leakage, and residues of elastica appears likely *(65)*. Indeed, in spiral arteries, which show incomplete transformation, a deficiency of intramural trophoblast and fibrinoid often co-exist. With regard to the possible dual origin of the intramural trophoblast, it is not certain in how far fibrinoid depo-

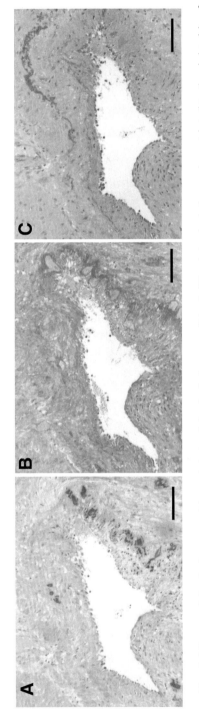

Fig. 9. Myometrial spiral artery with partial physiological change at 34 wk. Physiological change is restricted to the right side of the vessel, showing a thickened intima overlying the fibrinoid-embedded trophoblast. (**A**) Cytokeratin + hematoxylin and eosin; (**B**) periodic acid–Schiff; (**C**) Orcein staining, showing the presence of an elastica layer at the unconverted upper side of the vessel. (Bar = 100 μm.)

sition may be exclusively associated with endovascular trophoblast. Indeed, the use of a PAS counterstain in placental bed biopsies immunolabeled with cytokeratin has demonstrated PAS positive fibrinoid material associated with occasional perivascular trophoblast within the myometrium (JNB; **Fig. 6**).

The classical histological picture of a spiral artery near term is that of a vessel showing few structural features except a "glassy" ground substance with a few embedded cells. Application of PAS staining reveals a brilliant pink staining of this "fibrinoid," contrasting it with the pale embedded cells, which can be shown to be trophoblastic by cytokeratin-immunostaining. The typical PAS staining of the fibrinoid also facilitates the detection of partial physiological change in spiral arteries. The fibrinoid-containing areas of the vessel wall have lost both their vascular smooth muscle and their elastica, resulting in an irregular wavy outline (**Fig. 4**). It should be added here that physiologically changed spiral arteries near term possess a fully restored endothelial layer, although the misconception exists that in the course of pregnancy the endothelial layer is permanently replaced by endovascular trophoblast. Moreover, an additional subintimal layer, consisting of connective tissue with (myo)fibroblasts, may be formed between the endothelium and the fibrinoid layer, suggesting that a maternal tissue repair process takes place following trophoblast invasion (**Fig. 9**).

3.2.2.2. COMPLICATED PREGNANCIES

As alluded to in the introduction, placental bed research was initially very much focused on preeclampsia *(3)*, and for a long time, this was the only relatively well-studied pathological condition. It was increasingly recognized however, that in other pregnancy complications a spectrum of "preeclampsia-like" arterial defects might be present *(7,8,49,66–68)*. Therefore, in the following paragraphs, while different specific pathological changes are described, continuous reference will be made to preeclampsia as a primordial reference condition; however, it should be clear that similar vasculopathies might be present in other pathological situations. There is still a wide field of research to be explored.

The original observation that in preeclampsia physiological changes are restricted to the decidual spiral arteries and absent from the myometrial segments *(3)* (**Fig. 10**) brought excitement because of the implicit possibility of explaining the cause of preeclampsia. Sporadic observations in other hypertensive conditions of pregnancy strengthened the idea that the observed vascular defects in preeclampsia might be virtually pathognomonic for the disease *(69)*. Khong and colleagues *(12)* pointed out that the situation in preeclampsia may be even worse than originally thought, because in a proportion of spiral arteries, the decidual segments also showed failed invasion and absence of physiological change. Observations on intrauterine growth restriction (IUGR)

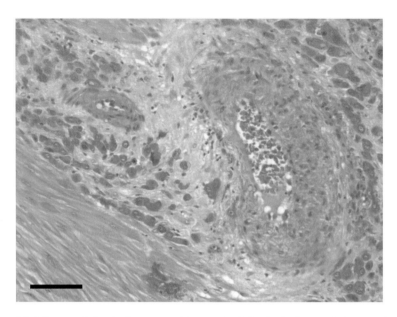

Fig. 10. Myometrial spiral artery without physiological change in a preeclamptic pregnancy at 27 wk. Although there is no indication of endovascular trophoblast invasion having taken place, plenty of interstitial trophoblast is present around the vessel. (Bar = 100 µm.)

pregnancies without hypertension represented the first difficulty with this black-and-white concept, however. Also, here defective physiological changes could be found in a proportion of cases, even in the decidual segments of the spiral arteries. Lack of vascular invasion in the decidua was observed in 50% of the hypertensive cases, but also in 30% of IUGR cases without hypertension *(13)*.

For a proper understanding of spiral artery changes in different pregnancy complications, all arterial structures in a placental bed biopsy should be identified (**Figs. 4–10**). To distinguish spiral from basal arteries, one can partly rely on their respective diameters of 200 µm vs less than 100 µm as indicated by Robertson and colleagues *(57)*, but there, difficulties always arise in classifying the intermediate 100- to 200-µm vessels. Noninvaded spiral arteries may show a "normal" arterial structure, which of course should be considered pathological because of the absence of physiological change. In such arteries, only the presence of fibrous glycoproteins, different in appearance from the amorphous fibrinoid of physiologically changed vessels, is revealed by PAS staining, whereas orcein staining often shows an intact elastica. On the other hand, such arteries may have undergone disorganization of the media, and elastica

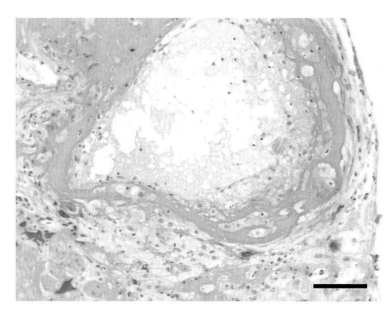

Fig. 11. Acute atherosis in a decidual spiral artery in a preeclamptic pregnancy at 29 wk. Several foam cells are present within the necrotic vessel wall. A few cytokeratin-positive perivascular trophoblastic cells or cell fragments are present. (Bar = 100 μm.)

staining may turn out to be weak and fragmented. The local presence of interstitial and perivascular trophoblast in addition to maternal infiltrating cells may play a role in this vascular disorganization. Also, various degrees of medial hyperplasia occur, which is possibly related to a hypertensive condition.

The most advertised defect in "noninvaded" spiral arteries is acute atherosis, a serious arterial lesion which was at one time assumed to be a possible pathognomonic feature of preeclampsia *(57)*, and which has been associated with placental infarcts *(21)*. The lesion is characterized by fibrinoid necrosis, lipophage (foam cell) infiltration, and the presence of inflammatory cells (**Fig. 11**). The three characteristics may occur in various degrees, the necrosis being the most frequently observed feature. In this context, the term "fibrinoid" is somewhat confusing, because it bears no relationship with the physiological fibrinoid of a trophoblast-invaded spiral artery. PAS staining of fibrinoid necrosis results in a more grayish-bluish color than the brilliant pink staining in a physiologically changed artery. Foam cells may be formed by lipid accumulation in smooth muscle cells *(70)*, but most of them are probably derived from infiltrating macrophages and often show a focal distribution. The macrophage-derived nature of the lipophages can be demonstrated by CD68 staining *(48,49)*. Early stages of atherosis may be more easily detected by applying lipoprotein(a) immunostaining *(71)*. The presence of cytokines such as tumor necrosis factor (TNF)-α *(72)* may support a potential lytic action of these cells towards invading trophoblast. Although in the past, the presence of trophoblast and atherosis were viewed as mutually exclusive, a painstaking perusal of large numbers of slides occasionally allows detection of physiologically changed arteries containing lipophages *(73)* and atherotic vessels showing remnants of cytokeratin-stained trophoblast *(8,48,49)*. Although atherosis is a striking vascular defect, its occurrence should not be exaggerated, and also Khong and Robertson *(74)* stated that in preeclampsia acute atherosis only occurs in a minority of vessels. It is not impossible that the extent of acute atherosis is related to the severity of the disease, and some observations suggest that there is a significantly higher incidence of acute atherosis in myometrial spiral arteries in patients with Hemolysis, Elevated Liver, Low Platelet (HELLP) syndrome (Pijnenborg and Hanssens, unpublished results).

Occasionally, also thrombosis can be seen in placental bed spiral arteries, although it is not a common finding. The presence of a thrombus often leads to stretching of the wall, which makes it difficult to recognize the vessel as an artery or a vein. However, if there is trophoblast in the wall, cytokeratin immunostaining allows identification of the vessel as spiral artery, which had previously undergone physiological change.

3.3. Quantitative and Qualitative Methods of Assessment

3.3.1. Interstitial Trophoblast

It is often striking how heavily a placental bed biopsy may be infiltrated by interstitial trophoblast, and one is tempted to believe that a paucity of invasion must have some clinical significance. Therefore, the exercise of quantifying this invasion would seem to be potentially rewarding.

In 8- to 18-wk hysterectomy specimens, a point-counting technique was used to determine volume densities of interstitial myometrial invasion in complete sections. The results of these measurements indicated a shift from an initial quadratic distribution (highest density at the center of the placental bed) to a quartic distribution from 10 wk onward, suggesting a ring-like maximal invasive zone around a less invasive center (**Fig. 12**). Because of this high variability of interstitial invasion throughout the placental bed, proper quantitation using biopsies derived from uncertain locations must always be problematical.

Evaluating the depth of invasion is also difficult, and even in properly oriented whole hysterectomy blocks individual variation occurs, which may partly be related to the contractile status of the myometrium. Following the seminal paper by Brosens and colleagues *(2)*, by convention one is accustomed to referring to "the inner third" of the myometrium as the invasion area. The question

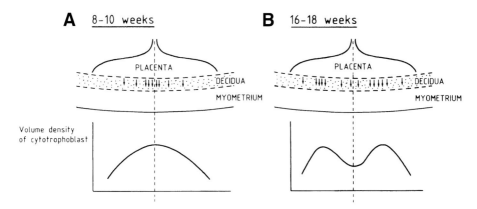

Fig. 12. Diagrams illustrating the distribution of interstitial trophoblast in the placental bed at 8–10 wk (**A**) and 16–18 wk (**B**). Arrows indicate probable pathways of interstitial invasion, showing a lateral shift at 16–18 wk. Reproduced from **ref. *19***, with permission.

which then arises is how deep this is in real distance and how the invasion depth is related to the anatomical composition of the uterine wall. A proper approach would be to define a real anatomical demarcation line between inner and outer myometrium, the existence of which is implied by the studies of J. J. Brosens and colleagues *(75)*. One might consider the level where radial arteries are splitting off into spiral arteries as the real limit of the inner myometrium, but this level is usually difficult to define on histological sections. Brosens and colleagues *(3)* stated that in normal pregnancies, the physiological changes of the myometrial spiral arteries "often reach the distal portions of the radial arteries." In some pregnancy complications, trophoblast invasion may occur beyond this level. Indeed, Khong and Robertson *(25)* observed in a few placenta accreta cases that physiological change extended into the radial and arcuate arteries deep in the myometrium. In hysterectomy specimens from severely anemic women, Kadyrov and colleagues *(22)* also showed deeper than normal invasion, whereas in the latter group invasion was deeper than in the preeclampsia cases. In their report, no indication is given of the position of the radial and spiral arteries, however. In the absence of objective criteria for defining deeper myometrial layers, it is not possible to evaluate the depth of invasion on biopsies, in which proper orientation of the tissue block vs the inner or outer uterine surface is usually not feasible.

Excluding the depth of invasion, placental bed biopsies may be scored for interstitial invasion to indicate high, moderate, or low invasion as a quick and easy approach. To our knowledge, such a scoring system never provided meaningful results. More objective counting methods can be applied, but so far, few data have been published in the literature. Pijnenborg and colleagues *(50)* counted trophoblast numbers within a randomly displaced reference frame in biopsies of normotensive and preeclamptic pregnancies, but the results were highly variable and the difference between the groups was not significant. In a different study, the area percentage of cytokeratin immunostaining was measured using a computerized image analysis system, and in this study on three randomly chosen decidual and myometrial fields, respectively, significantly less interstitial trophoblast was found in both decidua and myometrium of preeclamptic women *(76)*. There is, however, no reason why computer-assisted quantitation should yield more reliable data compared with a well executed manual counting. It is clear that such well randomized studies should be repeated in different centers using different collections of placental bed biopsies and executed according to rigorously defined parameters.

3.3.2. Assessment of Spiral Artery Changes

3.3.2.1. Individual Histological Features vs "Physiological Change"

The term "physiological change" *(2)* refers to the combination of tropho-blast cells within spiral artery walls, accumulated fibrinoid material, and loss of musculo-elastic tissue in the media. Although physiological change is present in variable degrees in a spiral artery depending on the proportion of the vessel wall circumference containing fibrinoid-embedded trophoblast and showing loss of medial smooth muscle and elastica, this has rarely been considered. Moreover, the degree of fibrinoid change does not always correspond with endovascular trophoblast invasion *(8)*. Thus, the assessment of physiological change as an entity *(26,77–79)* introduces the problem of defining which particular features constitute physiological change and how much weight should be attributed to each feature. Previous authors *(26,77–79)* have failed to take this into account. In particular, in pathological pregnancies, it remains possible that only some features of physiological change are abnormal and differences between abnormal and normal pregnancies would be missed if these features were not assessed separately.

3.3.2.2. Assessment of Individual Vessels vs "Overall Assessment" or Inclusion of One "Representative" Spiral Artery

Placental bed biopsies often contain more than one spiral artery. In previous studies, authors have made a subjective "overall assessment" of all spiral arteries for each case *(26,77,80)*, have included only one representative vessel per case *(30)* or have assessed spiral arteries individually *(8,10,49)*. An overall assessment can lead to underrepresentation of findings, which are present only in a minority of vessels, or to overreporting of rare but particularly striking abnormalities or artifacts, leading to bias. In fact, authors who made subjective overall assessments reported few or no placental bed spiral arteries with absent physiological changes in normal placental bed, whereas authors who systematically graded histological findings for separate spiral arteries *(8,10)* reported a larger proportion of unchanged spiral arteries. Selecting only one spiral artery as representative of the entire placental bed *(30)* is not valid in view of the reported variation in the proportion of myometrial spiral arteries affected by physiological change within one subject at term *(7,8)*. Observation of single features of spiral artery transformation in early pregnancy suggests an even larger variation *(10)*. Furthermore, changes may involve only isolated artery segments or a proportion of the vessel circumference *(2)*. Thus, it appears to be most appropriate to assess each spiral artery or spiral artery section individually. However, this approach can result in multiple observations in one individual, which, as a result of environmental and genetic confounders, cannot be regarded as independent, and thus cannot be analyzed with standard statistical tests, but require more complex statistical methods, such as the use of statistical models *(68)*.

3.3.2.3. Qualitative vs Quantitative Methods of Assessment of Spiral Artery Changes

1. Endovascular and intramural trophoblast. Intraluminal and intramural trophoblast cells are usually regarded as an entity *(80)* and, therefore, are assessed together *(10)*. However, there is evidence that these cells may represent two separate subgroups of extravillous trophoblast *(68)*. Whereas intramural trophoblast appears dendritic and expresses the α6β4 integrin pair, intraluminal trophoblast is rounded and α6β4 integrin-negative. Furthermore, there may be some merit in assessing intraluminal trophoblast quantitatively; an observational report suggested the failure of intraluminal trophoblast to form cohesive multicellular "plugs" in pregnancies complicated by preeclampsia *(82)*.

2. Media disruption. In a large series of predominantly non-placental bed decidua, spiral artery media was quantified using computerized micro-imaging by dividing (mathematically) the area of media by the external vessel diameter *(83)*. If applied to the placental bed, trophoblast cells and fibrinoid material interposed between medial smooth muscle cells would be likely to influence measurements. Furthermore, only round artery cross-sections can be analyzed using this approach and many spiral arteries would have to be excluded because of oblique or irregular cross sections, commonly detected in spiral arteries, which have undergone physiological change. Therefore, the semi-quantitative scale published by Pijnenborg and colleagues *(10)* of absent, mild, and severe medial changes appears to be a pragmatic approach.

3. Fibrinoid change. Although fibrinoid change makes a major contribution to the definition of physiological spiral artery change *(2)*, there are no published studies quantifying fibrinoid change and Pijnenborg and colleagues *(10)* also did not assess this feature. Meekins and colleagues *(8)* published a semi-quantitative assessment of fibrinoid including the grades "isolated, partial, and complete," depending on the proportion of fibrinoid with embedded intramural trophoblast cells in the vessel wall. However, in view of the observed discrepancy between fibrinoid and intramural trophoblast cells *(68)*, it would appear justified to assess these two features separately.

From this review of the literature, it is evident that authors have used a number of different methods to grade physiological spiral artery change. However, the comparison between normal and abnormal placental beds and between different studies would be made more meaningful if a common grading system was adopted.

4. Notes

Enormous progress has been made since the previous multicentric review was written on placental bed methodology *(11)*. Concerning biopsy techniques, the recent introduction of an ultrasound-guided approach *(28)* has allowed more ready access to samples from the first half of pregnancy. Meanwhile, insights in histology have been dramatically improved by the application of immunohistochemical techniques, an approach that was still in its pioneering stage 20 yr ago. Application of fast and less tiresome image analysis techniques with appropriate statistics may facilitate more extensive data collection on trophoblast invasion in the near future; moreover, computerized image analysis also facilitates studies of the relationship between several parameters. There is no doubt that also molecular techniques will increasingly be applied, including *in situ* hybridization and microarray analysis of individual cells obtained by laser microdissection.

The 1986 paper by Robertson and colleagues *(11)* concluded with a paragraph on "unanswered questions," and rereading this part provides a good exercise in modesty. They considered "elucidation of the promotional and controlling factors mediating the behavior of migratory extravillous trophoblast" as being "of prime importance." It must be said that in this field, enormous progress has been made during the last two decades, mainly based on the explosion of techniques for isolating and studying trophoblastic cells in vitro, ranging from isolated cells to tissue and organ cultures. Histology will, however, remain important as a guide to interpret cellular behavior observed in an artificial in vitro system. On the other hand, basic histological questions are still not fully answered, for example concerning the reality of the two-wave invasion and the extent of arterial invasion in normal and complicated pregnancies. We still do not understand the mechanisms of restricted physiological change in preeclampsia, particularly whether or not endovascular trophoblast invasion is inhibited at the very beginning, or is a secondary phenomenon, being initially normal but subsequently countered by maternal cells. Questions have arisen about the relationship of endovascular invasion to early intervillous blood flow *(84,85)*, which have forced us to rethink basic placental biology. Also on the clinical side, there are still many unanswered questions on pregnancy complications such as preeclampsia and IUGR. Refining methods for defining (categorizing) pregnancy complications will open up prospects for better management, but this should be backed up by an understanding of the placental bed. Therefore, it remains appropriate to end this chapter with the final sentence of Robertson's 1986 review, that "it is difficult to see how further progress can be made in the field of human placentation and its associated disorders without secure morphologic base."

References

1. Browne, J. C. M. and Veall, N. (1953) The maternal placental blood flow in normotensive and hypertensive women. *J. Obstet. Gyn. Br. Emp.* **60,** 141–148.
2. Brosens, I., Robertson, W. B., and Dixon, H. G. (1967) The physiological response of the vessels of the placental bed to normal pregnancy. *J. Path. Bact.* **93,** 569–579.
3. Brosens, I. A., Robertson, W. B., and Dixon, H. G. (1972) The role of spiral arteries in the pathogenesis of preeclampsia, in *Obstetrics and Gynecology annual* (Wynn, R., ed.). Appleton-Century-Crofts, New York: pp. 177–191.
4. Pijnenborg, R., Vercruysse, L., Hanssens, M., and Van Assche, F. A. (2003) Incomplete trophoblast invasion: the evidence, in *Pre-eclampsia* (Critchley, H., MacLean, A., Poston, L., and Walker, J., eds.). RCOG, London: pp. 15–26.
5. Sheppard, B. L. and Bonnar, J. (1976) The ultrastructure of the arterial supply of the human placenta in pregnancy complicated by fetal growth retardation. *Br. J. Obstet. Gynaecol.* **83,** 948–959.
6. Davey, D. A. and MacGillivray, I. (1988) The classification and definition of the hypertensive disorders of pregnancy. *Am. J. Obstet. Gynecol.* **158,** 892–898.
7. Pijnenborg, R., Anthony, J., Davey, D. A., et al. (1991) Placental bed spiral arteries in the hypertensive disorders of pregnancy. *Br. J. Obstet. Gynaecol.* **98,** 648–655.
8. Meekins, J.W., Pijnenborg, R., Hanssens, M., Van Assche, A., and McFadyen, I. R. (1994) A study of placental bed spiral arteries and trophoblast invasion in normal and severe pre-eclamptic pregnancies. *Br. J. Obstet. Gynaecol.* **101,** 669–674.
9. Pijnenborg, R., Bland, J. M., Robertson, W. B., Dixon, G., and Brosens, I. (1981) The pattern of interstitial trophoblastic invasion of the myometrium in early human pregnancy. *Placenta* **2,** 303–316.
10. Pijnenborg, R., Bland, J. M., Robertson, W. B., and Brosens, I. (1983) Uteroplacental arterial changes related to interstitial trophoblast migration in early human pregnancy. *Placenta* **4,** 397–414.

11. Robertson, W. B., Khong, T. Y., Brosens, I., De Wolf, F., Sheppard, B. L., and Bonnar, J. (1986) The placental bed biopsy: review from three European centers. *Am. J. Obstet. Gynecol.* **155,** 401–412.
12. Ramsey, E. M. (1982) *The placenta: human and animal.* Praeger, New York: p. 154.
13. Khong, T. Y., De Wolf, F., Robertson, W. B., and Brosens, I. (1986) Inadequate maternal vascular response to placentation in pregnancies complicated by pre-eclampsia and by small-for-gestational age infants. *Br. J. Obstet. Gynaecol.* **93,** 1049–1059.
14. Khong, T. Y. and Chambers, H. M. (1992) Alternative method of sampling placentas for the assessment of uteroplacental vasculature. *J. Clin. Pathol.* **45,** 925–927.
15. Zeek, P. M. and Assali, N. S. (1950) Vascular changes in the decidua associated with eclamptogenic toxemia of pregnancy. *Am. J. Clin. Path.* **20,** 1099–1109.
16. Salafia, C. M., Starzyk, K. A., Lage, J. M., Parkash, V., Vercruysse, L., and Pijnenborg, R. (1998) Lipoprotein(a) deposition in the uteroplacental bed and in basal plate uteroplacental arteries in normal and complicated pregnancies. *Trophoblast Res.* **11,** 377–387.
17. Boyd, J. D. and Hamilton, W. J. (1970) The Human Placenta. Heffer & Sons, Cambridge.
18. Burton, G. J., Jauniaux, E., and Waltson, A. L. (1999 Maternal arterial connections to the placental intervillous space during the first trimester of human pregnancy: the Boyd collection revisited. *Am. J. Obstet. Gynecol.* **181,** 718–724.
19. Pijnenborg, R., Dixon, G., Robertson, W. B., and Brosens, I. (1980) Trophoblastic invasion of human decidua from 8 to 18 weeks of pregnancy. *Placenta* **1,** 3–19.
20. Pijnenborg, R. (1990) Trophoblast invasion and placentation in the human: morphological aspects. Trophoblast Res. **4,** 33–47.
21. Brosens, I. and Renaer, M. (1972) On the pathogenesis of placental infarcts in pre-eclampsia. *J. Obstet. Gynaecol. Br. Cwlth.* **79,** 794–799.
22. Kadyrov, M., Schmitz, C., Black, S., Kaufmann, P., and Huppertz, B. (2003) Pre-eclampsia and maternal anaemia display reduced apoptosis and opposite invasive phenotypes of extravillous trophoblast. *Placenta* **24,** 540–548.
23. Dixon, H. G. and Robertson, W. B. (1958) A study of the vessels of the placental bed in normotensive and hypertensive women. *J. Obstet. Gyn. Br. Emp.* **65,** 803–809.
24. Hanssens, M., Pijnenborg, R., Vercruysse, L., and Van Assche, F. A. (1997) Adequacy of placental bed biopsies depends not only on sample-size. *Hypertension in Pregnancy* **16,** 165 (Abstract).
25. Khong, T. Y. and Robertson, W. B. (1987) Placenta creta and placenta praevia creta. *Placenta* **8,** 399–409.
26. Michel, M., Underwood, J., Clark, D. A., Mowbray, J. F., and Beard, R. W. (1989) Histologic and immunologic study of uterine biopsy tissue of women with incipient abortion. *Am. J. Obstet. Gynecol.* **161,** 409–414.
27. Michel, M. Z., Khong, T. Y., Clark, D. A., and Beard, R. W. (1990) A morphological and immunological study of human placental bed biopsies in miscarriage. *Br. J. Obstet. Gynaecol.* **97,** 984–988.

28. Robson, S. C., Simpson, H., Ball, E., Lyall, F., and Bulmer, J. N. (2002) Punch biopsy of the human placental bed. *Am. J. Obstet. Gynecol.* **187,** 1349–1355.

29. Ball, E., Robson, S. C., Lyall, F., Ayis, S., and Bulmer, J. N. (2001) Sporadic miscarriage is associated with abnormal trophoblast invasion into spiral arteries. *J. Soc. Gynecol. Invest.* **8(Suppl. 1),** 82A.

30. Gerretsen, G., Huisjes, H. J., and Elena, J. D. (1981) Morphological changes of the spiral arteries in the placental bed in relation to pre-eclampsia and fetal growth retardation. *Br. J. Obstet. Gynaecol.* **88,** 876–881.

31. von Wasielewski, R., Werner, M., Nolte, M., Wilkens, L., and Georgii, A. (1994) Effects of antigen retrieval by microwave heating in formalin-fixed tissue sections on a broad panel of antibodies. *Histochemistry* **102,** 165–172.

32. Hanssens, M., Vercruysse, L., Verbist, L., Pijnenborg, R., Keirse, M. J. N. C., and Van Assche, F. A. (1995) Renin-like immunoreactivity in human placenta and fetal membranes. *Histochem.Cell Biol.* **104,** 435–442.

33. Zhou, Y., Fisher, S. J., Janatpour, M., et al. (1997) Human cytotrophoblasts adopt a vascular phenotype as they differentiate. A strategy for successful endovascular invasion? *J. Clin. Invest.* **99,** 2139–2151.

34. Lyall, F., Bulmer, J. N., Kelly, H., Duffie, E., and Robson, S. C. (1999) Human trophoblast invasion and spiral artery transformation: the role of nitric oxide. *Am. J. Pathol.* **154,** 1105–1114.

35. Lyall, F., Barber, A., Myatt, L., Bulmer, J. N., and Robson, S. C. (2000) Hemeoxygenase expression in human placenta and placental bed implies a role in regulation of trophoblast invasion and placental function. *FASEB J.* **14,** 208–219.

36. Lyall, F., Simpson, H., Bulmer, J. N., Barber, A., and Robson, S. C. (2001) Transforming growth factor-beta expression in human placenta and placental bed in third trimester normal pregnancy, preeclampsia, and fetal growth restriction. *Am. J. Pathol.* **159,** 1827–1838.

37. Barber, A., Robson, S. C., Myatt, L., Bulmer, J. N., and Lyall, F. (2001) Heme oxygenase expression in human placenta and placental bed: reduced expression of placenta endothelial HO-2 in preeclampsia and fetal growth restriction. *FASEB J.* **15,** 1159–1168.

38. Simpson, H., Robson, S. C., Bulmer, J. N., Barber, A., and Lyall, F. (2002) Transforming growth factor beta expression in human placenta and placental bed during early pregnancy. *Placenta* **23,** 44–58.

39. Huppertz, B., Kertschanska, S., Demir, A. Y., Frank, H. G., and Kaufmann, P. (1998) Immunohistochemistry of matrix metalloproteinases (MMP), their substrates, and their inhibitors (TIMP) during trophoblast invasion in the human placenta. *Cell Tissue Res.* **291,** 133–148.

40. Phillips, R. J., Innes, B. A., Searle, R. F., Bulmer, J. N., and Robson, S. C. (2003) Use of laser capture microdissection and RT-PCR to study gene expression in heterogeneous, differentiating trophoblast populations. *J. Soc. Gynecol. Invest.* **10(Suppl. 2),** 398A.

41. Bulmer, J. N., Billington, W. D., and Johnson, P. M.(1984) Immunohistologic identification of trophoblast populations in early human pregnancy with the use of monoclonal antibodies. *Am. J. Obstet. Gynecol.* **148,** 19–26.

42. Khong, T. Y., Lanc, E. B., and Robertson, W. B. (1986) An immunocytochemical study of fetal cells at the maternal-placental interface using monoclonal antibodies to keratins, vimentin and desmin. *Cell Tissue Res.* **246,** 189–195.

43. Meekins, J. W., Pijnenborg, R., Hanssens, M., McFadyen, I. R., and Van Assche, F. A. (1994) Immunohistochemical identification of placental bed biopsies and the implications when studying the spiral artery response to pregnancy. *Hypertension in Pregnancy* **13,** 61–69.

44. Stiemer, B., Graf, R., Neudeck, H., Hildebrandt, R., Hopp, H., and Weitzel, H. K. (1995) Antibodies to cytokeratins bind to epitopes in human uterine smooth muscle cells in normal and pathological pregnancies. *Histopathology* **27,** 407–414.

45. Haigh, T., Chen, C.-P., Jones, C. J. P., and Aplin, J. D. (1999) Studies of mesenchymal cells from 1st trimester human placenta: expression of cytokeratin outside the trophoblast lineage. *Placenta* **20,** 615–625.

46. Robertson, W. B. and Manning, P. J. (1974) Elastic tissue in uterine blood vessels. *J. Path. Bact.* **112,** 237–243.

47. Cooper, K., Haffajee, Z., and Taylor, L. (1997) Comparative analysis of biotin intranuclear inclusions of gestational endometrium using the APAAP, ABC and the PAP immunodetection systems. *J. Clin. Pathol.* **50,** 153–156.

48. Hanssens, M., Vercruysse, L., Keirse, M. J. N. C., Pijnenborg, R., and Van Assche, F. A. (1995) Identification of 'renin'-containing cells in the choriodecidua. *Placenta* **16,** 517–525.

49. Hanssens, M., Pijnenborg, R., Keirse, M. J. N. C., Vercruysse, L., Verbist, L., and Van Assche, F. A. (1998) Renin-like immunoreactivity in uterus and placenta from normotensive and hypertensive pregnancies. *Eur. J. Obstet. Gynec. Reprod. Biol.* **81,** 177–184.

50. Pijnenborg, R., Vercruysse, L., Verbist, L., and Van Assche, F. A. (1998) Interaction of interstitial trophoblast with placental bed capillaries and venules of normotensive and pre-eclamptic pregnancies. *Placenta* **19,** 569–575.

51. DiFederico, E., Genbacev, O., and Fisher, S. J. (1999) Preeclampsia is associated with widespread apoptosis of placental cytotrophoblasts within the uterine wall. *Am. J. Pathol.* **155,** 293–301.

52. Lyall, F., Bulmer, J. N., Duffie, E., Cousins, F., Theriault, A., and Robson, S. C. (2001) Human trophoblast invasion and spiral artery transformation: the role of PECAM-1 in normal pregnancy, preeclampsia, and fetal growth restriction. *Am. J. Pathol.* **158,** 1713–1721.

53. Paffaro, V. A.Jr., Bizinotto, M. C., Joazeiro, P. P., and Yamada, A. T. (2003) Subset classification of mouse uterine natural killer cells by DBA lectin reactivity. *Placenta* **24,** 479–488.

54. Pongcharoen, S., Bulmer, J. N., and Searle, R. F. (2004) No evidence for apoptosis of decidual leucocytes in normal and molar pregnancy.*Clin. Exp. Immunol.* **138,** 330–336.

55. Bulmer, J. N., Wells, M., Bhabra, K., and Johnson, P. M. (1986) Immunohisto-logical characterization of endometrial gland epithelium and extravillous fetal tro-phoblast in third trimester human placental bed tissues. *Br. J. Obstet. Gynaecol.* **93,** 823–832.
56. Pijnenborg, R. (1998) The human decidua as a passage-way for trophoblast inva-sion. *Trophoblast Res.* **11,** 229–241.
57. Robertson, W. B., Brosens, I., and Dixon, G. (1975) Uteroplacental vascular pathology. *Eur. J. Obstet. Gynec. Reprod. Biol.* **5,** 47–65.
58. Pijnenborg, R., Vercruysse, L., Hanssens, M., and Van Assche, F. A. (2005) Tro-phoblast invasion in pre-eclampsia and other pregnancy disorders, in *Pre-eclamp-sia—Aetiology and Clinical Practice* (Lyall, L. and Belfort, M., eds.) Cambridge University Press, in press.
59. Proll, J., Blaschitz, A., Hartmann, M., Thalhamer, J., and Dohr, G. (1996) Human first-trimester placenta intra-arterial trophoblast cells express the neural cell adhe-sion molecule. *Early Pregnancy* **2,** 271–275.
60. Bulmer, J. N., Turnbull, E., Gilfillan, C., Innes, B., Lyall, F., and Robson, S. C. (1999) NCAM is expressed by endovascular and perivascular trophoblast through-out normal pregnancy. *Placenta* **20,** A14.
61. Cartwright, J. E., Kenny, L. C., Dash, P. R., et al. (2002) Trophoblast invasion of spiral arteries: a novel in vitro model. *Placenta* **23,** 232–235.
62. Weir, P. E. (1981) Immunofluorescent studies of the uteroplacental arteries in normal pregnancy. *Br. J. Obstet. Gynaecol.* **88,** 301–307.
63. Wells, M., Bennett, J., Bulmer, J. N., Jackson, P., and Holgate, C. S. (1987) Complement component deposition in uteroplacental (spiral) arteries in normal human pregnancy. *J. Reprod. Immunol.* **12,** 125–135.
64. Wells, M., His, B. L., Yeh, C. J., and Faulk, W. P. (1984) Spiral (uteroplacental) arteries of the human placental bed show the presence of amniotic basement mem-brane antigens. *Am. J. Obstet. Gynecol.* **150,** 973–977.
65. De Wolf, F., De Wolf-Peeters, C., and Brosens, I. (1973) Ultrastructure of the spiral arteries in the human placental bed at the end of normal pregnancy. *Am. J. Obstet. Gynecol.* **117,** 833–848.
66. Aardema, M. W., Oosterhof, H., Timmer, A., van Rooy, I., and Aardnoudse, J. G. (2001) Uterine artery Doppler flow and uteroplacental vascular pathology in nor-mal pregnancies and pregnancies complicated by pre-eclampsia and small for ges-tational age fetuses. *Placenta* **22,** 405–411.
67. Kim, Y. M., Chaiworapongsa, T., Gomez, R., et al. (2002) Failure of physiologic transformation of the spiral arteries in the placental bed in preterm premature rupture of membranes. *Am. J. Obstet. Gynecol.* **187,** 1137–1142.
68. Ball, E. (2004) *The control of human spiral artery transformation in sporadic early and late miscarriages.* PhD Thesis, University of Newcastle upon Tyne.
69. Brosens, I. (1977) Morphological changes in the utero-placental bed in pregnancy hypertension. *Clin. Obstet. Gynaecol.* **4,** 573–593.
70. De Wolf, F., Robertson, W. B., and Brosens, I. (1975) The ultrastructure of acute atherosis in hypertensive pregnancy. *Am. J. Obstet. Gynecol.* **123,** 164–174.

71. Meekins, J. W., Pijnenborg, R., Hanssens, M., McFadyen, I. R., and Van Assche F. A. (1994) Immunohistochemical detection of lipoprotein(a) in the wall of placental bed spiral arteries in normal and severe preeclamptic pregnancies. *Placenta* **15**, 511–524.

72. Pijnenborg, R., McLaughlin, P. J., Vercruysse, L., et al. (1998) Immunolocalization of tumour necrosis factor-alpha (TNF-alpha) in the placental bed of normotensive and hypertensive human pregnancies. *Placenta* **19**, 231–239.

73. McFadyen, I. R., Price, A. B., and Geirsson, R. T. (1986) The relation of birthweight to histological appearances in vessels of the placental bed. *Br. J. Obstet. Gynaecol.* **93**, 476–481.

74. Khong, T. Y. and Robertson, W. B. (1992) Spiral artery disease, in *Immunological Obstetrics* (Coulam, C. B., Faulk, W. P., and McIntyre, J., eds.) Norton, New York: pp. 492–501.

75. Brosens, J. J., de Souza, N. M., and Barker, F. G. (1998) Steroid hormone-dependent myometrial zonal differentiation in the non-pregnant human uterus. *Eur. J. Obstet. Gynecol. Reprod. Biol.* **81**, 247–251.

76. Naicker, T., Khedun, S. M., Moodley, J., and Pijnenborg, R. (2003) Quantitative analysis of trophoblast invasion in preeclampsia. *Acta Obstet. Gynecol. Scand.* **82**, 722–729.

77. Hustin, J., Jauniaux, E., and Schaaps, J. P. (1990) Histological study of the materno-embryonic interface in spontaneous abortion. *Placenta* **11**, 477–486.

78. Jauniaux, E., Zaidi, J., Jurkovic, D., Campbell, S., and Hustin, J. (1994) Comparison of colour Doppler features and pathological findings in complicated early pregnancy. *Hum. Reprod.* **9**, 2432–2437.

79. Khong, T. Y. and Ford, J. H. (1997) Lack of correlation between conceptual karyotype and maternal response to placentation. *Reprod. Fertil. Dev.* **9**, 271–274.

80. Khong, T. Y., Liddell, H. S., and Robertson, W. B. (1987) Defective haemochorial placentation as a cause of miscarriage: a preliminary study. *Br. J. Obstet. Gynaecol.* **94**, 649–655.

81. Benirschke, K. and Kaufmann, P. (1999) *Pathology of the Human Placenta.* Springer Verlag, Wien, New York: pp. 171–247.

82. Zhou Y., Damsky, C. H., and Fisher, S. J. (1997) Preeclampsia is associated with failure of human cytotrophoblasts to mimic a vascular adhesion phenotype. *J. Clin. Invest.* **99**, 2152–2164.

83. Morgan, T., Craven, C., Lalouel, J. M., and Ward, K. (1999) Angiotensinogen Thr235 variant is associated with abnormal physiologic change of the uterine spiral arteries in first trimester decidua. *Am. J. Obstet. Gynecol.* **180**, 95–102.

84. Hustin, J. and Schaaps, J. P. (1987) Echographic and anatomic studies of the maternotrophoblastic border during the first trimester of pregnancy. *Am. J. Obstet. Gynecol.* **157**, 162–168.

85. Jauniaux, E., Watson, A. L., Hempstock, J., Bao, Y. P., Skepper, J. N., and Burton, G. J. (2000) Onset of maternal arterial blood flow and placental oxidative stress. A possible factor in human early pregnancy failure. *Am. J. Pathol.* **157**, 2111–2122.

3

In Vitro Analysis of Trophoblast Invasion

John D. Aplin

Summary

Two methods are described for the study of human trophoblast invasion. When first-trimester placental villi are explanted on gels of a permissive extracellular matrix (ECM), a population of pure extravillous trophoblast cells grows out during the following several days from villous tips into the adjacent ECM. The outgrowths, which show a polarity and pattern of marker expression that replicates anchoring columns in vivo, may be used as the basis for preparation of small numbers of cells for gene expression studies, or for investigations of cell function and behavior. For quantitative studies, a standard trans-filter trophoblast migration experiment is described that starts from a homogeneous preparation of primary cells released from the tissue.

Key Words: Trophoblast; explant; placenta; cell migration; extracellular matrix; cell adhesion.

1. Introduction

Trophoblast invasion has received widespread attention as a critical component of placental development that is impaired in the common pregnancy pathologies of preeclampsia, intrauterine growth restriction, and spontaneous miscarriage *(1,2)*.

The most well established purpose of trophoblast migration is the remodeling of the maternal arterial supply, creating a low resistance circuit that allows sufficient blood to reach the fetus to accommodate the elevated growth rate required in later pregnancy. This occurs by loss of the spiral arterial mural musculoelastic matrix and its vascular smooth muscle cell population, with the conversion of the vessels to wide, passive channels *(3)*.

Immunologists have identified the interface between the extravillous trophoblasts and maternal uterine tissue as a key site of hemiallogeneic contact at which special mechanisms have evolved for fetal tolerance *(4)*. Conversely, mechanisms for the management of pregnancy failure must be available that ensure the survival of the mother. It has also interested tumor biologists as a mass cell migration that is highly regulated, terminating in late first trimester.

From: *Methods in Molecular Medicine, Vol. 122: Placenta and Trophoblast: Methods and Protocols, Vol. 2*
Edited by: M. J. Soares and J. S. Hunt © Humana Press Inc., Totowa, NJ

In the very early postimplantation stages, primate embryos develop invasive syncytiotrophoblast that excavates a site within the maternal stroma within which the hemochorial interface can be established *(5,6)*. This early syncytium is not to be confused with the syncytiotrophoblast of the placental villus. Such events are complete by 2–3 d after attachment and have not been widely studied. Within less than a week from implantation, the outermost boundary of the presumptive human placenta consists of a cytotrophoblast shell from which development occurs of an "invasive" or, more correctly, infiltrating cytotrophoblast population. In the following weeks, with growth of the conceptus, the shell becomes discontinuous and the periphery of the placenta consists of cytotrophoblast columns attached to anchoring villi *(2)*. The most proximal cytotrophoblast cells of the column, situated on the villous basement membrane, act as founders from which are generated the cell columns, from the distal aspects of which cytotrophoblasts break away to begin their infiltration. Cell proliferation ceases in the proximal column region so that the distal and migratory cells are uniformly postmitotic.

Once cytotrophoblast cells have escaped the shell or distal columns, migration occurs through the three-dimensional environment of the maternal decidual stroma, or into spiral arteries. Migration proceeds until approximately week 18 of pregnancy, by which time significant numbers of cytotrophoblast have passed the decidual–myometrial boundary and penetrated approximately one-third of the thickness of the myometrium. Some migratory cells eventually differentiate farther into placental bed giant cells, which are probably sessile. There is also evidence for substantial levels of apoptosis in the extravillous cell population in the placental bed *(7)*.

Trophoblast migration into maternal decidual stroma also occurs in a range of other species including monkeys, rats, mice, and guinea pigs, with very characteristic timing and anatomical patterns in each. There remains much to be learned about the control of trophoblast migration and how it may go wrong; discussion has been framed as a balance between an intrinsic developmental program in which extravillous trophoblast development and migration occur according to a time schedule that terminates in the late second trimester, and a maternal environment that acts either permissively, providing an environment within which the program can be played out, or has a more active role in the modulation of the program to ensure a successful outcome *(1)*. The extent to which maternal modulation occurs is clearly a function of environmental stress *(8,9)*.

The two methods described model distinct stages of human trophoblast migration: the development of cytotrophoblast columns and formation of anchoring sites from mesenchymal villi, and the migration of cytotrophoblasts that have escaped as single cells from these sites.

1.1. First-Trimester Villous Explants

According to a stochastic model of developing placental anchorage, branching morphogenesis in the villous tree leads to the tips of peripheral (mesenchymal) floating villi making contact with the surface of the decidual stroma *(10)*. In turn, this contact leads to local breakdown of syncytium (if present) and the stimulation of cytotrophoblast column formation. Such a process is reiterated in vitro when first trimester floating villi are allowed to adhere to a permissive extracellular matrix substrate. Gels of either collagen I or Matrigel can be used. Local proliferation of cytotrophoblast occurs during the first approximately 24 h in vitro in a burst, to generate a cell column. Cells then leave the cycle and reorganize over the following several days, growing out as an epithelial sheet across the surface of the collagen gel or invading the Matrigel in streams *(11)*. In contrast with their behavior in vivo, relatively few cytotrophoblasts detach to migrate singly. The sheet continues to expand for several days until it is one or two cells thick. There is evidence for paracrine support for this migration from the stroma, or autocrine stimulation, by insulin-like growth factor (IGF)-I *(12)*. Partial pressure of oxygen is a key variable that may alter trophoblast phenotype *(13,14)*. Its physiological relevance is based on the step increase in local oxygen tension at the maternal–fetal interface occurring at about 11 wk gestation. Thus, it is recommended that, for tissue obtained prior to 11 wk, an environment of 2–3% oxygen be used to reproduce physiological conditions. For later tissue, 6% oxygen is a good approximation to the physiological level. If medium changes and factor additions can be carried out in a fully oxygen-controlled enclosure, this option should be chosen as exposure to atmospheric oxygen, however brief, leads to a prolonged increase in the dissolved oxygen level in culture medium.

A significant fraction of first trimester specimens obtained at pregnancy termination will be abnormal and destined to miscarry. Fetal dysmorphia is an obvious diagnostic, but abnormalities can manifest in an abnormal karyotype, mosaicism, or infection with cytomegalovirus or other pathogens. Though few papers have included screening for karyotype, virus, or fetal anatomical abnormality, these options should be considered *(15,16)*. Dating of the tissue should be as precise as possible, as cell phenotypes may vary with gestation. One method that is useful in late first trimester, and independent of clinical data, relies on examination of cartilage condensation in fetal digits under a stereomicroscope. The system is amenable to studies of growth factor, matrix or protease effects, antibody-mediated blocking of cell surface events such as adhesion, or antisense strategies *(9,11,17–20)*. A more general review of placental explant methodology and the uses to which it can be put *(21)* may be consulted in concert with the present account.

1.2. Trans-Filter Cytotrophoblast Migration

This is a widely used experimental model for studying the phase of migration when single cells move through the decidual or myometrial environment *(22,23)*. It can be used quantitatively providing good quality control is in place. The most appropriate starting population is a purified primary first trimester cytotrophoblast cell suspension (described later). If prepared by light trypsinization, the majority of the cells are cytotrophoblasts dissociated from columns—the subsyncytial villous cytotrophoblast population requires a more stringent protocol for efficient release. It is essential that there be minimal contamination by connective tissue cells that may migrate or proliferate during the assay period *(24)*. It is important to recognize that even in experienced laboratories, cytotrophoblast are not unequivocally identifiable by morphological criteria. Cytokeratin 7 is a useful positive marker and vimentin a good one for identifying contaminating cell populations. Sound experimental protocol requires that, because a minor vimentin-positive population of contaminants may proliferate or migrate faster than trophoblast, confirmation of identity of migrated cells be carried out by immunostaining at the end of the assay. To date, this has rarely been done. Evidence of proliferation in primary normal cytotrophoblast isolates after 30 h in vitro should be treated with suspicion.

2. Materials

2.1. First-Trimester Villous Explant

1. Tissue: tissue may be obtained at medical or surgical termination in first or second trimester. Most centers require informed patient consent. Medical terminations usually produce an intact placenta (*see* **Note 1**). Surgical terminations by suction produce placental fragments that require separation from fetal and decidual tissue.
2. Culture medium: explants are grown in a 1:1 mixture of Ham's F12 and Dulbecco's modified Eagle's medium (DMEM) with glutamine (5 mM), antibiotics (e.g., 100 µg/mL streptomycin or 50 µg/mL gentamycin, 100U/mL penicillin), and HEPES (15 mM). Antifungal agent (e.g., 2.5 µg/mL amphotericin B [fungizone]) is added during tissue washing. 10X DMEM and 7.5% sodium bicarbonate are used for preparing collagen gels. Reagents can be obtained from Sigma Chemical Co. (St. Louis, MO), Invitrogen (Carlsbad, CA).
3. Petri dishes and multiwell plates are from Corning Costar (Corning, NY).
4. Extracellular matrix (ECM) substrate: rat tail collagen type I (BD Biosciences, San Jose, CA), Matrigel (BD Biosciences), type 1A collagenase (Sigma).
5. RNA analysis: RNALater (Ambion Inc., Austin, TX); TriReagent (Sigma).
6. Transwell filter inserts (8-µm pore size, 24-well plate format, Corning Costar). A 96-well plate format is available from Chemicon (Temecula, CA).

3. Methods

3.1. First-Trimester Villous Explant

3.1.1. Culture Medium

Cultures are routinely carried out in incubators containing 5% CO_2 and varying oxygen partial pressure as required. Outgrowth also occurs in medium containing 10% fetal calf serum.

3.1.2. Tissue Handling

1. Tissue is transferred to the laboratory as quickly as possible and suspended in serum-free culture medium (SFM): DMEM-Ham's F12; containing antibiotics (penicillin and streptomycin or gentamycin) and antifungal (amphotericin B) (AAM) in 9 cm bacterial grade plastic Petri dishes.
2. Transfer pieces of placenta to a fresh Petri dish containing sufficient SFM/AAM for immersion. (*see* **Notes 2–5**) Wash the separated tissue with several changes of medium.

3.1.3. Matrix Substrates

3.1.3.1. COLLAGEN

Collagen gels may be prepared the day before the experiment or at least 1 h beforehand. Storing gels for a longer time period may result in deterioration, indicated by a stringy appearance. For a 12-well plate, 1 mL of collagen type I is required. Ideally, the collagen concentration should be more than 3 mg/mL. Gels become less firm with storage time of the collagen, and more dilute stock solutions tend to have a shorter shelf life. If more than 3–4 mL of collagen are to be used, then it is recommended that it be prepared in separate 1- to 2-mL batches to ensure even mixing. For best results, use collagen, 10X medium, and sodium bicarbonate directly from the fridge.

1. For one plate: withdraw 1 mL of collagen from the container using a 1-mL syringe and needle.
2. Discard the needle before transferring to a 1.5-mL Eppendorf tube (this prevents the introduction of air bubbles).
3. Add 100 µL of 10X DMEM and mix carefully with a disposable pastette, taking care not to introduce bubbles (solution is a yellow color).
4. Add approx 200 µL of 7.5% sodium bicarbonate to neutralize the collagen and cause it to set (the color changes from yellow to pink).
5. Again, mix carefully with a pastette as the solution will set from the bottom.
6. Use the pastette to transfer 1 drop (approx 80 µL) to the center of each well of the plate. Avoid including air bubbles.
7. The culture plate can either be left in the hood or carefully transferred to a 5% CO_2 incubator. The collagen should take approx 10 min to gel.

8. Add culture medium to each well to cover the gel and incubate the plate in a humid box at 37°C in a CO_2 incubator until required.
9. Gels can alternatively be set using ammonia. This is accomplished by making up the solution as above and spotting into plates, which are then placed inside a box. A few drops of ammonia are placed on a small Petri dish inside the box, which is then sealed and incubated for 15–30 min at 37°C. Care must be taken not to disturb the collagen droplets and cause them to spread—they will be more fluid than in the normal method—and not to let the gels dry out. After setting, the gels are incubated as before in a box free from ammonia vapor.
10. Volumes may be increased for setting up multiple explants in larger dishes. For example, for protein or mRNA studies, several dozen explants are required, and these may be set up as an explant "array" in large Petri dishes coated uniformly with ECM.

3.1.3.2. MATRIGEL

1. Matrigel should be prepared 24 h prior to setting up explant cultures. Matrigel sets at room temperature, therefore all preparation should be performed on ice or at 4°C.
2. Frozen (–20°C) aliquots of Matrigel should be defrosted overnight at 4°C.
3. Pipet tips and culture plates should also be precooled to 4°C to prevent premature gelling.
4. Mix 1 mL of Matrigel in a 1.5-mL Eppendorf tube with 100-µL of 10X DMEM in a 1.5-mL Eppendorf tube and start the gelling process by adding 200 µL of 7.5% sodium bicarbonate ensuring complete mixing before placing a drop of approx 80 mL in the center of each culture well.
5. Incubate the culture plates at 37°C for 10–15 min and then cover the gel in 1 mL of SFM, and store in a sealed humid box at 4°C until required.
6. Alternatively, Matrigel can be diluted 1:10 in cold SFM and this solution used to coat tissue culture plastic at 37°C for 1 h. Excess Matrigel is then removed. The resultant thin layer supports a thinner outgrowth giving advantages over the three-dimensional gel support for microscopy and imaging.

3.1.4. Explant Method

3.1.4.1. SELECTION OF TISSUE

Using small scissors, cut away terminal portions (~2–3 mm; 5–10 mg wet weight) of the villous tree. Selected portions (*see* **Note 6**) are transferred to a drop of culture medium in a Petri dish until enough material has been collected.

3.1.4.2. EXPLANT ATTACHMENT

1. Once the placental tissue has been dissected into appropriately sized pieces, preformed gels can be drained of medium. During incubation, they will have contracted slightly and become firm, aiding tissue attachment. If explanting onto

drops of substrate in wells, use fine forceps to transfer one piece of villous tissue to each well (*see* **Note 7**). Attachment can be facilitated by centrifuging plates using a swing-out rotor (200g for 1 min).

2. Following placement, cover each piece of tissue with 20 µL of prewarmed SFM and incubate at 37°C in 5% CO_2 in a humid box for 3–12 h (*see* **Note 8**). Following this initial period, cultures are gently immersed in 1 mL of SFM, directing the pipet to the side of the culture well to avoid detachment of the tissue from the gel. At this stage, growth factors, bromodeoxyuridine, or adhesion-modulating antibodies may be added to the explant in the SFM at suitable concentrations. The culture plate is carefully transferred back to the humid box in the incubator (*see* **Note 9**).

3.1.4.3. CYTOTROPHOBLAST OUTGROWTH

Cytotrophoblast column outgrowth and subsequent cell migration from gel-attached villi is monitored daily using low and high power whole mount microscopy. For daily comparisons of column growth, low-power image capture is recommended (**Fig. 1**). The area of outgrowing cells is very variable, being highly dependent on the size of the initial villus–gel contact (*see* **Notes 10** and **11**).

3.1.4.4. RECOVERY OF CYTOTROPHOBLASTS

1. Removal of tissue from the surface of a collagen gel leaves a pure population of extravillous cytotrophoblast at the surface. Removal of villous tissue can be accomplished with minimal loss of extravillous trophoblasts by pulling gently with fine forceps or trimming with small sprung scissors.
2. To release the adherent cytotrophoblast outgrowth, first wash three times with phosphate-buffered saline (PBS), then incubate with 100 µg/mL collagenase (Sigma type 1A) at 37°C.
3. Cytotrophoblast cells are released from the collagen by a 10-min incubation at 37°C. Gentle agitation by pipetting can aid cell release.
4. Cells should then be pelleted by centrifugation at 100g for 10 min at 4°C, and washed twice with PBS to remove all traces of collagenase. Cells can be replated on Matrigel for further culture.

3.1.4.5. PREPARATION OF RNA FROM EXTRAVILLOUS TROPHOBLAST

Cells released as above can be taken into a standard RNA purification protocol. In this case collagenase should be reconstituted in diethylpyrocarbonate (DEPC)-treated sterile PBS. However, it is more convenient to use RNALater.

1. Wash the explants three times with PBS and add cold reagent (*see* **Note 12**).
2. Then the outgrowths may be teased out of the gel and transferred to a tube containing RNALater.
3. Tissue and cells thus preserved may be stored at 4°C for at least a week, or at –80°C for longer before continuing the procedure, without loss of RNA.

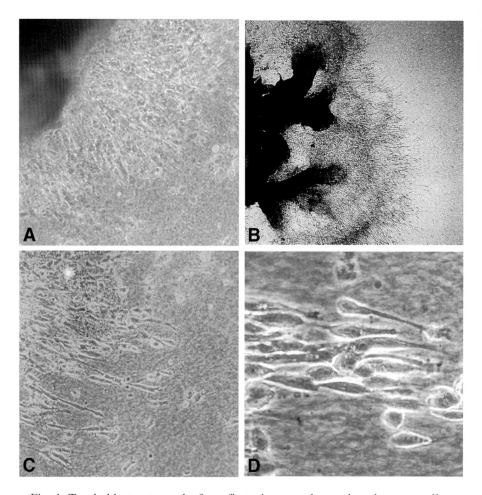

Fig. 1. Trophoblast outgrowths from first trimester placental explants on collagen gel. **(A)** Multilayered early outgrowth, 2 d. **(B)** Later outgrowth, 6 d. Note that outgrowths from different villous tips have merged to form a shell-like structure. Outgrowths are now only one or two cell layers thick. **(C,D)** Elongated and rounded cells at the periphery.

4. Continue by homogenizing the tissue into a dissociation medium such as TriReagent, and follow the manufacturer's instructions to obtain RNA. As a guide to quantity, 2–3 mL of TriReagent may be used for 150 explants, producing 60–80 µg total RNA from the villi and 30–40 µg from the cytotrophoblast outgrowths.

3.1.4.6. Whole-Mount Staining Protocol for Placental Explant Cultures

1. Wash cultures gently in PBS two times.
2. Fix using 1 mL methanol or 4% formaldehyde/PBS or 4% paraformaldehyde/PBS for 30 min at room temperature.
3. For methanol, replace the first solution immediately with a second aliquot (*see* **Note 13**). Wash three times with PBS. If formaldehyde or paraformaldehyde were used as fixatives, treat with methanol for 30 min to permeabilize the cells for localization of intracellular antigens.
4. Staining is carried out conveniently by trimming away excess gel matrix, detaching and transferring whole explants with their surrounding and underlying matrix to 0.6-mL Eppendorf tubes (*see* **Note 14**).
5. Incubate overnight (at least) at 4°C in a blocking solution of 4% BSA/PBS. Include 0.02% sodium azide if the plates are to be kept longer. Incubate in first antibody diluted in 4% BSA/PBS. Concentration, temperature (4°C to 37°C) and time (30 min to overnight) depend on the antibody and should be determined empirically. For short incubations, the volume can be restricted to 100 μL by repeatedly pipetting the solution over the explant, preventing it from drying out.
6. Wash in PBS, then overnight on a platform shaker in PBS/BSA. Incubate for 30 min to 2 h in fluorescent-tagged second antibody diluted in PBS/BSA. Plates should be wrapped in foil.
7. Wash in several changes of PBS using a platform shaker (3–24 h). Cultures can be inspected under the inverted microscope to monitor the removal of background fluorescence in the gel. Keep the plates in the dark throughout.
8. Counterstain nuclei using propidium iodide (PI) at 5 μg/mL in PBS for 10 min. PI is made up in water or PBS as a stock solution of 5 mg/mL.
9. Wash further in PBS, then spread the explant and its surrounding ECM gel out in the correct orientation on a glass slide under a dissecting microscope.
10. Mount in a water-compatible hardening mountant such as Histotec—this encapsulates the explant in a fluorescence-compatible polymer so that coverslipping is unnecessary. Leave to set in the dark overnight.

3.2. Trans-Filter Cytotrophoblast Migration

1. Primary trophoblast cells are prepared from first trimester placenta (*see* Chapter 17 of Volume I).
2. Cells are washed and resuspended in a 1:1 mixture of Ham's F12 and DMEM with glutamine and antibiotics as described previously (*see* **Note 15**).
3. If matrix-precoated filter inserts have not been purchased, coat with 10-fold diluted Matrigel, collagen I (30 μg/mL) or fibronectin (20 μg/mL).
4. Add the cell suspension (1 mL containing 5×10^5 cells per 15-mm well in a 24-well plate) and incubate at 37°C/5% CO_2 and a defined oxygen tension for times up to 72 h. Forty-eight hours is often an appropriate single time point at which to make measurements.

5. Remove inserts from the wells, wash in PBS and fix (ice-cold methanol or alde-hyde fixatives can be used, depending on the staining protocol) for at least 20 min at –20°C.

6. Filters should be washed twice in PBS then stained in haematoxylin solution for 5 min, or taken into an immunocytochemistry protocol.

7. Cells may be removed from the top of the insert membrane by gentle scraping using a cotton-wool bud. A scalpel may be used to cut out the filter for mounting. Select fields randomly in the microscope for counting. It is normal to count approx 10 × 10 fields or 250 cells; a statistical test will establish the number of fields required to differentiate a control from a test experiment.

4. Notes

1. Caution is required in case of pharmacological effects on the tissue. Normally, an antiprogestin such as RU486 is used along with a prostaglandin. There may be effects on receptors in the placenta.

2. For easier recognition and optimal viability, tissue should be washed and sepa-rated as soon as possible. Careful washing is particularly important for suction termination material, to remove excess blood, clots and other contaminants. After washing, discard fragments of placenta that contain clots, however small.

3. The amount of tissue obtained varies with gestational age: at 6 wk, the placenta is a disk of approx 4 cm in diameter, whereas at 12 wk, it is as much as three times this size.

4. Placenta expands in suspension to give a characteristic seaweed-like appearance. Under the stereomicroscope, some but not all villi are obviously vascularized. Chorioamnion is evident from late first trimester as a thin avascular sheet. Decidua is also present as sheets of vascular tissue lacking a villous appearance. A useful visual marker for decidua is its characteristic pattern of expanded capillary sinu-soids close to the surface of the sheet. Broken vascular elements are usually prominent at the edges of the tissue.

5. Placental tissue may be stored at 4°C overnight in serum-free culture medium prior to explanting.

6. These should be clusters of villi including several branches, which may be either trimmed from the placental periphery under a dissecting microscope or checked afterwards for suitability using the microscope. Observe the frond like structure of the villi after gentle teasing out with fine forceps. If the mesenchymal (termi-nal) villi appear elongated and stringy to the naked eye, then success of attach-ment and outgrowth tends to be low.

7. Use a portion that includes an intermediate villus with several mesenchymal branches emanating from it. Carefully tease the branches out over the gel sur-face, taking care not to score the gel. Alternatively, leave the medium in the well and add the selected villous tissue to the medium. Then carefully drain the medium from the well, thus gently lowering the tissue onto the collagen drop. If correct placement does not occur, use a pastette and a minimal volume of medium to gently lift and place the villous tissue onto the drop. This method avoids potential

scoring of the collagen gel. The villous termini should be arranged to extend radially over the surface of the gel drop.

8. At 12 h initial outgrowth may sometimes be seen using a high magnification phase contrast objective. Attachment may be indicated by the appearance of the subtle early signs of radial stress lines of bundled collagen in the gel. After a further 12 h, initial outgrowth from viable attached terminal villi structures should be readily apparent.

9. If tissue becomes detached when medium is added or during the overnight incubation that follows, then reattachment can be attempted by draining the well and repositioning the explant. However, repositioned tissue often has poor viability and is likely to detach again as well as exhibiting delayed growth characteristics.

10. The extent of outgrowth is highly variable, appearing to depend on the area of initial attachment of the villous tip. A variably sized population of founder cells is generated by proliferation of villous stem cells during the first approx 24 h, and the postmitotic cell column then rearranges to produce an outgrowing sheet. Outgrowth is limited to the tips of the villi but cells from adjacent tips may merge to form a shell-like structure surrounding the explant.

11. This method is suitable for morphological approaches such as cell behavior studies by time lapse microcinematography, or localization by immunochemical or in situ hybridization. Explants can be produced on matrix-coated filters commonly used for cell migration studies (see method below). In this case cytotrophoblasts growing out from explanted tissue cross the filter. Quantitative approaches are rendered difficult by the variation in size (cell number), and to a lesser extent, speed of outgrowth from a given site.

12. Treatment makes the tissue slightly brittle so that mechanical separation of residual villi from the cytotrophoblast outgrowth occurs more easily.

13. Methanol fixation gives the best-defined nuclear staining. Cultures should be kept as little time as possible before staining.

14. At this stage cultures can be trimmed under the dissecting microscope with a small pair of scissors. Take care not to damage the gel surface. If floating villi are removed, there is less likelihood of damaging the culture during processing.

15. Cell viability is affected by the composition of the substrate and culture medium. Additionally, the observed rate of migration will be affected by apoptotic loss. Culture on Matrigel prevents apoptosis and experiments can be done in the absence of serum or serum supplement. Other substrates may require the addition of 1–10% fetal calf serum or a serum replacement.

References

1. Aplin, J. D. (1991) Implantation, trophoblast differentiation and haemochorial placentation: mechanistic evidence in vivo and in vitro. *J. Cell Sci.* **99**, 681–692.
2. Vicovac, L. and Aplin, J. D. (1996) Epithelial-mesenchymal transition during trophoblast differentiation. *Acta Anatomica* **156**, 202–216.
3. Pijnenborg, R., Dixon, G., Robertson, W. B., and Brosens, I. (1980) Trophoblastic invasion of human decidua from 8 to 18 weeks of pregnancy. *Placenta* **1**, 3–19.

4. Hunt, J. S. (2002) Major histocompatibility antigens in reproduction, in *The Endometrium* (Aplin, J. D., Glasser, S. R., Giudice, L., and Tabibzadeh, S., eds.). Taylor and Francis, London: pp. 405–415.

5. Aplin, J. D. (2000) The cell biological basis of human implantation. *Bailliere's Best Practice Res. Clin. Obstet. Gynaecol.* **14,** 757–764.

6. Aplin, J. D. (2003) Implantation, in *The Encyclopedia of Hormones* (Simpson, E., ed.). Academic, San Diego: pp. 289–297.

7. Kaufmann, P., Black, S., and Huppertz, B. (2003) Endovascular trophoblast invasion: implications for the pathogenesis of intrauterine growth retardation and preeclampsia. *Biol. Reprod.* **69,** 1–7

8. Arck, P. C. (2001) Stress and pregnancy loss: role of immune mediators, hormones and neurotransmitters. *Am. J. Reprod. Immunol.* **46,** 117–123

9. Bauer, S., Pollheimer, J., Hartmann, J., Husslein, P., Aplin, J. D., and Knöfler, M. (2004) Tumor necrosis factor-alpha inhibits trophoblast migration through elevation of plasminogen activator inhibitor-1 in first-trimester villous explant cultures. *J. Clin. Endocrinol. Metab.* **89,** 812–822.

10. Aplin, J. D., Jones, C. J. P., Haigh, T., Church, H. J., and Vicovac, L. (1998) Anchorage in the developing placenta: an overlooked determinant of pregnancy outcome? Hum. Fertil. **1,** 75–79.

11. Aplin, J. D., Haigh, T., Jones, C. J. P., Church, H. J., and Vicovac, L. (1999) Development of cytotrophoblast columns from explanted first trimester placental villi: role of fibronectin and integrin $\alpha 5\beta 1$. *Biol. Reprod.* **60,** 828–838.

12. Lacey, H., Haigh, T., Westwood, M., and Aplin, J. D. (2002) Mesenchymally-derived IGF-I provides a paracrine stimulus for trophoblast migration. *BMC Dev. Biol.* **2,** 5.

13. Genbacev, O., Zhou, Y., Ludlow, J. W., and Fisher, S. J. (1997) Regulation of human placental development by oxygen tension. *Science* **277,** 1669–1672.

14. Aplin, J. D. (2000) Hypoxia and human placental development. (commentary). *J. Clin. Invest.* **105,** 559–560.

15. Polliotti, B. M., Sheikh, A., Subbarao, S., et al. (1998) HIV-1 infection of human placental villous tissue in vitro. *Trophoblast Res.* **12,** 205–244.

16. Fisher, S., Genbacev, O., Maidji, E., and Pereira, L. (2000) Human cytomegalovirus infection of placental cytotrophoblasts in vitro and in utero: implications for transmission and pathogenesis. *J. Virol.* **74,** 6808–6820.

17. Bilban, M., Ghaffari-Tabrizi, N., Hintermann, E., et al. (2004) Kisspeptin-10, a KiSS-1/metastin-derived decapeptide, is a physiological invasion inhibitor of primary human trophoblasts. *J. Cell. Sci.* **117,** 1319–1328.

18. Caniggia, I., Taylor, C. V., Ritchie, J. W. K., Lye, S. J., and Letarte, M. (1997) Endoglin regulates trophoblast differentiation along the invasive pathway in human placental villous explants. *Endocrinology* **138,** 4977–4988.

19. Coppock, H. A., White, A., Aplin, J. D., and Westwood, M. (2004) Matrix metalloprotease-3 and -9 proteolyse insulin-like growth factor binding protein-1. *Biol. Reprod.* **71,** 438–443.

20. Leach, R. E., Kilburn, B., Wang, J., Liu, Z., Romero, R., and Armant, D. R. (2004) Heparin-binding EGF-like growth factor regulates human extravillous cytotrophoblast development during conversion to the invasive phenotype. *Dev. Biol.* **266,** 223–237.

21. Miller, R. K., Genbacev, O., Turner, M. A., Aplin, J. D., Caniggia, I., and Huppertz, B. (2005) Human placental explants in culture: approaches and assessments. *Placenta,* **26,** 439–448.

22. Librach, C. L., Werb, Z., Fitzgerald, M. L., et al. (1991). 92-kD type IV collagenase mediates invasion of human cytotrophoblasts. *J. Cell Biol.* **113,** 437–449.

23. Damsky, C. H., Librach, C., Lim, K. H., et al. (1994) Integrin switching regulates normal trophoblast invasion. *Development* **120,** 3657–3666.

24. Haigh, T., Chen, C., Jones, C. J., and Aplin, J. D. (1999) Studies of mesenchymal cells from 1st trimester human placenta: expression of cytokeratin outside the trophoblast lineage. *Placenta* **20,** 615–625.

4

An In Vitro Model of Trophoblast Invasion of Spiral Arteries

Judith E. Cartwright and Mark Wareing

Summary

Extravillous trophoblasts invade the uterine wall (interstitial invasion) and the spiral arteries (endovascular invasion), replacing the cells of the vessel wall and creating a high-flow, low-resistance vessel. We describe a model to allow the interactions between the invading trophoblast cells and the cells of the spiral artery to be directly examined. Unmodified (nonplacental bed) spiral arteries are obtained from uterine biopsies at Caesarean section. Fluorescently labeled trophoblasts (either primary first-trimester extravillous trophoblasts or an extravillous trophoblast cell line) are seeded on top of artery segments embedded in fibrin gels (to study interstitial invasion) or perfused into the lumen of arteries (to study endovascular invasion). Trophoblasts are incubated with the vessels for different periods prior to cryosectioning. Both interstitial and endovascular interactions/invasion can be detected and immunohistochemical analyses carried out. This novel method is useful in an area where in vitro studies have been hampered by the lack of suitable models directly examining cellular interactions during invasion.

Key Words: Extravillous trophoblast; invasion; spiral artery; interstitial; endovascular; in vitro model.

1. Introduction

Remodeling of the uterine arteries is a key event in early pregnancy. In the first trimester of pregnancy, a subpopulation of fetal trophoblast cells, the extravillous trophoblast, invade the uterine wall (interstitial invasion) and its blood vessels (endovascular invasion) as far as the myometrial segments. In the uterine spiral arteries the trophoblasts interdigitate between the endothelial cells, replacing the endothelial lining and most of the musculoelastic tissue in the vessel walls. This creates a high-flow, low-resistance circulation that maximizes maternal blood flow to the placental villi at the maternal–fetal interface.

Immunohistochemical data suggest that trophoblasts bind to and migrate along the luminal surfaces of the endothelium and transiently coexist on the

From: *Methods in Molecular Medicine, Vol. 122: Placenta and Trophoblast: Methods and Protocols, Vol. 2*
Edited by: M. J. Soares and J. S. Hunt © Humana Press Inc., Totowa, NJ

walls of partially modified spiral arteries before replacing the endothelium and remodeling the vessel *(1–3)*. There is contrasting evidence as to whether trophoblasts themselves are important in arterial remodeling. Although it has been suggested that some changes in the decidual vessels occur independently of trophoblasts *(4)* as part of the maternal response to pregnancy, there is also strong evidence to suggest that invasive interstitial trophoblasts prepare the decidual spiral arteries for endovascular trophoblast migration *(5–7)*. The invasive trophoblast may play an important role in inducing further changes either by interactions or factors produced by the interstitial trophoblast or by direct cellular interactions of the endovascular trophoblast with the cells of the vessel that they subsequently replace.

Little is known as to how these processes are regulated in normal pregnancies; however, failure to remodel the spiral arteries is associated with pregnancies complicated by preeclampsia and intrauterine growth restriction *(8)*. The importance of interactions between trophoblasts and the vascular cells of the spiral arteries, which may account for these differences in remodeling, have yet to be determined in normal or complicated pregnancies.

Studies of spiral arteries have been confined primarily to immunohistochemical analysis of placental bed biopsies *(9–12)* whereas in vitro studies have been hampered by the lack of suitable models to directly examine cellular interactions during invasion. Here we describe an in vitro model of spiral artery invasion and remodelling, developed using spiral artery explants, extravillous trophoblast cell lines, and primary cytotrophoblasts *(13)*. In addition to the methods we describe later, another useful model has been recently described *(14)* which uses co-cultures of villous explants with sections of decidual tissue.

In our model, fluorescently-labeled trophoblasts are either perfused into dissected spiral arteries (to model endovascular invasion) or cultured with the vessels (to model interstitial invasion). A number of factors can be studied using this model, including the interactions between trophoblasts and vascular cells *(15)*, alteration of expression of markers during invasion, the effect of growth factors and oxygen tension on invasion *(16)*, and the cellular and molecular events occurring during vascular remodeling *(17)*. In addition, invasion of non-placental bed spiral arteries from preeclamptic and growth-restricted pregnancies can be compared with arteries from normal pregnancies at similar gestational age.

2. Materials

1. Cell culture and isolation medium: Ham's F10, Dulbecco's modified Eagle's medium (DMEM)-Ham's F12, L-glutamine, penicillin, streptomycin, trypsin/ethylenediamine tetraacetic acid (EDTA), and fetal calf serum (FCS) were obtained from Sigma-Aldrich, Poole, Dorset, UK. Large vessel growth medium was ob-

tained from TCS Biosciences Ltd., Buckingham, UK. Hank's balanced salt solution was obtained from Gibco, Paisley, UK. Trypsin solution and DNAse were from Roche Diagnostics, Mannheim, Germany. Matrigel™ was obtained from BD Biosciences, Bedford, MA, USA.

2. Fluorescent probes: CellTracker™ Probes were obtained from Molecular Probes, Leiden, The Netherlands.

3. Dissection buffer is made fresh on the day of the experiment using Purite (Purite Ltd, Thame, Oxon, UK) ultrapure water (PSS:119 mM NaCl, 25 mM NaHCO$_3$, 4.69 mM KCl, 2.4 mM MgSO$_4$, 1.6 mM CaCl$_2$, 1.18 mM KH$_2$PO$_4$, 6.05 mM glucose, 0.034 mM EDTA). The solution is gassed with 95% air/5%CO$_2$ and adjusted to pH 7.4 with NaOH before sterilization by filtration using a 0.2-μm Millipore filtration system (Appleton Woods Ltd., Birmingham, UK).

4. Dissection dishes: tissue is dissected in 45-mL evaporating dishes (Scientific Laboratory Supplies [SLS], Nottingham, UK) that have been filled to a depth of 1 cm with Sylgard (World Precision Instruments Ltd., Stevenage, Herts, UK). Dishes are wiped clean prior to the experiment with 2% Virkon (SLS), rinsed with deionized water and finally with 100% ethanol and dried in a sterile Class II cabinet.

5. Dissection equipment: tissue is pinned out in the dissection dishes using 25-gauge × 16-mm syringe needles (SLS). Dissection is performed using Dumont No. 5 watchmaker forceps (two pairs) and mini-vannas dissection scissors (Fine Science Tools, Heidelberg, Germany) with the aid of a binocular dissection microscope. We use an Olympus SZ series microscope with an integrated illumination source (Olympus UK, Ltd., Southall, Middlesex, UK) with ×10 eyepieces (maximum magnification of ×40 allowing sufficient accuracy without loss of depth perception which can occur at higher magnifications). This is suitable for both dissection and mounting of the arteries onto the cannulae for subsequent perfusion.

6. Perfusion equipment: equipment for perfusion can be obtained from either Danish Myotechnologies (Aarhus, Denmark) or Living Systems Incorporated (Burlington, VT, USA). For trophoblast perfusion experiments we use the Living Systems equipment consisting of a CH/1 chamber connected to a PS/200/Q pressure servo and peristaltic pump. Additionally, we have found that Living Systems can tailor their equipment to the individual needs of the researcher (www.livingsys.com). Silk suture is also obtained from Living Systems Inc.

7. Pipets: pipet glass for the manufacture of cannulae can be obtained from Clark Electromedical Incorporated (part of Harvard Apparatus Limited, Edenbridge, Kent, UK). We use the GC120-10 borosilicate glass capillary tubing (1.2-mm outer diameter × 0.69-mm inner diameter). Pipets are manufactured on a Narishige microelectrode puller (PP-830; Olympus UK, Ltd., Southall, Middlesex, UK). Glass is cut to size with a miniature glasscutter (SLS).

8. Tubing: solvent resistant silicone tubing can be obtained from a number of sources. We use tubing with a bore of 0.89 mm and a wall of 0.838-mm thickness (Altec, Alton, UK).

9. Fibrin gels: fibrinogen (bovine, >95% clottable) and thrombin were obtained from Sigma-Aldrich and aprotinin (Trasylol) was obtained from Bayer, Germany.

10. Cryosectioning and immunohistochemical reagents: Cryo-M-Bed embedding compound was obtained from Bright Instrument Company Ltd, Huntingdon, Cambs, UK. Paraformaldehyde, the liquid-repellent pen, goat serum and mouse immunoglobulin (Ig)G isotype control were from Sigma-Aldrich. Antibody to human von Willebrand Factor (vWF) and rabbit Ig control were from DAKO, Denmark. Monoclonal antibody to human smooth muscle actin (clone 1A4) was from Lab Vision (UK) Ltd., Newmarket, UK. Biotinylated anti-rabbit IgG and anti-mouse IgG antibodies, fluorescein-streptavidin and Vectashield mounting medium were from Vector Laboratories Inc., Burlingame, CA, USA.

11. Fluorescent microscopy: an Olympus IX70 inverted fluorescence microscope (Olympus UK, Ltd., Southall, Middlesex, UK) linked to a cooled charge-coupled device (CCD) camera (Hamamatsu Photonics UK, Welwyn Garden City, Herts, UK) was used. Images were analysed using Image Pro Plus software (Media Cybernetics UK, Wokingham, Berkshire, UK).

3. Methods

3.1. Trophoblast Cultures

We have used either a first-trimester extravillous trophoblast-derived cell line (SGHPL-4 cells) or primary first-trimester cytotrophoblasts in these models and have observed similar effects *(13)*.

1. SGHPL-4 cells are cultured in Hams F10 containing 2 mM L-glutamine, 100 µg/mL penicillin and 100 U/mL streptomycin and supplemented with 10% (v/v) FCS (*see* **Note 1**).

2. Primary cytotrophoblasts are isolated from late first trimester placental tissue obtained at elective termination of apparently healthy pregnancies. Informed consent is obtained and local ethical committee approval is in place. Tissue (approx 6 g) is washed thoroughly in Hank's balanced salt solution, chopped with scissors then washed twice more. The tissue is resuspended in trypsin (0.125%) and DNase (1 mg/mL) and incubated for 35 min at 37°C. The cells are harvested and the enzymatic treatment is repeated. Tissue pieces are removed by filtration (sterile 100-µm pore nylon mesh) and the trypsin is neutralized using medium with 10% (v/v) FCS. Cells are loaded on a Percoll gradient and, after centrifugation at 1800g for 30 min, cells are collected from the 30–45% range. Cells are pelleted by centrifugation at 350g, resuspended in serum-free medium (DMEM-Ham's F12) and plated on Matrigel-coated flasks (5–6 mg/mL) for 24 h (*see* **Note 2**).

3. Trophoblasts (SGHPL-4 cells or primary cytotrophoblasts) are labeled with CellTracker Orange CMTMR probe (*see* **Note 3**). Cells are incubated with normal medium containing 5-µM probe for 30 min at 37°C. The medium is then replaced with fresh medium and incubated for another 30 min at 37°C.

4. Cells are detached using trypsin/EDTA and resuspended at 5×10^6 cells/mL in large vessel growth medium in a bijou container (*see* **Note 4**).

3.2 Dissection of Spiral Arteries From Decidual/Myometrial Biopsies

1. Decidual/myometrial biopsies are obtained from normal pregnant women who had uncomplicated pregnancies, undergoing elective lower segment Caesarean section at term for reasons such as breech presentation. Informed consent is obtained and local ethical committee approval is in place. Small 1-cm × 1-cm biopsies are taken from the upper lip of the incision prior to closing the uterus. The biopsy is placed in a sterile container containing PSS, stored on ice and transported immediately to the laboratory.

2. Dissection is performed in sterile conditions in a Class II laminar flow cabinet. We routinely wear gloves and a mask to perform the dissection. Surfaces of the microscope, the dissection dish, and instruments are wiped with 100% ethanol prior to use. The biopsy is transferred to the sterile dissection dish and bathed in fresh PSS dissection buffer. Myometrial and decidual surfaces are identified and the biopsy is oriented so that the decidual surface is uppermost. The corners of the biopsy are pinned to the Sylgard using sterile 25-gauge needles. The biopsy is washed twice and the surface gently cleaned free of blood using the blunt end of pair of forceps. Care should be taken not to damage or overstretch the tissue. The biopsy should be kept wet with PSS throughout the dissection.

3. Spiral arteries are identified by dissection of the decidual connective tissue away from the vascular tissue. The connective tissue can be gently lifted, separated with forceps, and the tissue searched until a spiral artery is identified (*see* **Note 5**). Once an artery is successfully identified, the surrounding tissue is carefully dissected using forceps and mini-vannas scissors. Care must be taken not to stretch the vessel or touch the vascular smooth muscle (except for at the very end of the section being dissected). It is usually best to work methodically along one side of the artery to separate the arterial wall from the surrounding interstitium. The specimen can then be rotated and more tissue dissected away from the artery, i.e., working around the artery in a clockwise or counter-clockwise direction. In this way, the artery is carefully separated out from the surrounding tissues. Care should be taken when dissecting along the vessel to identify any side-branches that may occur. We usually identify side-branches, isolate their ends from the main vessel, and dissect the side-branch out once the major vessel has been removed. For endovascular perfusion experiments, the arteries are dissected so that they consisted of only the arterial wall. To facilitate the investigation of interstitial invasion, the arteries are isolated with a small amount of surrounding tissue present.

4. When a 3- to 4-mm section of vessel is dissected from the surrounding tissue, one end of the artery is held with forceps and the vessel is cut free from the biopsy and placed in a bijou container with PSS.

3.3. Perfusion Chamber Preparation

The following methods describe setting up the CH/1 perfusion chamber and PS/200/Q Pressure Servo and will have to be adapted if other perfusion equipment is used. The setup of the equipment is illustrated in **Fig. 1**. All experiments are carried out in a Class II laminar flow cabinet.

1. Glass cannulae are prepared prior to the experiment (*see* **Note 6**). Pipets are pulled, visualised using the dissecting microscope and then clipped to an approx 80-μm tip using forceps.

2. The screws holding the perfusion chamber PTFE cannula arms in position (proximal arm attached to the micrometer and distal cannula arm) are loosened and the arms are rotated up out of the bath. The Allen screws on each arm are loosened to allow the glass cannulae to be inserted into the grooved holder.

3. Tubing (3–4 cm in length) is attached to the nipples at the proximal and distal end of the bath. This will be a tight fit, but must be secure.

4. The blunt end of a prepared glass cannula is cut approx 2 cm from the tip and the blunt end is flamed. This prevents the glass cutting into the silicone tubing. Using forceps, the cannula is placed in the groove on the distal cannula holder with the sharpened tip pointing towards the proximal end of the bath and the Allen screw is tightened. Holding the PTFE part of the arm, the silicone tubing is eased onto the blunt end of the cannula. The PTFE cannula arm is rotated so that the glass cannula is positioned above the center of the window in the bottom of the bath and the screws on the cannula arm are tightened. This holds the cannula securely in place. This is repeated to place a glass cannula into the proximal (micrometer) cannula arm.

5. The sharpened tips of the cannulae must be aligned. The tips of the cannulae are visualized (under ×30–40 magnification) and moved closer together using the micrometer. Alignment is performed using the screws that hold each PTFE cannula arm in place. With the micrometer (proximal) cannula on the left, the back screw is loosened and the arm rotated. This moves the glass tip in the vertical plane. The screw is tightened, the near screw loosened and the arm rotated in the horizontal plane. Minor adjustments in the horizontal and vertical planes are made in this way until the tip is aligned with the distal cannula.

6. A 5-mL syringe with ethanol is attached to the distal cannula. The three-way tap is opened and ethanol gently pushed through the cannula, then the tap is closed, the syringe removed, and replaced with a syringe containing sterile water and the process repeated to flush the ethanol out of the system. The syringe is finally replaced with one containing sterile PSS and the process repeated to fill the cannula/tubing/tap. This proximal cannula is cleaned and filled in the same manner. The bath is rinsed several times to remove traces of ethanol and then filled with 10 mL of sterile PSS.

7. The PS/200/Q pressure servo and peristaltic pump is switched on and set to flow (rate is set relatively low at around 2). Ethanol is perfused through the tubing and out through the pressure transducer attachment. After 2 min, sterile distilled water is perfused through for a few min to remove the ethanol.

8. Sterile PSS is perfused through the system for a few min. Care must now be taken to ensure that there are no air bubbles in the system, as this will affect the assessment of intraluminal pressure (*see* **Note 7**).

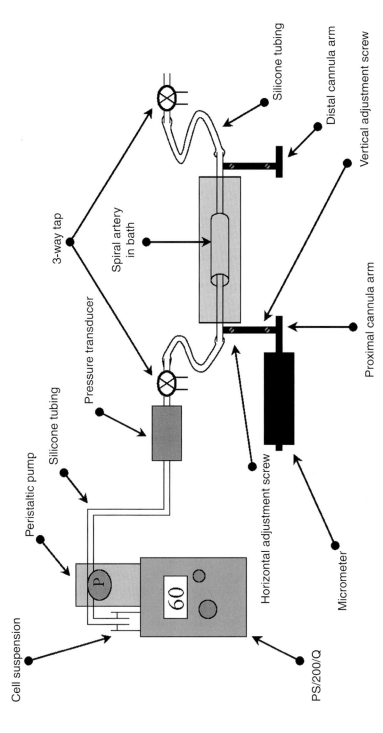

Fig. 1. Schematic representation of the perfusion setup using a CH/1 chamber connected to a PS/200/Q pressure servo and peristaltic pump (Living Systems Inc.).

Cell suspension

Peristaltic pump

Silicone tubing

Pressure transducer

3-way tap

Spiral artery in bath

Silicone tubing

Distal cannula arm

Vertical adjustment screw

Proximal cannula arm

Horizontal adjustment screw

Micrometer

PS/200/Q

65

9. The pressure transducer is attached to the three-way tap at the proximal end of the bath; the tap is opened and PSS is run through the system. Flow should be observed from the proximal cannula tip using the microscope. If the tip is blocked, forceps can be used to carefully break the tip and free the blockage. If this fails, the cannula will need to be replaced starting again from **step 4**.

3.4. Endovascular Perfusion of Trophoblasts into Isolated Spiral Arteries

1. The pump and tubing are primed with the media containing trophoblast cells prior to mounting the dissected artery on the cannula. The tubing is placed into the bijou containing the fluorescently-labeled trophoblast cell suspension. It is important that the cells are resuspended frequently to avoid clumping. A small air bubble should be introduced between the PSS already in the tubing and the cell suspension; this prevents mixing of the solutions and subsequent dilution of the cells but will not be perfused through the vessel. The cell suspension is now run through the tubing until cells are close to the tip of the cannula.

2. Having the bath oriented with the proximal end nearest the researcher aids in manipulation and mounting of the vessel. Two silk ties are placed around the cannulae away from the tip, one around the distal and one around the proximal cannula (*see* **Note 8**). An artery is carefully picked up by the very end using forceps. The artery is eased onto the tip of the distal cannula and gently moved up the cannula so that there is sufficient tissue over the glass to allow the tie to be securely attached (*see* **Note 9**). The thread is moved over the end of the vessel and tied thus securing the vessel to the distal cannula. A 5-mL syringe filled with PSS is attached to the three-way tap at the distal end. While visualizing the artery down the microscope, a small volume of PSS is slowly pushed through the vessel. This will displace any blood left in the artery and will open the other end of the artery, permitting easy mounting onto the proximal cannula. If there are any holes/small branches in the artery segment, these will also be visible (*see* **Note 10**). Using the micrometer, the tip of the proximal cannula is moved close enough to the distal cannula to permit the artery to be mounted without stretching or pulling the artery off the distal cannula.

3. Before mounting the artery onto the proximal cannula, the remaining PSS is slowly pushed out of the cannula tip using the perfusion pump (set on flow). The pump is kept running until the small air bubble and a very small amount of cell suspension come out of the tip. The flow is switched off and the artery placed onto the proximal cannula using forceps. The artery is tied in place with the thread. The micrometer can be used to straighten the artery (if required) taking care not to over-stretch the vessel.

4. After ensuring that the distal tap is closed, the perfusion pump is switched to "pressure." The control unit is in automatic mode and the pressure adjust dial is used to slowly increase the pressure until it reads 60 mmHg. The artery may need to be straightened slightly using the micrometer at this stage. The system is switched to "manual" and the readout is noted. If the vessel has no side branches or leaks and the ties are secure, the readout will remain at 60 mmHg and the

pump will not turn. If the pressure reading falls, or the pump continues to push fluid into the system, then the artery will need to be monitored (*see* **Note 11**). The system is then switched back to "automatic".

5. Once an artery has been successfully pressurized, the distal tap is opened. The pump should slowly push cells through the vessel and into the distal cannula, while the pressure is maintained at 60 mmHg. Progress of the flow can be monitored visually down the microscope. The artery is perfused for 30–60 s (approx 5×10^4 cells perfused into each artery, depending on the rate of flow through the artery). The distal tap is closed, the distal end of the artery moved off the cannula, and the artery immediately sealed by tightening the knot. This is repeated at the proximal end. The knotted thread at each end of the perfused vessel prevents the cells from leaking out.

6. The pump is turned off and the artery is placed in a bijou containing culture medium until the fibrin gels are prepared.

7. The experimental design may mean that different treatments of trophoblast cells (for example in the presence of function-blocking antibodies) are being perfused through the equipment. It is therefore crucial that all tubing is rinsed well with PSS between perfusions. Sterile distilled water followed by ethanol then more water should be perfused through the equipment at the end of the experiment.

3.5. Preparation of Fibrin Gels

Fibrin gels are prepared as previously described *(17)*.

1. Bovine fibrinogen is dissolved in phosphate-buffered saline (PBS) at 2.5 mg/mL and 200 U/mL aprotinin is added. The solution is filter sterilised through a 0.2-μm filter. Thrombin is added at 0.625 U/mL to induce clotting.

2. The solution is quickly added to wells of a 24-well tissue culture plate (200 μL/well) and allowed to set for 1 min. The perfused and tied arteries are placed carefully on top of the semi-set gel (1/well). They should not sink into the gel but will be anchored in place as the gel sets fully. When the gel has set (after approx 10 min) culture medium is added to the wells to cover the vessels. The plates are then incubated at 37°C in a humidified atmosphere of 5% CO_2 in air for the required time (*see* **Note 12**).

3.6. Interstitial Invasion Experiments

1. Vessels are dissected as described above but with a small amount of surrounding interstitium left around the vessel. Following dissection, the vessels are perfused with media and pressurization is assessed. Spiral arteries that successfully maintain pressure have their ends tied off (to prevent trophoblasts entering the vessel endovascularly) prior to immobilization.

2. The arteries are immobilized in fibrin gels. Vessels are submerged just below the surface of the fibrin gel as it sets. Once set, fluorescently labeled trophoblasts (as described previously) are resuspended at 10^5 cells/mL in large vessel growth medium and seeded on top of the preparation (5×10^4 cells in total) and incu-

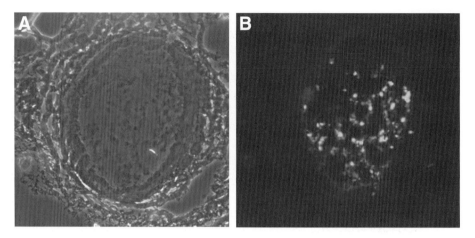

Fig. 2. Phase contrast (**A**) and fluorescent (**B**) images of a non-placental bed spiral artery perfused with Cell Tracker™-labeled SGHPL-4 cells. The vessel was frozen and cryosectioned immediately after perfusion and illustrates that fluorescently labeled trophoblasts can be successfully perfused into the lumen of the vessel.

bated for up to 5 d. We have previously shown that trophoblasts will invade fibrin gels while remaining viable in this environment for >5 d *(17,18)*.

3. It is possible to combine the experiments to study endovascular and interstitial invasion (*see* **Note 13**).

3.7. Cryosectioning of Perfused Spiral Arteries

1. The segments of spiral artery are carefully removed from the fibrin gels after the experiment, immediately placed in embedding compound, snap-frozen, and stored at –80°C. It is important that the orientation of the artery in the embedding compound is noted and that it does not become crumpled during this procedure.
2. Cryostat sections are cut (5–10 μm) of the whole length of vessels orientated so that transverse sections of the vessel are taken. The sections are screened by fluorescence microscopy for the presence of fluorescent trophoblasts in the lumen or the arterial wall (as seen in **ref.** *13* and **Fig. 2**) and the sections stored at –80°C for up to 3 mo.

3.8. Immunohistochemistry of Spiral Artery Sections

The methods detailed below can be used to detect the endothelium (by staining for the endothelial marker vWF) and the smooth muscle cells (by staining for smooth muscle actin; **Fig. 3**) but will need to be optimised for antibodies from different sources or for detection of other markers on the vascular cells or

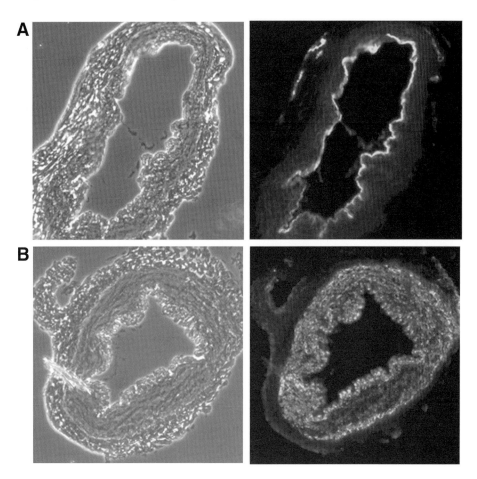

Fig. 3. Phase contrast and fluorescent images of spiral arteries perfused with culture medium illustrating the detection of intact endothelium by staining for von Willebrand factor (**A**) and smooth muscle cells by staining for smooth muscle actin (**B**).

invading trophoblasts (*see* **Note 14**). Detection of the endothelium and smooth muscle layer can be useful in studies of vessel remodelling or to identify the location of fluorescent trophoblasts that have invaded *(13,15)*.

1. Sections are removed from storage at –80°C and equilibrated to room temperature for 30 min. A ring is drawn round the arteries using a liquid-repellent slide marker pen to form a well for the antibodies.
2. Sections are fixed with 4% (w/v) paraformaldehyde in PBS for 10 min, washed three times with PBS for 5 min, and permeabilized in 0.2% (v/v) Triton-X100/PBS for 5 min.

3. Following one wash with PBS, slides are incubated with 10% (v/v) goat serum in PBS for 20 min to block non-specific binding. Blocking serum should be derived from the same species in which the secondary antibody is raised. This and the subsequent antibody incubations take place at room temperature in a humidified chamber.

4. Following three washes with PBS for 5 min, slides are incubated for 1 h with rabbit anti-human von Willebrand Factor or rabbit Ig control at 14.25 µg/mL in PBS/1.5% goat serum or mouse anti-smooth muscle actin at 1 µg/mL or mouse IgG isotype control at 1 µg/mL in PBS/1.5% goat serum. A volume of 50–100 µL is sufficient to cover the artery sections.

5. Slides are washed three times with PBS and then incubated for 45 min with biotinylated goat anti-rabbit Ig antibody or biotinylated goat anti-mouse Ig antibody at 7.5 µg/mL in PBS/1.5% goat serum.

6. After three washes with PBS, slides are incubated with fluorescein-streptavidin at 15 µg/mL in PBS for 15 min, washed six times in PBS, and Vectashield mounting medium added.

7. Sections are examined by fluorescence microscopy and digital images are captured using a CCD camera. Images are overlayed and the location of invaded trophoblasts determined (by comparison with the location of the endothelium and smooth muscle layer) using Image Pro Plus software. The extent of invasion *(13)* and the integrity of the endothelial *(15)* and smooth muscle layers can thereby be assessed.

4. Notes

1. SGHPL-4 cells are a well-characterized cell line derived from primary human first-trimester extravillous trophoblasts and retain many features of normal extravillous trophoblast including expression of cytokeratin-7, BC-1, CD9, hPL, and human leukocyte antigen (HLA)-G *(17,19–21)*.

2. Studies by Tarrade et al., 2001 *(22)* have shown that isolated cytotrophoblasts grown on Matrigel will differentiate into cells with an extravillous phenotype.

3. It is important to avoid thiol-containing buffers when preparing the CellTracker probes. The probes pass through the cell membrane but once inside the cell undergo a reaction with intracellular thiols that makes them cell-impermeant. We routinely use CellTracker Orange CMTMR probe to fluorescently label trophoblast cells and the cells retain their fluorescence through cell divisions and for at least 5 d. We have also successfully used CellTracker Green CMFDA in these experiments but have found CellTracker Blue labeling is less robust and the cells are more difficult to detect in the vessels.

4. Cells should be detached when the perfusion equipment has been prepared and the arteries are dissected. It is crucial that the cells are resuspended well and are not clumped otherwise they may block the cannula during perfusion. We found that detachment of trophoblast cells with Versene was not as satisfactory and a single cell suspension was not obtained.

5. Spiral arteries can be identified in a number of ways. Occasionally, arteries are visible projecting vertically up through the surrounding tissue. In this case the arterial lumen can be easily identified, especially if there is blood still remaining in the lumen of the vessel. Blood can also occasionally be displaced upon gentle manipulation of the surrounding connective tissue using forceps, thus allowing the identification of the open end of a vessel. Arterial walls can also be identified in a similar fashion. Upon gentle stretching of the sample, connective tissue tends to become translucent. Arterial smooth muscle tends to retain its dense whiteness.

6. Glass cannulae are made from the borosilicate glass using a Narishige standard vertical pipette puller. We coat the glass with Sigmacote® (Sigma) prior to pulling which produces a thin film inside the glass and aids in reducing the number of blocked cannula. We routinely use a two-stage pull to produce our cannulae. The first pull, a short, approx 2-mm drop, produces a short shoulder on the cannula. The second pull (free drop) produces the sharp tip portion of the cannula. Each machine and element will have their own individual resistance and heating characteristics and will therefore have to be optimized until the correct shape of cannula is produced.

7. Small air bubbles will cause problems when assessing whether the vessel is capable of maintaining an imposed intraluminal pressure and will affect endothelial integrity if perfused through the vessel. Gently massaging the tubing or flicking the tubing while holding vertically can remove air bubbles. Bubbles usually seed at junctions in the tube or in three way taps and connectors. Bubbling can be minimized using excess fluid on connection of the parts of the system. For example, before joining the pressure transducer to the three-way tap at the proximal end of the bath, use a syringe primed with PSS to fill the connector with solution; movement of the needle during filling can ensure that bubbles do not adhere to the plastic. Leave a prominent meniscus and finally attach the transducer using a twisting motion.

8. A small, approx 1-cm length of silk thread is cut from the roll and placed onto a piece of adhesive tape. Silk ties are prepared by splitting the silk into its individual threads. An individual thread is then crossed over itself to form a small loop that can be left attached to the tape ready for use. Prior to use, the tape and thread is wiped with ethanol to maintain sterility.

9. When manipulating arteries, it is best to only touch the very end of the tissue with forceps. This will minimize the tissue damage and these areas should be in the area crushed by the ties. Thus the handling of the tissue should not affect the experimental outcome. Occasionally, the physical cutting of the artery will seal the end of the vessel. If this is the case we use two pairs of forceps to open the end of the artery segment by gently stretching the tissue. The tip of the cannula can also be used to open the end of the arteries that have become sealed.

10. If the artery has a hole, it is sometimes possible to adjust the artery so that the hole is past the area that will be tied to the cannula. If this is not the case, then a new artery segment will need to be mounted.

11. If any artery fails to pressurize, visualize the segment and check for holes in the wall. If there are obvious side-branches, it may be possible to adjust the artery segment without completely removing the artery from the system, especially if the side-branch / hole is close to the ties. If there are no obvious side-branches, it may be that the ties are not tight enough to prevent fluid leakage. Simply tighten the ties and re-test the pressurization. If the artery segment continues to fail to pressurize, it may be that there is a leak in the system. Check the system by eye for air bubbles or leaks (especially at the connectors). If this does not work the artery will have to be removed and another segment placed on the system.

12. Depending on the experimental design the vessels can be incubated in the presence of different stimuli (for example growth factors), under different oxygen tensions and for different lengths of time. It is a good idea to carry out an initial time-course to ensure that changes are not missed. We have detected changes in vascular cells as a result of endovascular invasion as early as 20 h, with invasion apparent between 20 h and 5 d. Interstitial invasion experiments may require a longer time course than endovascular experiments.

13. Interstitial and endovascular experiments can be combined. The vessels are dissected with a small amount of surrounding tissue present, perfused endovascularly, then incubated with trophoblast as described in the interstitial experiments. It may prove more difficult to mount and perfuse a vessel with some surrounding tissue present but it is possible, with some patience. The only significant problem is the visualization of the tip of the cannula, to ensure that it is correctly placed within the vessel lumen and that the wall of the vessel is undamaged by the cannula insertion. The trophoblasts will need to be labelled with different CellTracker probes so that they can be distinguished. Depending on the fluorescent microscope available this may limit the subsequent immunohistochemical analysis.

14. It is possible to identify markers on the invaded trophoblasts and on the vascular cells of the spiral arteries, for example adhesion molecules, apoptotic proteins *(15)*, and so on. The immunohistochemical protocols will have to be optimised according to the specific antibodies used.

Acknowledgments

The authors would like to thank Sandra V. Ashton, Guy St.J. Whitley, Philip R. Dash, Ian P. Crocker, Louise C. Kenny, Glenn Ferris, John D. Aplin, and Philip N. Baker for their participation in the development of procedures associated with these models. This work was supported by The British Heart Foundation.

References

1. Pijnenborg, R., Dixon, G., Robertson, W. B., and Brosens, I. (1980) Trophoblastic invasion of human decidua from 8 to 18 weeks of pregnancy. *Placenta* **1,** 3–19.
2. Enders, A. C. and Blankenship, T. N. (1997) Modification of endometrial arteries during invasion by cytotrophoblast cells in the pregnant macaque. *Acta Anatom.* **159,** 169–193.

3. Zhou, Y., Damsky, C. H., and Fisher, S. J. (1997). Preeclampsia is associated with failure of human cytotrophoblasts to mimic a vascular adhesion phenotype. One cause of defective endovascular invasion in this syndrome? *J. Clin. Invest.* **99,** 2152–2164.

4. Craven, C. M., Morgan, T., and Ward, K. (1998). Decidual spiral artery remodelling begins before cellular interaction with cytotrophoblasts. *Placenta* **19,** 241–252.

5. Pijnenborg, R., Bland, J. M., Robertson, W. B., and Brosens, I. (1983). Uteroplacental arterial changes related to interstitial trophoblast migration in early human pregnancy. *Placenta* **4,** 397–413.

6. Blankenship, T. N. and Enders, A. C. (1997). Trophoblast cell-mediated modifications to uterine spiral arteries during early gestation in the macaque. *Acta Anatom.* **158,** 227–236.

7. Kam, E. P. Y., Gardner, L., Loke, Y. W., and King, A. (1999). The role of trophoblast in the physiological change in decidual spiral arteries. *Human Reprod.* **14,** 2131–2138.

8. Brosens, J. J., Pijnenborg, R., and Brosens, I. A. (2002). The myometrial junctional zone spiral arteries in normal and abnormal pregnancies: a review of the literature. *Am. J. Obstet. Gynecol.* **187,** 1416–1423.

9. Lyall, F., Barber, A., Myatt, L., Bulmer, J. N., and Robson, S. C. (2000). Hemeoxygenase expression in human placenta and placental bed implies a role in regulation of trophoblast invasion and placental function. *FASEB J.* **14,** 208–219.

10. Lyall, F., Hayman, R. G., Ashworth, J. R., Duffie, E., and Baker, P. N. (1999). Relationship of cell adhesion molecule expression to endothelium-dependent relaxation in normal pregnancy and pregnancies complicated with preeclampsia or fetal growth restriction. *J. Soc. Gynecol. Invest.* **6,** 196–201.

11. Genbacev, O., Joslin, R., Damsky, C. H., Polliotti, B. M., and Fisher, S. J. (1996). Hypoxia alters early gestation human cytotrophoblast differentiation/invasion in vitro and models the placental defects that occur in preeclampsia. *J. Clin. Invest.* **97,** 540–550.

12. Zhou, Y., Fisher, S. J., Janatpour, M., et al. (1997). Human cytotrophoblasts adopt a vascular phenotype as they differentiate. A strategy for successful endovascular invasion? *J. Clin. Invest.* **99,** 2139–2151.

13. Cartwright, J. E., Kenny, L. C., Dash, P. R., et al. (2002). Trophoblast invasion of spiral arteries: a novel in vitro model. *Placenta* **23,** 232–235.

14. Dunk, C., Petkovic, L., Baczyk, D., Rossant, J., Winterhager, E., and Lye, S. J. (2003). A novel in vitro model of trophoblast-mediated decidual blood vessel remodeling. *Lab. Invest.* **83,** 1821–1828.

15. Ashton, S. V., Whitley, G. St J., Dash, P. R., et al. (2005) Uterine spiral artery remodeling involves endothelial apoptosis induced by extravillous trophoblasts through Fas/FasL interactions. *Arterioscler. Thromb. Vasc. Biol.* **25,** 120–108.

16. Crocker, I. P., Wareing, M., Ferris, G. R., et al. (2005) The effect of vascular origin, oxygen, and tumour necrosis factor alpha on trophoblast invasion of maternal arteries in vitro. *J Pathol.* **206,** 476–485.

17. Cartwright, J. E., Holden, D. P., and Whitley, G. S. (1999). Hepatocyte growth factor regulates human trophoblast motility and invasion: a role for nitric oxide. *Br. J. Pharmacol.* **128,** 181–189.

18. Lash, G. E., Cartwright, J. E., Whitley, G. S., Trew, A. J., and Baker, P. N. (1999). The effects of angiogenic growth factors on extravillous trophoblast invasion and motility. *Placenta* **20,** 661–667.

19. Choy, M. Y., Whitley, G., and Manyonda, I. T. (2000). Efficient, rapid and reliable establishment of human trophoblast cell lines using poly-L-ornithine. Early Pregnancy **2,** 124–143.

20. Choy, M. Y. and Manyonda, I. T. (1998). The phagocytic activity of human first trimester extravillous trophoblast. *Human Reprod.* **13,** 2941–2949.

21. Shiverick, K. T., King, A., Frank, H., Whitley, G. S., Cartwright, J. E., and Schneider, H. (2001). Cell culture models of human trophoblast II: trophoblast cell lines—a workshop report. *Placenta* **22,** S104–S106.

22. Tarrade, A., Lai Kuen, R., Malassine, A., et al. (2001). Characterization of human villous and extravillous trophoblasts isolated from first trimester placenta. *Lab. Invest.* **81,** 1199–1211.

III

ANALYSIS OF UTEROPLACENTAL IMMUNE CELLS AND THEIR FUNCTIONS

5

In Vivo Models for Studying Homing and Function of Murine Uterine Natural Killer Cells

B. Anne Croy and Xuemei Xie

Summary

Decidualization of the mouse and human uterus is accompanied by the influx of large numbers of natural killer lymphocytes (uterine natural killer [uNK] cells). Adoptive cell transfer to mated, alymphoid mice is a general model suitable for analysis of homing, differentiation and function of the uNK cell lineage. Simultaneous transfer of two cell populations, tagged with different fluorescent tracker dyes, permits in vivo analysis of key mechanisms regulating lymphocyte homing and is described. uNK cells are central to initiation of spiral arterial modification (i.e., structural changes that increase capacity of the blood supply channels leading to the placenta). Quantitative histological techniques for identification, localization, and enumeration of uNK cells, as well as for assessment of spiral artery modification and microdomain size within mouse implantation sites are also included.

Key Words: Adoptive cell transfer; decidua; fluorescent cell tracking; histology; image analysis; mouse pregnancy; spiral arteries.

1. Introduction

During pregnancy in mice (19 d, counting from a copulation plug as gestation day [gd] 0.5), large numbers of transient granulated lymphocytes that belong to the natural killer (NK) cell lineage, appear mesometrially in the uterus. These cells become numerous on gd 6; divide rapidly until gd 11 and then die. Maximum uterine (u)NK cell numbers are present between gd 10–12. Near term, only one-tenth of the peak population remains, and this is shed with the placenta. The immediate postpartum uterus lacks terminally differentiated uNK cells *(1,2)*. During our studies of the lineage and functions of pregnancy-associated uterine lymphocytes, we histologically examined implantation sites from mice genetically ablated for NK cells. We noted that the major branches of the uterine arteries passing through midgestation decidua basalis (DB) in NK cell-deficient mice were unusually thick walled. Subsequent studies revealed that these arteries, called decidual spiral arteries (SA), failed to undergo preg-

From: *Methods in Molecular Medicine, Vol. 122: Placenta and Trophoblast: Methods and Protocols, Vol. 2*
Edited by: M. J. Soares and J. S. Hunt © Humana Press Inc., Totowa, NJ

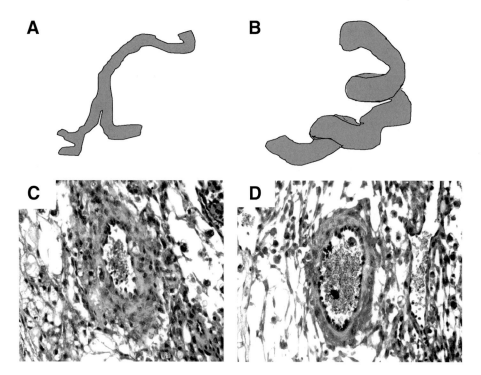

Fig. 1. Tracings of spiral artery lumens from ultrastructural images of maternal arterial casts from a natural killer (NK) cell-deficient **(A)** and a normal **(B)** mouse at gestational day (gd) 12 are presented *(6)*. Typical histological differences between SA in uterine natural killer (uNK) cell-deficient **(C)** and uNK cell competent **(D)** are shown and represent transverse sections through vessel regions illustrated in **(A,B)**. The artery in **(C)** is more similar to branches of the uterine artery in a virgin mouse than it is to the normal, pregnancy-modified artery in **(D)**. The differences can be described by morphometric measurements at midgestation of lumen area, which is greater in normal mice, and wall thickness, which is less in normal mice. Hematoxylin and eosin × 400.

nancy-associated modifications that are normally completed in mice between gd 9 and 10 *(3–6)*. SA modification is a series of structural changes that results in loss of vascular smooth muscle coat, dilation of the lumen and elongation **(Fig.1)**.

To conclude that destabilization of SA or their sensitization to other destabilizing mechanisms was indeed a function of uNK cells, beneficial effects from reconstitution of NK cells in pregnant, lineage-incompetent mice was required. This was achieved initially using intravenous inoculation of bone marrow cells from mice of *scid/scid* genotype (severe combined immunodeficient [SCID]; T-cell and B-cell-deficient) into virgin NK cell-deficient females who were later mated *(3)*. Subsequently, uNK cell reconstitution of NK cell-deficient females has been achieved using all lymphoid tissues and pregnant as well as nonpregnant recipients *(7)*. A very useful general model emerged from these experiments in which in vivo regulation of uNK cell precursor homing and differentiation is assessed by quantitation of graft-derived uNK cells within different subcompartments of implantation sites in mice genetically deficient in NK cells *(8)*. Further, functional capability of the graft-derived uNK cells can be assessed. This is achieved by morphometric measurements of SA in histological sections from pregnant, reconstituted mice at gd 10–12. Our protocol for in vivo evaluation of molecules regulating homing of uNK precursor cells is described, as well as the morphometric procedures for assessing uNK cell numbers and function at midgestation. The homing studies are based upon intravenous delivery of a 1:1 mixture of cells from two sources, each tagged with a different fluorochrome. Subsequently, the ratio of the cell populations is measured in selected organs at specific times. Our example will compare splenocytes from C57Bl/6 mice to splenocytes from mice genetically-deleted for L-selectin, the key receptor involved in the initial lymphocyte–endothelial cell interactions that promote egress of naïve lymphocytes from the circulation *(9)*. The model is applicable, however, to comparison of any two populations, even from the same donor mouse. Reciprocal labeling of cell populations has confirmed that the dyes used do not influence this assay *(10)* (*see* **Notes 1** and **2** for additional suggestions for use of the model).

2. Materials

2.1. Homing Studies

2.1.1. Mice

1. Two strains of donor mice, each at gd 5. One strain represents the normal state (i.e., the congenic control, such as C57Bl/6); the other, the experimental group (i.e., genetically modified mice such as L-selectin$^{o/o}$) (*see* **Note 3**).
2. Recipient, NK cell-deficient mice at gd 6, such as alymphoid recombinase activating gene (RAG)-2$^{o/o}$/common cytokine receptor chain γ (γc)$^{o/o}$ (*see* **Note 4**). In our studies, one donor of each genotype is usually prepared for each available plugged recipient (*see* **Note 5**).

2.1.2. Preparation of Spleen Cell Suspensions

1. 60×15 mm sterile plastic Petri dishes.
2. Sterile plungers from 3-mL syringes.
3. Sterile 200-μm stainless steel mesh screens.
4. Sterile 15-mL conical centrifuge tubes.
5. Sterile tissue culture medium such as RPMI1640 (Sigma-Aldrich, St. Louis, MO), supplemented with 5% fetal bovine serum.

6. Sterile dissection instruments.
7. Sterile 0.1 *M* phosphate-buffered saline (PBS), pH 7.4.
8. Sterile erythrocyte lysis buffer, such as 0.15 *M* ammonium chloride and 10 m*M* KHCO$_3$ erythrocyte lysis buffer (ACK).
9. 1% Trypan blue in 0.1 *M* PBS (Sigma-Aldrich).

2.1.3. Labeling and Infusion of Spleen Cells

1. Sterile 7-amino-4-chloromethylcoumarin (CMAC), a dye fluorescing blue (Molecular Probes, Inc., Eugene,OR).
2. Sterile 5-chloromethylfluorescein diacetate (CMFDA), a dye fluorescing green (Molecular Probes).
3. RPMI 1640 base solution without supplement.
4. Sterile anhydrous dimethylsulfoxide (DMSO).
5. Sterile 1-mL syringe and 26- to 30-gage needles.
6. Skin disinfectant such as 70% alcohol.
7. Sterile lucite mouse restrainer for intravenous inoculations.
8. Laminar flow hood, autoclaved microisolator cages, sterile gloves (if using immune deficient mice).
9. Infrared heat lamp to warm the tails of the mice.

2.1.4. Perfusion Supplies

1. 30- to 40-mL syringe.
2. Butterfly 21-gage needle with 1-mm diameter tubing (Abbott Laboratories, Queenborough, UK).
3. 4% paraformaldehydehyde (PFA) in 0.1 *M* PBS with 0.1 *M* sucrose (Fisher Scientific, Pittsburgh, PA).
4. Dissection tray with sides, lined by absorbent material.

2.1.5. Collection of Frozen Tissues for Cryostat Sectioning

1. Isopentane (Fisher Scientific).
2. Liquid nitrogen.
3. 10- × 10- × 5-mm cryomolds (Tissue Tek, Miles Inc. Elkhart, IN).
4. O.C.T. compound (Tissue Tek).
5. Cryostat.
6. 25- × 75- × 1-mm frosted end, positively charged glass histology slides.
7. Coverslips for histology slides (22 mm × 60 mm).
8. Aqua Poly/Mount (Polysciences, Inc. Warrington, PA).
9. Aluminum foil, labels, and marker pens suitable for cryostorage labeling.

2.1.6. Microscope

Compound fluorescence microscope equipped with eyepiece micrometer, image analysis software and filters suitable for CMAC (absorbance 354 nm, emission 466 nm) and for CMFDA (absorbance 492 nm, emission 516 nm) (*see* **Note 6**).

2.2. Studies of uNK Cell Numbers and Functional Actions Promoting Spiral Arterial Modification

2.2.1. Mice

Mated, gd 10–12 mice. These mice may have endogenous NK cells (i.e., C57Bl/6, SCID) or be NK cell deficient mice with or without transplanted precursor cells. Transplants may come from fertile, infertile or sterile mutant mice or from strains showing fetal lethality, if fetuses survive to gd 8–10 when cells from the aortic/gonadal/mesonephric region or fetal liver can be recovered for transplant *(11–13)* (*see* **Note 7**). For reconstitution studies, infused cells are normally obtained from a single tissue source and not prelabeled with tracking dyes. Infusion of 2×10^7 to 1×10^8 cells is done five or more days before euthanasia. This allows time for cell division and for expression of functional activity morphologically.

2.2.2. Perfusion Supplies (see **Subheading 2.1.4.**)

2.2.3. Tissue Embedding and Microscopy Supplies

1. Paraffin (melting point 50–54°C, for best results, use at temperatures above 56°C, Fisher Scientific).
2. Rotary microtome.
3. 25- × 25- × 10-mm embedding rings.
4. 25- × 25- × 10-mm embedding molds (Electron Microscopy Sciences, Washington, PA).
5. 25- × 75- × 1-mm frosted-end, positively charged glass histology slides.
6. Coverslips for histology slides (22 mm × 60 mm).
7. Compound microscope equipped with image analysis software.

2.2.4. Staining With Hematoxylin and Eosin (H&E)

1. Harris' hematoxylin (Sigma-Aldrich).
2. Alcoholic eosin (Sigma-Aldrich).
3. 70%, 95% and 100% ethanol (Fisher Scientific).
4. Xylene or one of its substitutes (Fisher Scientific).
5. Permount (Fisher Scientific).

2.2.5. Staining With Periodic Acid-Schiff Reagent

1. Periodic acid (Fisher Scientific).
2. Schiff reagent (Fisher Scientific).
3. Sulfurous acid (Fisher Scientific).
4. Harris' hematoxylin (Sigma-Aldrich).
5. 70%, 95%, and 100% ethanol.
6. Xylene or one of its substitutes (Fisher Scientific).
7. Permount (Fisher Scientific).

2.2.6. Reagents for Dolichos biflorus Agglutinin Lectin Histochemistry

1. Wash buffer of 0.05 M phosphate-buffered saline (PBS, pH 7.4).
2. 0.05 M Tris-buffered saline (TBS; pH 7.4).
3. 30% H_2O_2.
4. 1% bovine serum albumin in 0.05 M PBS (pH 7.4).
5. Biotinylated *Dolichos biflorus* agglutinin (DBA) lectin (Sigma-Aldrich) diluted 1:150.
6. 0.1 M N-acetyl-D-galatosamine.
7. Streptoavidin–peroxidase complex (Sigma-Aldrich).
8. Diaminobenzidine (DAB;, Sigma-Aldrich).
9. Harris' hematoxylin (Sigma-Aldrich).
10. 70%, 95%, and 100% ethanol.
11. Xylene or one of its substitutes.
12. Permount (Fisher Scientific).

3. Methods

The methods outlined as follows describe isolation of spleen cells, fluorochrome labeling of spleen cells and their inoculation into pregnant, alymphoid mice, harvesting of tissues from cell transfer recipients for cryostat sectioning and homing studies, harvesting of tissues from cell transfer recipients for paraffin processing histochemical staining for assessment uNK cell numbers and functions, quantitative histological measurements, and statistical recommendations for data analyses.

3.1. Isolation of Spleen Cells

1. Spleens are dissected from each euthanized donor mouse. If multiple donors of the *same* gd and *same* genotype are available, spleens may be pooled. For each genotype independently, freshly removed spleens are placed onto a 200-μm mesh screen in a 60 × 15-mm Petri dish containing 3 mL prewarmed (37°C) RPMI 1640 and minced finely with scissors. The pieces of spleen are mechanically dissociated with a 3-mL syringe plunger to push them, using a circular motion, gently through the stainless steel mesh into the Petri dish. The resulting cell suspension is transferred by pipet into a 15-mL conical tube and suspended in 5 mL RPMI 1640. The procedure is repeated for the second genotype of mouse.
2. Centrifuge each cell suspension (300g, 10 min, 20°C) and discard the supernatants. Resuspend each pellet in 5 mL RPMI 1640, wash the cells again, and discard the supernatants.
3. Resuspend each pellet in room temperature ACK, using 1 mL per spleen, *immediately* vortex *gently* for 10 s, add PBS to fill the tube, and centrifuge (300g, 10 min, 20°C). Discard the supernatants and wash the pellets twice with PBS. Resuspend each pellet in 1 mL *serum-free* RPMI 1640 and determine the cell concentrations and viability using a hemocytometer and trypan blue dye exclusion or other appropriate procedure.

3.2. Fluorochrome Labeling of Spleen Cells and Their Inoculation

1. Dilute the two dye stock solutions (10 mM CMAC or CMFDA) to final working concentrations in serum-free RPMI 1640 and prewarm these solutions to 37°C. Usually, 1×10^7 to 1×10^8 cells are labeled per mL of diluted dye. For studies with tissue recovery within 72 h, 0.5–5 µM is an optimal labeling concentration for the dyes. For studies with cell recovery from hosts after 72 h, 5–25 µM of labeling dye must be used. One cell suspension is labeled with each dye (30 min, 37°C, 5% CO_2), using the same cell number and the same dye concentration for each labeling.
2. Centrifuge the cell suspensions (300g, 10 min, 20°C), discard the supernatants, and incubate the cells in pre-warmed, serum-free RPMI 1640 (30 min, 37°C, 5% CO_2).
3. Centrifuge the cell suspensions (300g, 10 min, 20°C), discard the supernatants, and wash the pellets twice with PBS. Resuspend each pellet in 1 mL of PBS and determine cell concentration and viability using a hemocytometer and trypan blue dye exclusion or other appropriate procedure.
4. Mix equal numbers of viable, differentially fluoresceinated splenocytes together (i.e., equal numbers of each genotype) in a volume of PBS appropriate for inoculation for the number of recipients available in the experiment. We routinely use 3.75×10^7 cells of each genotype in a total inoculum of 150 µL.
5. Place each gd 6 alymphoid RAG-2$^{o/o}$/γc$^{o/o}$ recipient into an approved, disinfected restrainer in a clean laminar-flow bench. Warm the tail, if needed, by placing the mouse briefly under a heat lamp and inoculate the cell mixture into the lateral tail vein. Record, *exactly*, the time of the inoculation for each recipient.

3.3. Harvesting of Tissues From Cell Transfer Recipients for Cryostat Sectioning and Homing Studies

1. Euthanize recipients, using CO_2, at the planned specific times following their inoculation. (Lymphocyte trafficking to the decidualized uterus can be detected within 30 min and followed, in sequential animals, for at least 72 h.) *Immediately* place the cadaver into a small dissection tray lined with absorbent material and open the ventral abdomen, enter the thoracic and abdominal cavities, and begin perfusion fixation using freshly prepared PFA. Fixative, in a 30- to 50-mL syringe, is slowly perfused through a butterfly needle into the dorsal aorta of the mouse. Approximately 3 mL will be given during the first minute, at a constant slow flow rate; then, the right atrium is incised to permit drainage after 1 min of perfusion. The remaining fixative will be delivered much more slowly over a period of 15 min (i.e., ~1 mL/30 s). Uterus, spleen, liver, intestine, kidney, lung, and other organs of interest are then removed (*see* **Note 8**), placed into a vessel containing PFA and further fixed in the dark for 1 h. Using as little illumination as safe procedure will permit, remove the fixed organs from PFA into prelabeled cryomolds and snap-freeze them in isopentane in a liquid nitrogen bath for 30 s. Wrap frozen tissues in foil, label, place in sealed plastic storage containers, and store at –80°C.

2. Frozen specimens are moved to a cryostat, cut at 10-µm in thickness, and mounted on glass histology slides. Place mounted slides in a holding tray and cover the top with foil to reduce excitation of the dyes by ambient light until cutting is completed. The slides are placed into processing holders, moved into distilled water for 5 min in the dark, then coverslipped using Aqua PolyMount. If the slides cannot be examined immediately, they can be covered with foil and refrigerated in the dark for up to 6 mo. Slides are examined at 100–200× magnification using an ultraviolet fluoresence microscope equipped with a 1-mm^2 ocular grid. Cells of each color are scored per mm^2 of tissue as depicted in **Fig. 2**. For small tissues, such as gd-6 uterus, scoring may be reported per section. Routinely, we count the number of homed cells in 50 sections from each tissue. The mean number of cells of the control genotype is divided by the mean number of cells of the experimental genotype to establish the ratio of cells of the two colors and describe the homing behavior of the test cells as normal (ratio of 1:1), deficient (ratio >1:1) or targeted (ratio <1:1) to each organ in comparison with the normal cells. In these assays, many cells are found in lung. Lung, however, contains the first capillary bed the cells reach after tail vein injection and cells located there represent a combination of trapping, clearance, and homing. Results for all other organs represent homing. For true homing studies to lung, injection of the left ventricle is required for samples collected between 0 and 24 h If tail vein injection is used, collection of lung samples should not be made before 24 h have elapsed *(14)*.

3.4. Harvesting of Tissues From Cell Transfer Recipients for Paraffin Embedding and Histological Study of uNK Cell Numbers and Function

1. For this procedure, spleen cell suspensions are prepared from only one genotype of donor mouse and infused intravenously at 10^7 to 10^8 cells in 200 µL per mated (gd 0) alymphoid mouse. Usually, the donor mouse is deficient in the function of a gene of interest, pregnant at gd 3–5, and used as one donor for each available recipient *(11)*.

2. Recipient mice are euthanized between gd 10 and 12 using CO_2 followed by perfusion through the dorsal aorta (*see* **Subheading 3.3.1.**) The uterus is removed intact after perfusion, leaving some of the mesentery attached as a landmark. The uterus is then transected between the implantation sites (**Fig. 3A**) and the implantation sites are further fixed in PFA (4°C, 6 h; if studying specimens less than gd 10, this incubation should be reduced to 2 h). The implantation sites are next moved into PBS for 15 min and then transferred to 70% ethanol at 4°C until processed (*see* **Note 9**).

3. For embedding, cut each implantation site into two equal parts mid-saggitally (**Fig. 3B**) and automatically process them into paraffin using a commercial tissue processor. At an embedding station, put the two halves of the same implantation site cut side down at the bottom of the mold. Place an embedding ring on the mold, fill with molten paraffin and chill. This will place the central portion of the implantation site, the region of interest, at the cutting face of the paraffin block (**Fig. 3C**). Ideally, six viable implantation sites from three dams (i.e., two implan-

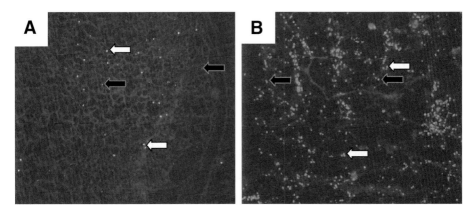

Fig. 2 (*see* companion CD for color version). Photomicrographs showing sections of uterus ×200 (**A**) and spleen ×200 (**B**) from a gd 6 recombinase activating gene (RAG)-2$^{o/o}$/γc$^{o/o}$ recipient 2 h after transfer of a 1:1 mixture of 7-amino-4-chloro-methylcoumarin (CMAC)-labeled splenocytes from gd 5 L-selectin$^{o/o}$ mice (stippled arrow indicates blue cells) and 5-chloromethylfluorescein diacetate (CMFDA)-labeled splenocytes from gd 5 B6 mice (white arrow indicates green cells). The mean ratio of B6 to L-selectin$^{o/o}$ cells in the uterus at 2 h was 1.45 and that in the spleen was 1.32, indicating an L-selectin mediated homing deficit to both tissues at this time point.

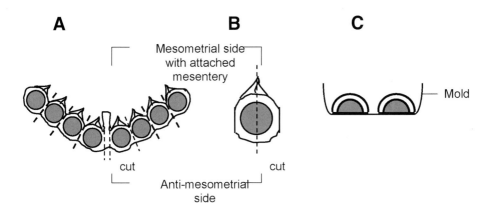

Fig. 3. Diagram showing separation of fixed implantation sites (**A**), their mid-sagittal transverse cutting (**B**) and embedding position (**C**).

tation sites per dam) should be examined. If not available, six implantation sites from two dams (i.e., three implantation sites per dam) can be used. Dying implantation sites must be excluded from these analyses. Section the embedded implantation sites serially at 7-µm thickness using a rotary microtome, mount

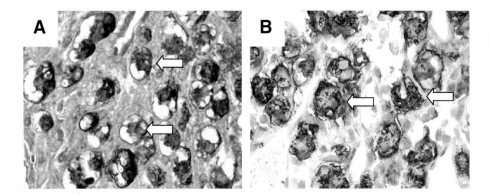

Fig. 4. Photomicrograph showing uterine natural killer (uNK) cells (arrows) in implantation sites from gestational day (gd) 12 C57Bl/6 mice. (**A**) shows periodic acid–Schiff (PAS)-stained cells in MLAp. (**B**) shows *Dolichos biflorus* agglutinin (DBA) lectin stained cells in decidua basalis (DB) under ×1000 magnification. Cells in MLAp are less mature and generally smaller than cells in DB *(17)*.

the sections onto labeled 22 × 33 mm glass slides and dry the slides overnight on a 42°C hot plate.

3.5 Histochemical Staining for Assessment of uNK Cell Numbers and Function

1. Periodic acid–Schiff (PAS) reaction *(1,15)* is used for tissues that will be assessed for uNK cell numbers. It gives prominence to the cytoplasmic granules of uNK cells (**Fig. 4A**). Other cells, such as trophoblast, are PAS positive. *Only* granulated lymphocytes should be scored as uNK cells. PAS is recommended when large numbers of slides must be stained.

2. DBA lectin reacts with both the plasma membrane and cytoplasmic granules of uNK cells (**Fig. 4B**). Endothelium is the only other reactive cell type in mouse implantation sites. DBA lectin staining is currently the reaction of choice over immunostaining for identification of mouse uNK cells *(16,17)*. Reagent costs may limit use of DBA lectin when large numbers of specimens are being evaluated. For DBA lectin staining, routine procedures are used to deparaffinize and rehydrate tissue sections mounted on glass slides. Specimens must then remain moist. 0.05 *M* PBS, pH 7.4 is used throughout the staining procedure. Sections are washed three times in PBS for 5 min each. Then endogenous peroxidases are inactivated using 1% H_2O_2 in PBS at room temperature for 30 min. This is followed by three further 5-min washes in PBS and blocking with 1% BSA in PBS for 30 min at room temperature. Biotinylated DBA lectin (1:150) in PBS with 1% BSA, is applied and the slides are incubated overnight in a humid chamber at 4°C. The following day, slides are washed three times for 5 min each using PBS and then incubated with streptavidin-peroxidase complex in PBS for 60 min at

room temperature. Slides are washed three times in PBS and then three times in 0.05 M TBS (pH 7.4), 5 min per wash, and incubated with 0.1% diaminobenzedine tetraoxide in 0.05 M TBS with 0.3% H_2O_2, at room temperature for approx 5 min. It is best to observe color development under a microscope. To terminate color development, the slides are washed three times in distilled water, then lightly counterstained with Harris' hematoxylin, dehydrated, and permanently mounted.

To establish specificity of the reaction, a control slide in which binding of DBA lectin is blocked by its specific sugar ligand should be included in each staining run. This is accomplished by adding 0.1 M N-acetyl-D-galactosamine to the lectin solution used for the overnight incubation at 4°C.

3. H&E staining *(15)* is used for tissues that will be used for measurements of area of the mesometrial lymphoid aggregate of pregnancy (MLAp), DB, placenta, and blood vessels. uNK cells have faint eosinophilic granules in H&E stained specimens and can be easily overlooked. Masson's trichome staining can be used if arterial walls are the only structures of interest *(15)*.

3.6. Quantitative Histological Measurements

1. Enumeration of uNK Cells. Using PAS or DBA-stained material, select a well prepared section estimated to be at the very center of the implantation site. The uterine artery will clearly enter from the mesentery into the implantation site in this section. Mark the glass below this section with a permanent marker. Then select ten more sections for each implantation site. We usually select both placental halves in each seventh section in the series and mark below these sections with a marker. This leaves >40 μm between sections that will be measured, a distance exceeding the diameter of one small to medium sized cell. This avoids duplicate counting of individual uNK cells as does scoring only uNK cells in which the nucleus is clearly visible. uNK cells are counted at 400× magnification, in the central part of the MLAp and DB on each selected section using a 1-mm² ocular grid. UNK cells are recognized by their PAS- or DBA lectin-reactive cytoplasmic granules. Usually, the nucleus located to one side of the cell and not centrally. Blood vessel spaces are excluded (**Fig. 5**). If enumeration of uNK cells found in vessel lumens is desired (approx 10% of the population *[8]*), the perfusion step must be omitted.

2. To obtain the ratio of Vessel Area to Lumen Area for the SA, 11 H&E-stained sections are selected and marked as indicated under **Subheading 3.6.1.** The SAs are in the central DB. There may be twenty cross-sectioned arterial segments in each tissue section. Select SA cut as closely as possible to circular shapes (**Fig. 6A**). Trace, with the computer-drawing tool, the endothelial surface of the vessel and calculate the area this line encloses. That is the lumen area (L). Next, trace the stroma-associated, external smooth muscle coat of the vessel and calculate the area of this shape. This is the vessel area (W) (**Fig. 6B**). Ratios maybe presented a W/L or L/W. Alternatively, maximum vessel diameter to maximum lumen diameter can be measured (**Fig. 6C**). We undertake these measurements at 400× magni-

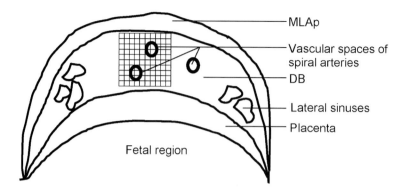

Fig. 5. Diagram showing micrometer grid placement for enumeration of uterine natural killer (uNK) cells. To adjust counts to represent cells/mm^2 of decidualized tissue (X) and exclude regions of vascular space (Y, total number of grid squares occupied by vessel lumen regions), the following formula is used: X = total cells counted/(number of grids – Y × 1 mm^2/100)

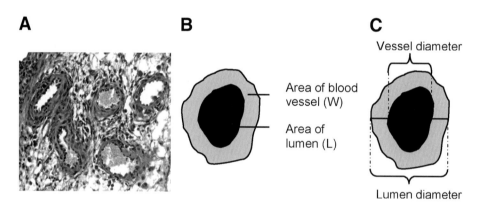

Fig. 6. Analysis of uterine spiral arteries (SA). **(A)** is a photomicrograph of an hematoxylin and eosin (H&E)-stained SA cut in five cross sections. The diagrams show the measurements made and averaged over 66 sections to calculate the total vessel area and its lumen area **(B)** or the maximum diameter of the vessel and of its lumen **(C)**.

fication and employ Optimas image analysis software, version 6.2 (Optimas Corporation, Bothwell, MA, USA) (*see* **Note 10**).

3. To measure the surface area of the MLAp, DB, and placenta, use the same H&E-stained sections selected under **Subheading 3.6.2.** With the computer drawing tool, delineate the MLAp by drawing along the outer muscle layer of the uterus

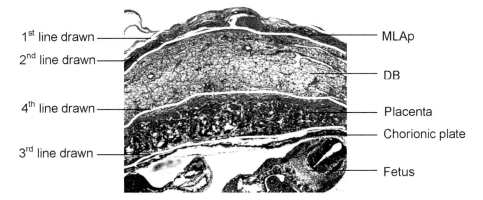

Fig. 7. Photomicrograph of C57Bl/6 gestational day (gd)-10 implantation site showing the placement of the computer drawing tool for calculation of the areas of the MLAp, decidua basalis (DB), and placenta. Measurements are made on 11 sections per implantation site and a total of at least 6 implantation sites collected on the same gestation day from different dams is used.

and along the partially disrupted circular smooth muscle layer. The area between these two lines is the surface area of the MLAp. Next, delineate the placenta by drawing along the surface closest to the fetus (**Fig. 7**) where the chorion and yolk sac attach. Then draw a line along the trophoblast giant cell layer. The area between these two lines is the midplacental surface area. The area in the middle of the implantation site, defined between the circular smooth muscle line and the trophoblast giant cell line, is then calculated. This area represents the central decidua basalis. We make these measurements at 25× magnification and use Optimas image analysis software, version 6.2 (Optimas Corporation, Bothwell, MA, USA) for drawing and analysis.

3.7. Statistical Recommendations for Analyses of These Types of Data

SigmaStat (Version 2.03) can be used for statistical analyses. Graphs can be produced using Excel (MS Office). Comparisons between groups are performed using the One-way Analysis of Variance (ANOVA) multiple comparison test (SAS Version 8; SAS Institute, Cary, NC, USA). Statistical significance is set at $p < 0.05$.

4. Notes

1. Because RAG-$2^{o/o}$/$\gamma c^{o/o}$ mice are alymphoid, they accept transplants of human cells and tissues. The trafficking of dye-tagged human blood NK cells into the decidua and other tissues of pregnant RAG-$2^{o/o}$/$\gamma c^{o/o}$ has been successful (B. A. Croy, X. Xie, S. Bashar and M.van den Heuvel, unpublished). CMAC is our preferred dye for single-label studies.

2. This approach is not restricted to cell inoculation but has been successful in two studies addressing molecules affecting spiral artery modification *(4,18)*. Intraperitional or intravenous injections of mouse recombinant interferon gamma or human $\alpha2$ macroglobulin were given to pregnant RAG-$2^{o/o}$/$\gamma c^{o/o}$ mice once daily for 6 d, commencing on gd 6. On gd 12, the mice were euthanized and implantation sites prepared by wax embedding and studied morphometrically as described under **Subheadings 3.6.2.** and **3.6.3.**

3. The homing studies we conduct employ cells from mice of two distinct genotypes. A similar approach is valid for comparison of different organs from a single donor or cells from the same organ from genetically identical donors killed at different gestational stages.

4. The preferred mouse for these studies is the RAG-$2^{o/o}$/$\gamma c^{o/o}$. This strain, available from Taconic, Germantown, NY, has a total deficit in uNK cells as well as good health and fertility under barrier husbandry conditions. At least 70% of mice with copulation plugs who are then injected either intravenously or intraperitoneally carry viable litters at midgestation study points.

5. The outlined homing study approach employs three strains of pregnant mice. This is greatly facilitated if the investigator conducts vaginal examination of the females prior to their pairing with males, to ensure the females are in estrus. Visual examination should be adequate but vaginal smears could be used to confirm the opinion formed by visual examination *(19,20)*.

6. The recommended dyes are those we use routinely but other fluoresent tags are useful for short term, cell homing studies. These include CFS-E (Molecular Probes), which also permits calculation of cell division, if analyses are conducted by flow cytometry, calcein-AM (Molecular Probes) and PKH26 (Sigma) *(21,22)*.

7. It is possible to reconstitute NK cells in RAG-$2^{o/o}$/$\gamma c^{o/o}$ from mice with fetally-lethal genetic modifications, if the mutant mice survive to gd 8–10 when the aortic/gonadal/mesonephric region *(12)* or fetal liver *(13)* can be dissociated and transplanted. All NK cells in the host will be derived from the engrafted fetal hematopoietic cells. Adult, reproductively sterile mice, such as estrogen receptor knockout (ERKO), can also be used as donors of lymphocyte progenitors *(11)*.

8. If recipients of transferred, dye-labeled cells are immune competent, study of lymph nodes, especially the iliac lymph center draining the pelvic cavity and its contents including the uterus, is recommended. Lymph nodes cannot be identified routinely in RAG-$2^{o/o}$/$\gamma c^{o/o}$ recipients.

9. Do not remove the placenta and fetus from the implantation site for studies of uNK cells. Much of the important information for the study of these cells is occurring in the wall of the uterus. Leave the entire implantation site intact, when possible. For times after gd 12, complete infiltration of paraffin is sometimes not successful. To study these time points, open the uterus antimesometrially, remove the fetus and prepare the implantation site with the placenta attached to the uterine wall. *Cut*, rather than pull, the fetus off of the placenta to avoid artifactually misshaping the placenta.

10. Visual inspection of the SA is often misleading. Morphometry *must* be used to evaluate whether modification is occurring. In this chapter, we illustrated extremes. In other strains of mice, such as CXCR3$^{o/o}$ and FCR$\gamma^{o/o}$/CD3$\xi^{o/o}$, partial modification of SA occurs that can only be assessed by careful morphometric measurements.

Acknowledgments

We thank the staff of the Ontario Ministry of Agriculture, Food, and Rural Affairs (OMAFRA) Animal Isolation facility for their dedicated care of our immune-deficient mouse colony, Dr. J. P. Di Santo, Paris France for providing the foundation RAG-2$^{o/o}$/γc$^{o/o}$ breeding stock and Drs. S. Chantakru, Faculty of Veterinary Medicine, Kasetsart University, Bangkok, Thailand and A. Ashkar, Faculty of Medicine, McMaster University, Hamilton, Canada for their contributions to development of these models. Our research program is supported by the Natural Sciences and Engineering Research Council, Canada, OMAFRA and the Canada Research Chairs Program.

References

1. Peel, S. (1989) Granulated metrial gland cells. *Adv. Anat. Embryol. Cell Biol.* **115,** 1–112.
2. Delgado, S. R., McBey, B. A., Yamashiro, S., Fujita, J., Kiso, Y., and Croy, B. A. (1996) Accounting for the peripartum loss of granulated metrial gland cells, a natural killer cell population, from the pregnant mouse uterus. *J. Leukoc. Biol.* **59,** 262–269.
3. Guimond, M. J., Wang, B., and Croy, B. A. (1998) Engraftment of bone marrow from severe combined immunodeficient (SCID) mice reverses the reproductive deficits in natural killer cell-deficient tg epsilon 26 mice. *J. Exp. Med.* **187,** 217–223.
4. Ashkar, A. A., Di Santo, J. P., and Croy, B.A. (2000) Interferon gamma contributes to initiation of uterine vascular modification, decidual integrity, and uterine natural killer cell maturation during normal murine pregnancy. *J. Exp. Med.* **192,** 259–270.
5. Ashkar, A. A., Black, G. P., Wei,Q., et al. (2003) Assessment of requirements for IL-15 and IFN regulatory factors in uterine NK cell differentiation and function during pregnancy. *J. Immunol.* **171,** 2937–2944.
6. Croy, B. A., Esadeg, S., Chantakru, S., et al. (2003) Update on pathways regulating the activation of uterine Natural Killer cells, their interactions with decidual spiral arteries and homing of their precursors to the uterus. *J. Reprod. Immunol.* **59,** 175–191.
7. Chantakru, S., Miller, C., Roach, L. E., et al. (2002) Contributions from self-renewal and trafficking to the uterine NK cell population of early pregnancy. *J. Immunol.* **168,** 22–28.
8. Chantakru, S., Kuziel, W. A., Maeda, N., and Croy, B. A. (2001) A study on the density and distribution of uterine Natural Killer cells at mid pregnancy in mice

genetically-ablated for CCR2, CCR 5 and the CCR5 receptor ligand, MIP-1 alpha. *J. Reprod. Immunol.* **49,** 33–47.

9. Kadono, T., Venturi. G. M., Steeber, D. A., and Tedder, T. F. (2002) Leukocyte rolling velocities and migration are optimized by cooperative L-selectin and intercellular adhesion molecule-1 functions. *J. Immunol.* **169,** 4542–4550.

10. Xie, X., Kang, Z., Anderson, L. N., He, H., Lu, B., and Croy, B. A. (2005) Analysis of the contributions of L-selectin and CXCR3 in mediating Leukocyte homing to pregnant mouse uterus. *AJRI* **53,** 1–12.

11. Borzychowski, A. M., Chantakru, S., Minhas, K., et al. (2003) Functional analysis of murine uterine natural killer cells genetically devoid of oestrogen receptors. *Placenta* **24,** 403–411.

12. Samson, S. I., Richard, O., Tavian, M., et al. (2003) GATA-3 promotes maturation, IFN-gamma production, and liver-specific homing of NK cells. *Immunity* **19,** 701–711.

13. Colucci, F., Soudais, C., Rosmaraki, E., Vanes, L., Tybulewicz, V. L., and Di Santo, J. P. (1999) Dissecting NK cell development using a novel alymphoid mouse model: investigating the role of the c-abl proto-oncogene in murine NK cell differentiation. *J. Immunol.* **162,** 2761–2765.

14. Fidler, I. J., and Nicolson, G. L. (1976) Organ selectivity for implantation survival and growth of B16 melanoma variant tumor lines. *J. Natl. Cancer Inst.* **57,** 1199–1202.

15. Sheehan, D. C. and Hrapchak, B. B. (eds.) (1987) *Theory and Practice of Histotechnology.* Battelle, Columbus, OH.

16. Stewart, I. J. and Webster, A. J. (1997) Lectin histochemical studies of mouse granulated metrial gland cells. *Histochem. J.* **29,** 885–892.

17. Paffaro, V. A. Jr., Bizinotto, M. C., Joazeiro, P. P., and Yamada, A. T. (2003) Subset classification of mouse uterine natural killer cells by DBA lectin reactivity. *Placenta* **24,** 479–488.

18. He, H., McCartney, D. J., Wei, Q., et al. (2005) Characterization of a murine alpha 2 macroglobulin gene expressed in reproductive and cardiovascular tissue. *Biol. Reprod.* **72,** 266–275.

19. Champlin, A. K., Dorr, D. D., and Gates, A. H. (1973) Determining the stage of the estrous cycle in the mouse by the appearance of the vagina. *Biol. Reprod.* **8,** 491–494.

20. Branson, F. H., Dagg, C. P., and Snell, G. D. (1966) Reproduction. In *Biology of the Laboratory Mouse, Second Edition* (Green, E.R., ed.). McGraw Hill, New York: pp. 187–204.

21. Venturi, G. M., Tu, L., Kadono, T., et al. (2003) Leukocyte migration is regulated by L-selectin endoproteolytic release. *Immunity* **19,** 713–724.

22. D'Ambrosio, D. and Sinigaglia, F. (2004) *Cell Migration in Inflammation and Immunity, Methods and Protocols.* Humana, Totowa, NJ.

6

Immune and Trophoblast Cells at the Rhesus Monkey Maternal–Fetal Interface

Thaddeus G. Golos, Gennadiy I. Bondarenko, Edith E. Breburda, Svetlana V. Dambaeva, Maureen Durning, and Igor I. Slukvin

Summary

To promote the use of the nonhuman primate model for the study of the cellular and molecular biology of maternal–fetal interactions and placental development during early pregnancy, we have developed protocols for the isolation and characterization of placental trophoblasts and decidual immune cells from the rhesus monkey. In this chapter, we provide protocols for trophoblast and decidual immune cell isolation, phenotyping of isolated cells by flow cytometry, and analysis of placental and decidual tissues by immunohistochemistry. Information on antibodies for these analyses are also provided, which is an important consideration when attempting to use anti-human antibodies for the study of nonhuman primates.

Key Words: Rhesus monkey; pregnancy; immune tolerance; placenta; HLA-G; MHC; decidua; NK cell; macrophage; flow cytometry.

1. Introduction

Nonhuman primates represent important models for the investigation of human physiology, and this is particularly true in pregnancy, where nonprimate mammals generally have limitations in form and sometimes function of the placenta and the fetal membranes. On the other hand, human and, in particular, Old World nonhuman primates share many characteristics of the maternal–fetal interface, which make Old World nonhuman primates particularly appropriate models for human placental and decidual biology (1–3) (see Note 1). The placenta is the first organ to undergo differentiation and morphogenesis and to become functional in mammalian development. The interaction of fetal and maternal systems is carried out at multiple levels, from the endocrine control of maternal corpus luteum function by placental chorionic gona-

From: *Methods in Molecular Medicine, Vol. 122: Placenta and Trophoblast: Methods and Protocols, Vol. 2*
Edited by: M. J. Soares and J. S. Hunt © Humana Press Inc., Totowa, NJ

dotropin *(4)*, to the adhesion of the embryonic trophectoderm to the uterine epithelium and subsequent invasion of the endometrium by differentiating placental trophoblasts *(5,6)*. We have been studying the differentiation of rhesus monkey villous cytotrophoblasts and the (putative) interactions of the fetal placenta with maternal immune cells resident within the decidua *(2,3,7,8)*.

An important advance in research in trophoblast biology was the development of a relatively straightforward basic protocol for the isolation of villous cytotrophoblasts from human term placentas *(9)*. Subsequent modifications have improved the purity of available trophoblast preparations *(10)*. Shortly thereafter, protocols were also reported similar to this basic protocol for the isolation of villous cytotrophoblasts from rhesus monkey villous tissues *(11,12)*. An updated detailed protocol is provided herein. At the time that these protocols were developed, it was not widely recognized that the rhesus monkey placental syncytiotrophoblasts, in contrast to the human placenta, expressed high levels of nonclassical major histocompatibility complex (MHC) class I molecules *(7,13)*. This has now also been shown for the baboon as well *(14)*. Thus, in addition to placental endocrine function, the study of villous trophoblasts is an important component of current research into maternal–fetal immune interactions in nonhuman primate models.

The maternal counterpart to primate placental MHC class I expression is the novel population of decidual nonspecific immune cells, namely decidual natural killer (NK) cells (large granular lymphocytes) and macrophages. The presence of decidual dendritic cells remains controversial *(16–18)*, although there is no question that decidual immune cell dendritic cell-specific intercellular adhesion molecule (ICAM)-grabbing nonintegrin (DC-SIGN) expression is readily detectable. Whether DC-SIGN-positive cells are actually decidual dendritic cells or macrophages remains to be defined. In general, the protocol for decidual dispersion is similar to that for placental dispersion. Although mechanical disruption of human decidual tissue in the first trimester is sufficient to liberate decidual NK cells *(19)*, in our initial experiments enzymatic treatment was necessary with the rhesus monkey decidua *(8)*.

Because most labs have their own methods for immunostaining, and these methods are also discussed elsewhere in this book, we have summarized below special conditions or considerations, which we have found to be important for immunohistochemistry (IHC) studies of the rhesus monkey maternal-fetal interface. The antibodies for leukocyte markers and the W6/32 and 25D3 antibodies DO NOT recognize their respective antigens in paraffin-embedded materials, in our hands. It is possible that appropriate antigen-specific epitope retrieval methods could be established, but we have not had success in our efforts in this area.

2. Materials

2.1. Trophoblast Isolation: Have Ready the Day Before

1. Two diethylpyrocarbonate (DEPC)-treated and siliconized autoclaved 250-mL flasks.
2. Autoclaved tools—medium forceps and curved scissors (two sets of each).
3. 3 × 50-mL polypropylene tubes each containing 500,000 U Trypsin, (cat. no. T-4665, [approx 50 mg, varies by lot]) and 10 mg DNAse (cat. no. D-5025), both from Sigma, St Louis, MO.
4. 3 × 15-mL tubes each containing 10 mg DNAse.
5. 500 mL sterile Dulbecco's modified Eagle's medium (DMEM) (Invitrogen, Carlsbad, CA, cat. no. 31053-028).
6. Sterile DMEM/10% fetal calf serum (FCS; Sigma).
7. 500 mL sterile phosphate-buffered saline (PBS).
8. Sterile 10-mL syringes, 6-μm Acrodisc filters, pipets.
9. Percoll (Amersham Biosciences, Sweden, Cat. No. 17-0891-01) gradients 50% to 5% (diluted in PBS, sterile).
10. Sterile calcium/magnesium-free Hank's balanced salt solution (HBSS) (CMF; Invitrogen, cat. no. 14180-061).
11. Opti-Mem medium (if transfecting the same day) (Invitrogen, cat. no. 22600-050).
12. Freezing medium (for cells in DMEM media). Total volume of 40 mL: 24 mL of heat-inactivated (HI) FCS, 14 mL of DMEM culture medium (without FCS), 2 mL of dimethylsulfoxide (DMSO) (added last). Filter freezing media and pour into a 50-mL centrifuge tube. Store at 4°C.

2.2. Preparation of Stripped FCS

1. HBSS-CMF with 0.9% NaCl (400 mg KCl, 60 mg KH_2PO_4, 96 mg Na_2HPO_4, 9 g NaCl).
2. Dextran (Pharmacia, cat. no. 17-0280-01).
3. Norite A activated charcoal (Sigma, cat. no. C5260).

2.3. Decidual Leukocyte Isolation: Have Ready the Day Before

1. Sterile (autoclaved) siliconized 250-mL glass Erlenmeyer flask.
2. Autoclaved tools—forceps and scissors.
3. 150-mL bottle top filter, 5-mL disposable syringes, Acrodiscs.
4. One 50-mL tube with enzyme mixture: 60 mg collagenase IV (Sigma, cat. no. C-5138) and 10 mg DNAse (Sigma, cat. no. D-5025).
5. Three 15-mL tubes each containing 10 mg DNAse.
6. Sterile PBS.
7. Sterile PBS containing $CaCl_2$ (100 mg/L), $MgCl_2$ (47 mg/L), 10 mM HEPES, pH 7.4 (CM-PBS) (Invitrogen-Gibco, cat. no. 21300-025).
8. Sterile RPMI-1640 medium.
9. Ficoll-Paque.

10. Culture medium: sterile RPMI 1640 medium supplemented with 2 m*M* L-glutamine, 10% FCS, penicillin-streptomycin (from 100X stock, Invitrogen-Gibco), sodium pyruvate (from 100X stock, Invitrogen-Gibco), nonessential amino acids (from 100X stock, Invitrogen-Gibco), 2-mercaptoethanol ($5 \times 10^{-5} M$ final from sterile stock) *(8)*.
11. 100-mm cell culture dishes (BD Biosciences, Bedford, MA, Falcon cat. no. 353803); T-75 flasks (Corning Life Sciences, Acton, MA, cat. no. 430641).
12. 4% paraformaldehyde in PBS.
13. Recombinant human interleukin (IL)-2, 0.5×10^6 U/mL (R&D Systems, Minneapolis, MN).
14. Purified phytohaemagglutinin (PHA), 1 mg/mL (Abbott Laboratories, Abbott Park, IL).
15. Monoclonal antibodies recognizing CD3, 8, 14, 20, 56, 64, Human Leukocyte Antigen (HLA)-DR, DC-SIGN (BD-Pharmingen, San Diego, CA), corresponding monoclonal immunoglobulin (Ig) isotype controls, rat anti-mouse antibodies (**Table 1**).

2.4. NK Cell Sorting and Culture

1. PBS/2% FCS.
2. 15-mL plastic tubes.
3. Antibodies for cell surface markers: fluorescein isothiocyanate (FITC)-, phycoerythrin (PE)-, and allophycocyanin (APC)-conjugated mouse Ig isotype controls, anti-CD56-FITC, anti-CD3-PE, anti-CD8-APC.
4. Culture medium: sterile RPMI 1640 medium supplemented with 2 m*M* L-glutamine, 10% FCS, penicillin-streptomycin (from 100x stock, Invitrogen-Gibco), sodium pyruvate (from 100X stock, Invitrogen-Gibco), nonessential amino acids (from 100X stock, Invitrogen-Gibco), 2-mercaptoethanol ($5 \times 10^{-5} M$ final from sterile stock) *(8)*.
5. Recombinant human IL-2, 0.5×10^6 U/mL (R&D Systems).
6. Purified PHA, 1 mg/mL (Abbott Laboratories).

2.5. Flow Cytometry of Tropohoblasts, Decidual and Peripheral Blood Immune Cells

1. PBS/2% FCS.
2. Fluorochrome-conjugated antibodies (**Table 1**).
3. 4% paraformaldehyde.

2.6. Immunohistochemical Analysis of Placenta and Decidua

1. 2% paraformaldehyde/PBS.
2. 9% sucrose/PBS; 20% sucrose/PBS.
3. Peel-A-Way disposable plastic tissue embedding molds (22 mm to 12 mm taper, Polysciences, Inc., Warrington, PA, cat. no. 18986).
4. OCT embedding compound.
5. Liquid nitrogen or isopentane/dry ice–ethanol bath.
6. Antibodies used for immunohistochemistry (**Table 2**).

Table 1
Monoclonal Antibodies Used for FlowCytometry Analysis
of Rhesus MonkeyPeripheral Blood and Placenta Cells (*see* Notes 8–10)

Antigen	Clone	Format	Major specificity	Supplier
CD3	SP34	PE	All T-cells	BD Pharmingen
CD8	RPA-T8	PE, APC	T-cytotoxic/supressor cells NK cells subset	BD Pharmingen
CD14	M5E2	PE, APC	Monocytes, macrophages	BD Pharmingen
CD16	3G8	PE	NK cells,monocytes	BD Pharmingen
CD20	2H7	PE	B-cells	BD Pharmingen
CD56	MY31 B159	PE, Cy-Chrome	peripheral blood: monocytes decidua: NK cells	BD Pharmingen
CD64	10.1	purified, FITC	Monocytes, macrophages	BD Pharmingen
CD83	HB15a	FITC	Mature DC (dendritic cells)	Immunotech
CD86	FUN1	FITC	Monocytes, DC, activated B cells	BD Pharmingen
DC-SIGN	DCN46	FITC	DC	BD Pharmingen
HLA-DR	G46-6	PE, PerCP-Cy5.5	B cells, monocytes, macrophages, DC	BD Pharmingen
HLA-E (Mamu-E)	MEM-E/06	purified	expressed on most nucleated cells	EXBIO Praha
Mamu-AG	25D3	hybridoma supernatant	Extravillous cytotrophoblast, villous syncytiotrophoblast	Golos laboratory
pan MHC class I	W6/32	FITC	expressed on most nucleated cells	SIGMA
Cytokeratin	C-11	FITC	permeabilized epithelial cells	SIGMA
EGF-R	EGFR.1	PE	many cells; villous cytotrophoblasts, column cytotrophoblasts	BD Pharmingen

NK, natural killer; PE, phycoerythrin; FITC, fluorescein isothiocyanate; DC, dendritic cell; DC-SIGN, dendritic cell-specific intercellular adhesion molecule (ICAM)-grabbing nonintegrin; HLA, human leukocyte antigen; MEM, modified Eagle's medium; MHC, major histocompatibility complex; EGF, epidermal growth factor; EGFR, epidermal growth factor receptor.

BD Pharmingen, San Diego CA, USA; Immunotech, Marseilles, France; EXBIO Praha, dist. by Axxora, Inc., San Diego CA, USA; Sigma, St. Louis MO, USA; Sigma-Aldrich, St. Louis MO, USA; Golos laboratory: contact golos@primate.wisc.edu

Table 2
Anti-Human and Anti-Rhesus Monoclonal Antibodies
Used for Immunohistochemistry (*see* Notes 9 and 10)

Antigen	Dilution	Clone	Major specificity	Supplier
CD 1a	1:50	SK9	Langerhans cells, cortical thymocytes, DCs	Becton Dickinson
CD 3	1:250	FN-18	All T-cells	BioSource
CD14	1:75	M5E2	Monocytes, macrophages	BD PharMingen
CD 56	1:50	MY31	NK-cells, peripheral monocytes	Becton Dickinson
CD 64	1:50	101	Monocytes, macrophages	BD PharMingen
CD 68	1:50	EBM11	Macrophages	DAKO
CD 83	1:50	HB 15a	Mature DCs	BD PharMingen
CD 83	1:50	HB 15e	Mature DCs	Immunotech
CD 86	1:50	GL1	DC (also some other leukocytes)	BD PharMingen
HLA-DR	1:75	G46-6	Monocytes, macrophages, DCs, B-lymphocytes, activated T cells	BD PharMingen
DC-SIGN	1:50	DCN 46	DC	BD PharMingen
DEC-205	1:100	NLDC-145	DCs/Interdigitating cells	Mater Med Res. Inst., AUS
IDO	1:150	10.1	Human IDO (indolamine 2, 3 dioxygenase)	Chemicon
Bovine LHβ (P)	20 µg/mL	518B7	hCG/mCG	Univ of California-Davis, USA
Mamu-AG	5–10 µg/mL	25D3	STB, EVT	Golos lab
MHC I	1 µg/mL	W6/32	STB	SIGMA
Vimentin	5 µg/mL	V6630	Villous mesenchyme	SIGMA
IGF-II	5 µg/mL	Goat	Syncytiotrophoblast	R&D Systems
Soluble Mamu-AG	5 µg/mL	I6G1	STB, VCTB	Dan Geraghty, Fred Hutchinson Cancer Center
β₂-microglobulin	1:1000 (rabbit)	A-072	STB. EVT	DAKO
EGF-R (P)	6.14 µg/mL	H11	STB, VCTB	DAKO
HLA-E	5 µg/mL	MEM-E/06	Native surface-expressed HLA-E	EXBIO
Cytokeratin (P)	1 µg/mL	CAM 5.2	Most epithelial cells, with the exception of stratified squamous epithelium	Becton Dickinson
Cytokeratin	62.5 ng/µL	CAM 5.2	Most epithelial cells, with the exception of stratified squamous epithelium	Becton Dickinson
Smooth Muscle Actin (P)	20 µg/mL	1A4	Smooth muscle cells of vessels	DAKO
Von Willebrand factor (P)	4.8 µg/mL	F8/86	Endothelial cells	DakoCytomation

STB, syncytiotrophoblast; EVT, extravillous trophoblast; VCTB, villous cytotrophoblast; DC, dendritic cell; NK, natural killer; DC-SIGN, dendritic cell-specific intercellular adhesion molecule (ICAM)-grabbing nonintegrin; MCH, major histocompatibility complex; IGF, insulin-like growth factor; MEM, modified Eagle's medium; HLA, human leukocyte antigen.

"P" in the Antigen column indicates suitable for staining paraffin sections; otherwise, frozen sections are recommended.

Becton Dickinson, San Jose CA, USA; BioSource, Camarillo CA, USA; DAKO, Carpinteria CA, USA; Chemicon, Temecula CA, USA; DakoCytomation, Carpinteria CA, USA; R&D Systems, Minneapolis MN, USA; Dan Geraghty: geraghty@fred.fhcrc.org; DEC-205: Professor Derek N.J. Hart: director@mmri.mater.org.au; UC-Davis, Professor Janet F. Roser: jfroser@ucdavis.edu

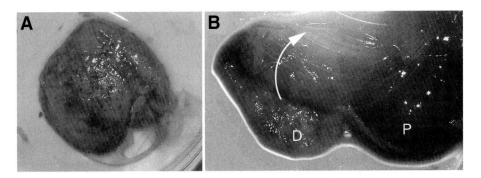

Fig. 1 (*see* companion CD for color version). (**A**) Appearance of the intact deciduas, placentas, and fetal membranes from day 50 of gestation. The maternal side of the decidua is visible in this photograph, with the placentas not visible since they are behind the maternal tissue. The translucent fetal membranes are at the upper left and lower right of the conceptus. (**B**) Partially separated decidua and placenta are visible at the left (arrow indicates the direction that the placenta has been peeled back to separate from decidua, **D**). The fetal face of the other placenta (P) appears at the right, with fetal blood vessels apparent on the chorionic plate.

3. Methods

3.1. Isolation and Culture of Villous Cytotrophoblasts

1. The placenta is collected aseptically at surgery into a plastic Petri dish, a sterile bacterial 100-mm dish or a tared sterile stainless bowl (if >50 d of age). Record total weight and number of placental discs. The entire conceptus can be carefully removed intact if the fetus is to be used. Rhesus monkeys usually have two placental discs.
2. Working in a sterile hood, remove fetal membranes from around the placentas. Through approx d 70 of pregnancy, the decidua will remain adherent to the placenta upon removal from the uterus. The decidua is the pale pink "grainy" tissue, the placenta is the darker red tissue attached directly to the fetal membranes (**Fig. 1**). Gently peel the deciduas from the placenta and place the decidua in a separate sterile dish (*see* **Subheading 3.2.** for decidual processing).
3. Rinse placental tissue with CMF to remove red blood cells.
4. Mince tissue very finely with sterile scissors and place in a siliconized flask. Before mincing, tissue can be set aside for histology or for RNA or protein isolation. Add approx 50 mL CMF to each flask, swirl to rinse tissue, slant flask for 5 min, remove CMF. Weigh clean, minced tissue (*see* **Note 2**).
5. Add 20 mL CMF to 50 mg trypsin/10 mg DNAse. Mix well by pipetting until dissolved. Sterile filter the enzyme solution through an Acrodisc filter and into flask containing the tissue. This can be done either with an Acrodisc and an attached syringe or Steriflip filter units.

6. Cover the flask with a double layer of sterile heavy-duty aluminum foil and shake in a rotary shaker at 60 rpm at 37°C for 20 min. Take care to ensure that the flask is well secured and does not spill or tip.

7. Add 5 mL CMF to a tube containing 10 mg DNAse and filter through Acrodisc into flask as above.

8. Shake at 37°C for an additional 10 min.

9. Place flask in slanted position in hood for 5 min to allow tissue to settle.

10. During shaking steps, start making gradient(s) in 50-mL polystyrene (clear) tubes. Two or three gradient tubes are typically prepared, depending on the total amount of tissue being dispersed. Add 3-mL aliquots of Percoll in layers very slowly down side of tube. Layers are 5% increments from 50% (bottom layer) to 5%. The interface between layers should be visible. Take care not to bump or jostle gradient tubes at any time during preparation or when layering cells.

11. Remove enzymatic digest supernatant, using a 9-in. sterile siliconized Pasteur pipet with bulb, taking care to avoid bringing up tissue fragments. Transfer supernatant into a polypropylene 50-mL tube and add 20 mL DMEM (calcium inactivates trypsin).

12. Pellet these cells at 240g for 10 min. Bring pellet up in 5 mL DMEM and place in incubator. Repeat the dispersion two more times with tissue remaining in the flask, each time recovering the supernatant and cells as in **steps 8** and **9**.

13. After recovering the cells from the last dispersion, add 15 mL CMF to the tissue in the flask, agitate to dissociate remaining cells from the tissue, and add that aliquot along with the supernatant from the third dispersion.

14. Combine all pellets together in the 5–10 mL from **step 12**. Gently resuspend cells to minimize damage.

15. Pipet the cell suspension carefully onto the Percoll gradient, using an automatic Pipetman pipettor fitted with a 10 mL pipet and slowly allow the suspension to drain onto the gradient with as little disturbance as possible to the top layer. Add a maximum of 5 mL suspension per gradient tube.

16. Load the tubes into a Sorvall RC-5B Plus floor centrifuge and spin at 1200g for 25 min, with the brake off to ensure that the gradient is not disturbed at stopping.

17. Trophoblasts are found in the second layer from the top (concentrated white layer of cells) (**Fig. 2**). Pipetting medium off from the top, recover and discard the first layer of debris, and then recover and transfer the second layer and surrounding medium into a clean 50 mL polypropylene tube. Add approximately four times the volume of DMEM to dilute out the Percoll. Spin at 240g for 10 min.

18. Bring up the pellet in 10 mL of DMEM. If there are obvious tissue fragments present, spin briefly (10 s) to pellet these fragments, transfer supernatant to a new tube, and count an aliquot of cells in a hemocytometer. Plate approx 5×10^4 to 1×10^5 cells/16-mm well, 5×10^5/35-mm dish, 2×10^6/60-mm dish (*see* **Notes 3** and **4**).

19. Freezing cells. Label one cryovial for every 2×10^6 cells to be frozen. Include the name of the cell line, the number of cells contained in the vial, the date, and your initials. Place the vials in the –20°C freezer for a few minutes to chill.

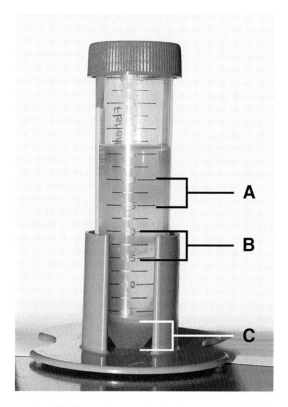

Fig. 2 (*see* companion CD for color version). Appearance of a Percoll gradient that has completed centrifugation. A broad cloud of debris (**A**) appears at the top, the band of enriched trophoblasts is in the central zone (**B**), and red blood cells have pelleted to the bottom of the tube (**C**). The gradations in color are due to the differential proportion of Dulbecco's modified Eagle's medium (DMEM) in the various layers of DMEM/Percoll through the gradient.

20. Aspirate off supernatant and add 1 mL of cold freezing medium to the cells for each vial that is to be frozen.
21. Resuspend and aliquot into the cold cryovials.
22. Immediately transfer to a styrofoam box and place at –80°C.
23. Transfer to liquid nitrogen (being careful not to thaw cells) 24 h to 2 wk later.
24. Thawing cells. Prior to removing cells from liquid nitrogen, have 15-mL centrifuge tubes ready with 5 mL of prewarmed media for each cell type.
25. Remove cells from liquid nitrogen and immediately thaw in a 37°C water bath by gently swishing back and forth until there is a little cube of frozen cells left.
26. Thoroughly wipe the vial in the hood with 100% ethanol.
27. Pipet cells gently with a 1 mL pipet and add dropwise to the prewarmed medium.

28. Pipet up and down gently several times to mix the cells in the culture medium, diluting the DMSO.
29. Spin as usual in the tabletop centrifuge for 5 min at 213*g*.
30. Re-suspend cells in fresh medium and plate.

3.2. Preparation of Stripped FCS (500 mL)

1. Add 0.5 g of Dextran and 5.0 g of Norite A to 1 L of HBSS-CMF with 0.9% NaCl (after adding charcoal, pH = 9.98).
2. Stir in cold room on stir plate for 4 h.
3. Spin in 50-mL polypropylene tubes in Sorvall centrifuge at room temperature for 5 min at 1390*g*.
4. Resuspend charcoal pellets with a total of 500 mL HI FCS. To heat-inactivate FCS, place in 56°C water bath for 45 min prior to adding to charcoal pellets. Do not filter; that will happen later.
5. Stir beaker *very slowly* overnight in cold room.
6. The following day, centrifuge at 4°C in Sorvall for 1 h at 6600*g*. Use 30-mL Corex tubes.
7. In hood, sterile filter serum and aliquot into sterile 50-mL tubes (approx 40 mL/tube). Label tubes as "HI Stripped FCS" along with the date, and initial. Store at –20°C.

3.3. Isolation, Characterization and Culture of Decidual Immune Cells

1. Dissolve collagenase IV/DNAse mixture in 60 mL of CM-PBS and filter through 150-mL bottle top filter.
2. Dissect decidua free of the placenta. Rinse decidua with PBS and weigh in a tared 100-mm culture dish.
3. Mince tissue very finely with scissors and place in flask.
4. Add 20 mL of collagenase IV/DNAse mixture.
5. Shake at 37°C for 20 min in a rotary shaker at 60 rpm.
6. Add 5 mL of PBS to a tube with 10 mg DNAse and mix well.
7. Filter the DNAse solution through an Acrodisc filter and add to the flask.
8. Shake at 37°C for 10 min in a rotary shaker at 60 rpm.
9. Place flask in slanted position in hood for 5 min to allow tissue to settle.
10. Take off supernatant without tissue fragments, transfer into a 50-mL tube, and add 20 mL of culture medium.
11. Spin at 240*g* for 10 min. Bring pellet up in 10 mL of culture medium and place in an incubator.
12. Repeat **steps 4–11** two more times with the remaining tissue.
13. Combine all pellets together, spin and resuspend with 50 mL of RPMI 1640.
14. Prepare two 50-mL tubes with 15 mL of Ficoll-paque.
15. Carefully layer 25 mL of the cell suspension onto Ficoll-paque.
16. Spin tubes at 240*g* for 30 min at 18–20°C in a Sorvall RC-5B floor centrifuge with the brake off.

17. Collect the total leukocytes from an interface between the Ficoll-paque and medium. Combine cells from two tubes and wash twice with 5 vol of RPMI 1640 medium.
18. Resuspend the cells in 25 mL of culture medium and count (*see* **Note 5**).
19. Decidual cells may be sorted by surface marker expression (discussed later), or alternatively monocytes/macrophages may be removed by adherence to plastic. For adherence selection, cells are plated at 1×10^6/mL into 100-mm dishes or T-75 flasks. Cells are maintained at 37°C overnight and nonadherent cells are recovered and can be sorted as below for further culture. The remaining adherent cells are primarily macrophages, with some contaminating decidual fibroblasts.

3.4. NK Cell Sorting and Culture

1. Decidual leukocytes are pelleted and re-suspended in PBS with 2% FCS at 10×10^6 cells/mL. Label five 15-mL tubes as below. Aliquot 50 μL of the cell suspension into each "compensation control" tube (1–4) and the rest of cells into the sort tube. Add appropriate antibodies using approx 8–10 μL of antibody (adjusting for supplier's recommendation) for control tubes and 30–80 μL for the sort tube (*see* **Note 6**). All reagents and sorting need to be done under sterile conditions if cells are to be subsequently cultured.
2. Mix and incubate for 30 min at 4°C in the dark.
3. Wash cells by adding 5 mL of PBS/2% FCS and centrifuge at 300*g* for 10 min.
4. Repeat washing step.
5. Resuspend cells in 0.5 mL of culture medium. For the sort tube, a cell density of approx 50×10^6/mL should not be exceeded. Keep cells on ice and in the dark until sorting.
6. Sort CD3–CD56+CD8+ cells. Spin and resuspend in 10 mL of culture medium with IL-2 at 500 U/mL. Place cells into a T-25 flask and add equal volume of feeder cells.
7. Culture cells at 37°C in 5% CO_2. Cells require feeding when medium has turned yellow. Set the flask vertically and allow cells to settle into the bottom. Remove 15 mL of medium from the flask (leave approx 5 mL), and add 15 mL of fresh medium with IL-2 and PHA. Check NK cell phenotype by flow cytometry when the cells have been expanded to required numbers.

3.5. Flow Cytometry of Trophoblasts and Decidual and Peripheral Blood Immune Cells

1. Prepare a single-cell suspension (isolated trophoblasts, decidual leukocytes or Ficoll-isolated peripheral blood leukocytes) and determine cell number.
2. Suspend cells in buffer (PBS + 2% FCS) at 10×10^6 cells/mL and transfer 50 μL (0.5 $\times 10^6$ cells)/tube to 12×75 mm round-bottom test tubes (in case of a large number of samples, it is possible to use U-bottom 96-microwell plates for staining).
3. Add fluorochrome-conjugated antibodies according to the manufacturer's recommendations (e.g., 10 μL per 0.5×10^6 cells for most of BD-PharMingen's antibodies). Appropriate controls are needed, including an unstained control, and an isotype-matched nonspecific antibody stained control (*see* **Note 7**).

4. Mix gently and incubate 30 min at 4°C in the dark.
5. Wash cells by adding 2–3 mL of buffer and centrifuge at 300g for 5 min.
6. Repeat washing step. For a 96-well plate, wash cells at least three times with 0.2 mL buffer.
7. Resuspend the cell pellet in 0.2 mL buffer and add 0.2 mL of 4% paraformaldehyde. Fixed cells can be stored 24–48 h at 4°C in the dark until analysis on a flow cytometer.

3.6. Immunohistochemical Analysis of Placenta and Decidua

1. Fix tissue fragments of <1 cm square in 2% paraformaldehyde in PBS for 2–4 h. If collecting early implantation sites, it is recommended to conduct whole body perfusion of the rhesus monkey with at least 1 L of fixative after flushing with 1 L of PBS to remove red blood cells from tissues. Bisect pregnant uterus (away from the implantation site if visualization is possible) and allow fixation for an additional 2–4 h.
2. Following fixation wash tissue samples twice in PBS or TBS (twice for 20 min). If preparing for *freezing*, proceed to **step 3**. If preparing for *paraffin* embedding, place tissue in 70% ethanol and proceed with dehydration and embedded.
3. Infuse sample in 9% sucrose in PBS (3–4 h), followed by infusion in 20% sucrose/PBS overnight at 4°C.
4. Blot tissue on paper towel to remove excess sucrose.
5. Place tissue in Peel-A-Way disposable plastic tissue embedding molds (22 mm to 12 mm taper).
6. Add embedding compound (OCT) and place on the cryostat chuck.
7. Freeze in liquid nitrogen or isopentane cooled in a dry ice and 100% ethanol bath.
8. Store at –80°C.

4. Notes

1. Investigators should consider further characterization of other nonhuman primate species for research in implantation and placental biology. Although the rhesus is an excellent model for pregnancy research, further development of primate models would be a significant advance in this area, to complement the progress already made with the baboon, as has been described elsewhere in this volume.
2. If storing minced tissue overnight for dispersion the following morning, add 1:1 vol:wt DMEM, wrap flasks with Parafilm and store at 4°C. The next morning, carefully pour tissue/DMEM mixture into 50-mL centrifuge tubes. Centrifuge at 213g in a tabletop centrifuge for 10 min to remove DMEM. Add 20 mL CMF to each tube, invert tube gently several times to wash, and spin again. Remove CMF, repeat wash. Proceed to isolation protocol. Expect 50–100% of the viable cell yield as with fresh tissues.
3. The yield of cells will be approx 3×10^6/g of tissue at day 36 of rhesus pregnancy [d 0 = day of ovulation, after the luteinizing hormone (LH) peak]. This yield is also typical through at least d 70 of pregnancy. At later pregnancy (i.e., term), the

yield is much more variable as the proportion of villous cytotrophoblasts/g tissue decreases substantially. Culture of rhesus cytotrophoblasts will promote their differentiation as evidenced by fusion into multinuclear syncytiotrophoblasts within 48–72 h (**Fig. 3**) *(12)*. Immunostaining of an aliquot of cells prepared by cytospin centrifugation should demonstrate >90% trophoblast identity (cytokeratin-positive, vimentin-negative). At this time in pregnancy, the rhesus placenta is secreting minimal chorionic gonadotropin *(15)*, so investigators should not use monkey chorionic gonadotropin secretion as an indicator of syncytiotrophoblast differentiation. However, progesterone secretion may be used, being sure to use FCS for culture, which has been stripped of steroids by treatment with dextran-coated charcoal.

4. There is a real need for a thorough phenotyping of extravillous trophoblasts and development of isolation procedures for specific subsets of rhesus trophoblasts. In particular, defining integrin expression throughout the nonhuman primate placental bed may provide insight into new isolation approaches.

5. We have found that whereas approx 70–80% of the isolated cells are decidual leukocytes with tissues from day 36 of pregnancy, only approx 20–30% of the cells from day-50 tissues are leukocytes (the balance are presumably stromal cells, although we have not formally confirmed this presumption). Thus, there is no significant advantage for decidual cell isolation to collect the larger tissues available at day 50.

6. Typical organization of controls and tests required for cell sorting rhesus decidual leukocytes.

   a. Isotype control—FITC-, PE-, and APC-conjugated mouse isotype Ig;
   b. CD56-FITC;compensation control tubes;
   c. CD3-PE;
   d. CD8-APC;
   e. Sort tube—CD56-FITC, CD3-PE, CD8-APC.

7. An alternate protocol for unlabelled primary antibody. Add selected unlabeled antibody (primary) according to the manufacturer's recommendations. Appropriate controls are needed as above. After incubation and washes, add the appropriate secondary fluorochrome-conjugated antibody according to the manufacturer's recommendations. Proceed as with **step 4** of the flow cytometry protocol (*see* **Subheading 3.5.**).

8. CD9 has been reported to be useful for negative selection of human villous cytotrophoblasts *(10)*, but in our experience it is not appropriate with rhesus placental cells.

9. There is a pressing need to develop rhesus-specific antibodies for decidual leukocytes as well as rhesus MHC class I molecules. Currently, human anti-CD marker reagents must be evaluated individually for their efficacy in the rhesus monkey, and often anti-human reagents are not suitable. Reagents specifically developed against rhesus molecules would be valuable tools for research as well as in vivo targeting of specific cell types.

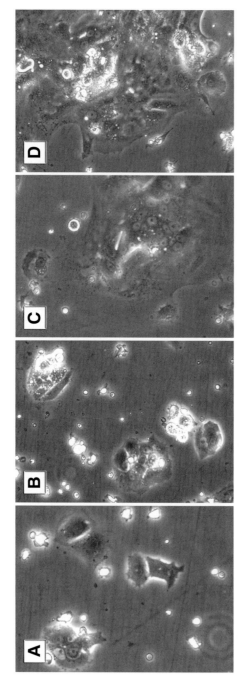

Fig. 3. Primary cultures of rhesus trophoblasts 24 h (**A,B**) or 48 h after (**C,D**) after plating. Within 24 h, there are individual cells that have initiated aggregation, and within 48 h there are numerous multinuclear syncytia that are evident.

10. Many antibodies that recognize human antigens are effective at recognizing their rhesus monkey counterparts, although in reality not many of them have been rigorously tested for cross-reactivity with purified or recombinant rhesus proteins. Thus, it is prudent when possible to confirm expression of a selected antigen by Western blot, by co-expression of additional markers by flow cytometry, or by immunohistochemistry of serial sections to confirm identity of positive cells.

Acknowledgments

We wish to thank the Veterinary, Pathology and Reproductive Services staff of the Wisconsin National Primate Research Center (WNPRC) for all procedures with animals, Eva Rakasz in the Immunology Service Unit at the WNPRC for assistance with flow cytometry and cell sorting, and Kathy Faren for excellent assistance in preparation of this manuscript. Rick Grendell and Behzad Gerami-Naini assisted with preparation of the figures. Supported by National Insitututes of Health (NIH) grants HD37120, HD34215, and RR14040 (T. G. G.), HD 044067 (I. I. S.), and P51-RR000167 (to the WNPRC).

References

1. Enders, A. C. and Schlafke, S. (1986) Implantation in nonhuman primates and in the human. *Comp Primate Biol., Reprod. and Dev.* **3,** 291–310.
2. Golos, T. G. (2003) Nonhuman primate placental MHC expression: a model for exploring mechanisms of human maternal-fetal immune tolerance. *Hum. Immunol.* **64,** 1102–1109.
3. Langat, D. K. and Hunt, J. S. (2002) Do nonhuman primates comprise appropriate experimental models for studying the function of human leukocyte antigen-G? *Biol. Reprod.* **67,** 1367–1374.
4. Munro, C. J., Laughlin, L. A., Tieu, J. and Lasley, B. L. (1997) Development and validation of an enzyme immunoassay for monkey chorionic gonadotropin. *Am. J. Primatol.* **41,** 307–322.
5. Genbacev, O. D., Prakobphol, A., Folk, R. A., et al. (2003) Trophoblast L-selectin-mediated adhesion at the maternal-fetal interface. *Science* **299,** 405–408.
6. Pijnenborg, R., Aplin, J. D., Ain, R., et al. (2004) Trophoblast and the endometrium-a workshop report. *Placenta* **25(Suppl),** S42–S44.
7. Slukvin, I. I, Lunn, D. P., Watkins, D. I. and Golos, T. G. (2000) Expression of the non-classical MHC Class I molecule Mamu-AG at implantation in the rhesus monkey. *Proc. Natl. Acad. Sci. USA* **97,** 9104–9109.
8. Slukvin, I. I., Watkins, D. I. and Golos, T. G. (2001) Phenotypic and functional characterization of rhesus monkey decidual lymphocytes: rhesus decidual large granular lymphocytes express CD56 and have cytolytic activity. *J. Reprod. Immunol.* **50,** 57–79.
9. Kliman, H. J., Nestler, J. E., Sermasi, E., Sanger, J. M., and Strauss III J. F. (1986) Purification, characterization, and in vitro differentiation of cytotrophoblasts from human term placenta. *Endocrinology* **118,** 1567–1582.

10. Douglas, G. C. and King, B. F. (1989) Isolation of pure villous cytotrophoblast from term human placenta using immunomagnetic microspheres. *J. Immunol. Methods* **119**, 259–268.

11. Douglas, G. C. and King, B. F. (1990) Isolation and morphologic differentiation in vitro of villous cytotrophoblast cells from rhesus monkey placenta. *In Vitro Cell Dev. Biol.* **26**, 754–758.

12. Golos, T. G., Handrow, R. R., Durning, M., Fisher, J. M. and Rilling, J. K. (1992) Regulation of chorionic gonadotropin-alpha and chorionic somatomammotropin messenger ribonucleic acid expression by 8-bromo-adenosine 3',5'-monophosphate and dexamethasone in cultured rhesus monkey syncytiotrophoblasts. *Endocrinology* **131**, 89–100.

13. Slukvin, I. I., Boyson, J. E., Watkins, D. I. and Golos, T. G. (1998) The rhesus monkey analogue of human lymphocyte antigen-G is expressed primarily in villous syncytiotrophoblasts. *Biol. Reprod.* **58**, 728–738.

14. Langat, D. K., Morales, P. J., Fazleabas, A. T., Mwenda, J. M. and Hunt, J. S. (2002) Baboon placentas express soluble and membrane-bound Paan-AG proteins encoded by alternatively spliced transcripts of the class Ib major histocompatibility complex gene, Paan-AG. *Immunogenetics* **54**, 164–173.

15. Hodgen, G. D. (1981) Primate chorionic gonadotropins: their comparative biological, immunologic, and chemical properties, in *Fetal Endocrinology* (Nathanielsz, P. W., ed.). Academic, New York: pp. 95–110.

16. Gardner, L. and Moffett, A. (2003) Dendritic cells in the human decidua. *Biol. Reprod.* **69**, 1438–1446.

17. Kammerer, U., Schoppet, M., McLellan, A. D., et al. (2000) Human decidua contains potent immunostimulatory CD83(+) dendritic cells. *Am. J. Pathol.* **157**, 159–169.

18. Breburda, E. E., Slukvin, I. I. and Golos, T. G. (2003) Immunohistochemical localization of DC-SIGN at the rhesus monkey maternal-fetal interface. *Placenta* **24**, A.39.

19. Ritson, A. and Bulmer, J. N. (1987) Extraction of leukocytes from human deciduas. A comparison of dispersal techniques. *J. Immunol. Meth.* **104**, 231–236.

20. Boyson, J. E., Iwanaga, K. K., Golos, T. G., and Watkins, D. I. (1997) Identification of a novel MHC class I gene, *Mamu-AG* in the placenta of primate with an inactivated *G* locus. *J. Immunol.* **159**, 3311–3321.

7

Methods for Isolation of Cells from the Human Fetal–Maternal Interface

Anita Trundley, Lucy Gardner, Jacquie Northfield, Chiwen Chang, and Ashley Moffett

Summary

During human pregnancy, fetal placental cells known as trophoblast invade into the uterine mucosal lining, coming into contact with maternal cells including a specialized population of leukocytes. In order to understand the interaction of maternal cells with trophoblast, it is useful to be able to isolate the various cell types from the fetal–maternal interface so that they may be characterized and co-cultured in vitro. This chapter details the methods we use in our laboratory for enrichment and/or purification of trophoblast cells, decidual leukocytes, decidual natural killer cells, decidual stromal cells, and decidual glandular epithelial cells from human first-trimester tissue samples.

Key Words: Human; pregnancy; purification; trophoblast; decidua; leukocytes; natural killer cells; stromal cells; glandular epithelium.

1. Introduction

Implantation of the developing embryo into the wall of the maternal uterus is a critical early stage of pregnancy. For the fetus to survive for 9 mo, it must adequately tap into its mother's metabolic resources. This is achieved through the formation of an invasive extra-embryonic tissue called the placenta *(1)*. The primary function of the placenta is to allow the exchange of nutrients and gases between the maternal and fetal circulations and it achieves this by invading into the wall of the uterus and eroding into maternal blood vessels.

The cells of the placenta are known as trophoblast and they can be subdivided into subpopulations according to their interaction with maternal tissues. Villous trophoblast form the outer layers of the chorionic villi and from the site of exchange between the fetal and maternal circulations. Extravillous trophoblast form at the proliferating tips of villous buds and become attached to the decidua. Cells from these buds disperse into the decidua as single, migratory

From: *Methods in Molecular Medicine, Vol. 122: Placenta and Trophoblast: Methods and Protocols, Vol. 2*
Edited by: M. J. Soares and J. S. Hunt © Humana Press Inc., Totowa, NJ

cells and are responsible for the invasion and conversion of the maternal spiral arteries into distensible vessels that maintain the flow of maternal blood to the placenta *(2)*.

Trophoblast cells have the potential to invade uncontrollably but the uterine lining is thought to prevent this. The uterine mucosa, which in pregnancy is known as the decidua, has several unique features compared to other mucosal layers. At the site of implantation it is known as decidua basalis, whereas elsewhere it is known as decidua parietalis. The decidua contains specialized stromal cells, glands, and endothelial cells, all of which are likely to be important for creating the correct milieu for trophoblast invasion *(3–5)*. The decidua also contains a large and unique complement of immune cells many of which come into direct contact with the trophoblast. This leukocyte population contains approx 10% T cells, 20% macrophages, and 70% CD56[+] decidual natural killer (NK) cells *(4)*. The exact functions of these maternal immune cells at the fetal interface and how they play a role in placentation are as yet unknown *(6,7)*.

In order to characterize the trophoblast and cells of the decidua and to study their interaction in vitro, it is necessary to be able to isolate the different cell types from whole tissues. In this chapter, we explain in detail the methods used in our laboratory for the isolation and culture of trophoblast, stromal, and glandular cells and decidual leukocyte populations from the first trimester of pregnancy. These methods will not be suitable for the isolation of cells at term, when the anatomical organisation of both the placenta and decidua is different.

The tissue used in our laboratory comes from first-trimester elective terminations of pregnancy. Ethical approval for the use of this material is provided by the Local Research Ethics Committee, Cambridge Health Authority, Addenbrooke's Hospital, Cambridge, United Kingdom and full consent is also obtained from the patients. Laboratories hoping to obtain such samples must also be fully aware of the health and safety implications of utilizing potentially unscreened human material. All work on human samples in our lab is performed in a designated containment level I tissue culture room and within class II microbiological safety cabinets. Persons working on such material are required to be immunized and shown to be protected against Hepatitis B. Initial tissue sorting is carried out in a dedicated plastic tray lined with paper to absorb spilled blood and plastic aprons are worn. Additional personal precautions taken during isolation protocols include the strict use of lab coats and the wearing of two pairs of gloves. The potential presence of infectious pathogens also has implications for waste disposal, spillages and culture of isolated cells. It is important that laboratories undertaking these isolations comply with their local safety and waste disposal regulations.

2. Materials

All lab plastics and instruments that come into contact with the tissue or cells are sterile. Unless otherwise indicated, media used are produced in-house to standard specifications.

2.1. Initial Tissue Sorting

1. 150-mm diameter Falcon Petri dishes.
2. Ham's F12.
3. RPMI (in-house preparation used for washing).
4. Large metal sieve with waste collection tray (Endecotts Ltd., London, UK).
5. Gauze: butter muslin cut to 200-mm squares to go in large metal sieve and then autoclaved to sterilize.
6. Forceps.
7. Scissors.
8. Magnetic stirrer.
9. Sterile magnetic fleas.
10. 250-mL sterile bottles.

2.2. Isolation of Trophoblast Cells

1. 0.2% trypsin, 0.02% ethylenediamine tetraacetic acid (EDTA). For 1 L: glucose 0.3 g (Sigma), NaCl 12 g, KCl 0.3 g, Disodium hydrogen orthophosphate (1.725 g), potassium dihydrogen orthophosphate 0.3 g (All from BDH Laboratory Supplies, Poole UK). Make up to 1 L with sterile water. Mix thoroughly on stirrer. Adjust pH to 7.4. Add 2 g trypsin (Difco, Trypsin 250) and 0.2 g EDTA (BDH Laboratory Supplies). Stir until dissolved. Leave overnight at 4°C. Then Filter-sterilize 75-mL aliquots into 100-mL bottles using 0.2-µm filters. Store at –20°C.
2. 150-mm diameter Petri dishes.
3. Scalpels.
4. Forceps.
5. Newborn calf serum (NCS) (Invitrogen-Gibco Corporation, Carlsbad, CA), heat-inactivated at 56°C for 60 min, cooled quickly in cold water, and then stored in aliquots at –20°C and, after opening, at 4°C for 1 mo.
6. Ham's F12/20% NCS.
7. Plastic funnel.
8. Gauze (**Subheading 2.1., step 5**). Cut to go in plastic funnel.
9. Lymphoprep™ (Nycomed, Oslo, Norway).
10. Sterile, 35-mm diameter Petri dishes.
11. Fibronectin (BD Biosciences, Bedford, MA). Add 1 mL of sterile water to 1 mg vial. Let stand for 30 min (do not mix). Store 20-µL aliquots at –70°C.
12. 35-mm fibronectin-coated dishes. Dilute 20 µL in 1 mL Ham's F12 and place in 35-mm Petri dish. Leave at room temperature for 45 min. For immediate use, pour off the fibronectin solution; otherwise, the dishes can be stored at –20°C for 2 wk.

2.3. Isolation of Decidual Leukocytes by Enzymatic Digestion

1. Fetal calf serum (FCS) (Invitrogen-Gibco Corporation), heat-inactivated and stored as for NCS above.
2. RPMI 1640 with L-glutamine (Sigma Chemical Company, St. Louis, MO), 10% FCS, and antibiotics (penicillin/streptomycin 100 U/mL and amphotericin-B 2.5 U/mL, Sigma). This culture medium will be referred to as RPMI 10% FCS in later sections.
3. Scalpels.
4. Forceps.
5. Collagenase Type V (10 mg/mL, Sigma). Dissolve 1 g of collagenase (cat. no. C 9263) in 100 mL RPMI 10% FCS. Make 5-mL aliquots and store at –20°C.
6. DNAse I (Sigma, cat. no. D5025): Dilute 15,000 U in 10 mL of RPMI and store 0.5-mL aliquots at –20°C.
7. 37°C incubator with roller.
8. 100-μm, 70-μm, and 40-μm cell filters (Becton-Dickinson Falcon).
9. Phosphate-buffered saline (PBS) with 2% FCS (as above) and 0.1% azide (Sigma).
10. Lymphoprep (**Subheading 2.3., step 9**).

2.4. Isolation of Decidual NK Cells

1. Ice.
2. MACS® buffer: PBS with 0.5% bovine serum albumin (BSA) (Sigma) and 2 mM EDTA (BDH Laboratory Supplies). Filter-sterilize through a 0.2-μm filter, de-gas under a vacuum, and autoclave to sterilize. Store at 4°C for 1 mo (*see* **Note 1**).
3. Human γ-globulins (Sigma) made up in PBS to 1 mg/mL. 1-mL aliquots can be stored at –20°C until use and then at 4°C for 1 mo.
4. CD56 MicroBeads (Miltenyi Biotec, Bergisch Gladbach, Germany).
5. 40-μm cell filter (previously described).
6. LS separation column and collection tubes (Miltenyi Biotec).
7. VarioMACS™ magnet (Miltenyi Biotec).
8. RPMI 10% FCS (**Subheading 2.3., step 2**).

2.5. Isolation of Decidual Stromal Cells

1. RPMI 10% FCS (**Subheading 2.3., step 2**).
2. Sterile scalpels.
3. 0.25% trypsin, 0.02% EDTA (**Subheading 2.2., step 1**).
4. Gauze (**Subheading 2.1., step 5**).
5. Lymphoprep (**Subheading 2.2., step 9**).

2.6. Isolation of Decidual Glandular Cells

1. RPMI 10% FCS (**Subheading 2.3., step 2**).
2. Sterile scalpels and forceps.
3. Collagenase Type V (**Subheading 2.3., step 5**).

4. 37°C incubator with roller.
5. Phase contrast microscope.
6. 100-μm cell filter (**Subheading 2.3., step 8**).

3. Methods

At several stages in these methods, investigators will be using sharp instruments on primary human material; it should be obvious that at such times, particular care must be taken to avoid injury and potential infection with human pathogens such as human immunodeficiency virus (HIV) and hepatitis C.

3.1. Initial Tissue Sorting

1. Prepare several large Petri dishes for tissue collection. For collection of trophoblast, the dish should contain approx 20 mL of Ham's F12 and for decidua the same volume of RPMI.
2. Place a metal sieve over a waste collection vessel and line with double thickness sterile gauze. Carefully empty the contents of the tissue collection bag into the gauze. Gently disaggregate large clots with sterile forceps and wash the tissue with large amounts of RPMI. Pick the pieces of decidua or villi into the appropriate dish of media. The villi are identifiable by their light pink color and when washed will have a frond-like/fluffy appearance. Pieces of decidua parietalis are generally grayer, smoother, and more solid in appearance. Membranes and pieces of tissue that are very bloody are avoided; it is important to minimize as much maternal blood contamination as possible, especially when isolating decidual leukocytes. Pieces of decidua that are more ragged and have flecks of yellow and haemorrhagic areas are likely to be decidua basalis-containing trophoblast cells. These tissues are generally discarded because they are too bloody; however, we do collect them if tissue sections from the implantation site are required.
3. Tissues can be pooled or retained as single samples depending on the experiment and how many cells are required (*see* **Note 2**). Samples are then placed in 250-mL bottles with a sterile magnetic flea and are covered in the appropriate media. Samples are stirred at moderate speed for 15 min in order to wash off as much residual blood as possible.

3.2. Isolation of Trophoblast Cells

1. Prewarm 20 mL of 0.25% trypsin in 0.02% EDTA to 37°C.
2. The washed villous tissue is placed in a clean large Petri dish and the cells are carefully separated from the denser, supporting connective tissue by gentle scraping with a scalpel blade. Any residual blood clots should either be cut from the villous tissue or removed with forceps. Membranous remnants are then discarded.
3. The warmed trypsin is poured onto the tissue and the suspension is placed in a sterile 100-mL bottle and stirred at 37°C for 8 min (*see* **Note 3**). The digestion is stopped by the addition of 20 mL Ham's F12 20% NCS.
4. The digested tissue is then filtered through double thickness gauze and the cells recovered as a pellet by centrifugation at 450g for 5 min. The pellet is soft at this stage, and care must be taken not to decant the pellet as well.

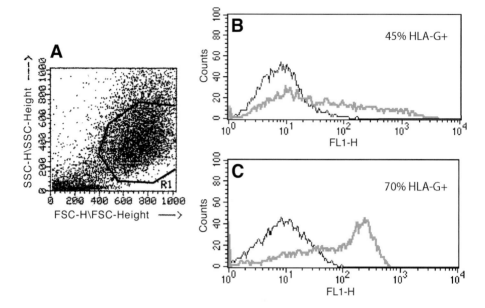

Fig. 1. Flow cytometric analysis of purified trophoblast. (**A**) Forward vs side-scatter analysis of freshly purified trophoblast cells showing the analysis gate R1. (**B**) Trophoblast cells before overnight incubation on fibronectin: 45% of cells collected through R1 are Human Leukocyte Antigen (HLA)-G+ (gray line) compared with an isotype control antibody (black line). (**C**) After overnight incubation on fibronectin, 70 % of cells collected through R1 are HLA-G+ (gray line) compared to the isotype control (black line).

5. The cell pellet is resuspended in 10 mL of Ham's F-12 and the cell solution is layered onto 10 mL of Lymphoprep (*see* **Note 4**). The tube is then centrifuged at 710*g* for 20 min with no brake.

6. After centrifugation, cells at the interface are collected and washed with 10 mL of Ham's F12 medium. At this stage, the preparation contains approx 50% Human Leukocyte Antigen (HLA)-G+ cells (**Fig. 1**) (*see* **Note 5** and **6**).

7. To remove placental macrophages (Hofbauer cells), the cell pellet is resuspended in 3 ml of Ham's F12 and incubated for 20 min at 37°C in a 35-mm Petri dish.

8. Nonadherent cells are collected and seeded onto a 35-mm fibronectin-coated dish overnight at 37°C. The next day, the adherent fraction is recovered and typically consists of approx 70–90% HLA-G+ cells (**Fig. 1**) (*see* **Notes 7** and **8**).

3.3. Isolation of Decidual Leukocytes by Enzymatic Digestion

1. Clean decidual tissue is finely minced (*see* **Note 9**) using surgical blades and residual blood clots are removed.

2. Ten grams of the minced tissue is placed in 20 mL of RPMI 10% FCS with 4 mL of collagenase, and 0.5 mL DNAse I (*see* **Note 10**). Digestion of the tissue is allowed to proceed for 1 h on a roller at 37°C (*see* **Notes 11** and **12**).
3. At the end of the incubation, 30 mL of RPMI 10% FCS is added and the mixture is left to stand for 5 min to allow undigested tissue to sediment.
4. The supernatant is decanted by aspiration and is passed sequentially through 100-μm, 70-μm, and 40-μm filters.
5. The filtrate is centrifuged at 450g for 5 min and the resultant cell pellet is resuspended in 15 mL of 1X PBS containing 2% FCS and 0.1% azide (*see* **Note 13**). This mixture is then overlaid onto 15 mL Lymphoprep and the tube is centrifuged at 710g for 20 min with no brake.
6. The cells at the interface are collected, washed in RPMI 10% FCS, and pelleted by centrifugation at 700g for 5 min. Leukocytes prepared in this way usually consist of 60–80% NK cells (CD56$^+$CD16$^-$), 5–15% CD14$^+$ macrophages, and 10–20% T-cells plus some nonleukocyte cells (**Fig. 2**) (*see* **Note 14**).

3.5. Isolation of Decidual NK Cells

CD56$^+$ decidual NK cells are further purified from decidual leukocytes by positive selection using CD56 antibody-coated magnetic MicroBeads and a magnet-assisted cell separation (MACS) protocol.

1. Decidual leukocytes are washed once in 20 mL ice-cold PBS centrifuged at 450g for 5 min and resuspended in MACS buffer with additional 0.05% human γ-globulins. 10^7 cells are resuspended in 100 μL of MACS buffer. CD56 MicroBeads are added at 20 μL per 10^7 cells and the mixture is incubated on ice for 20 min.
2. After the incubation, the cells are washed in 20 mL PBS, centrifuged at 450g for 5 min, and resuspended in cold MACS buffer at a concentration of 10^7 cells/mL. The cell suspension is then passed through a 40-μm cell filter to remove clumps, which might block the column and then kept on ice during the purification.
3. An LS separation column is positioned within the magnetic field of a VarioMACS magnet and a waste collection tube is placed beneath it. The column is equilibrated with 3 mL of MACS buffer.
4. The cell suspension is applied to the column 1 mL at a time (*see* **Note 15**). The column is then washed with 15 mL of ice-cold MACS buffer.
5. Bound cells are eluted out of the column by the addition of 6 mL of ice-cold MACS buffer followed by removal of the column from the magnet. The elution buffer is flushed gently into a collection tube using the plunger supplied (*see* **Note 16**). The suspension is then centrifuged at 450g for 5 min in order to pellet the cells. The cells are finally resuspended in RPMI 10% FCS. CD56$^+$ cells purified in this way are typically >95% pure (**Fig. 3**) (*see* **Notes 17–21**).

3.6. Isolation of Decidual Stroma

These cultures are not pure stromal cells but will contain glandular epithelial cells, small numbers of endothelial cells, and decidual leukocytes (*see* **Note 22**).

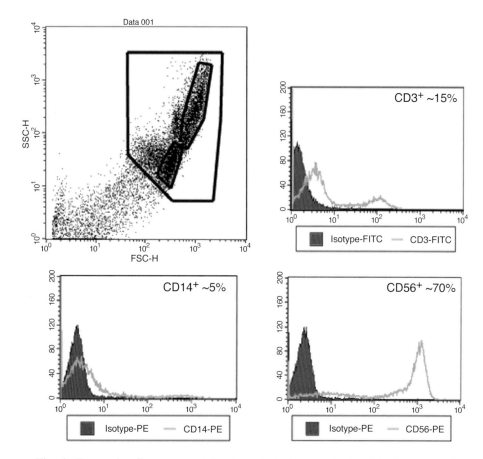

Fig. 2. Two-color flow cytometric characterisation of decidual leukocytes using monoclonal antibodies to the leukocyte differentiation antigens CD56-phycoerythrin (PE), CD14-PE, and CD3-fluorescein isothiocyanate (FITC) **(A)** Forward vs side-scatter of freshly isolated decidual leukocytes. Gate R1 contains all cells, Gate R2 contains mainly CD14+ macrophages and stromal cells, and Gate R3 contains predominantly lymphocytes. Cells in Gate R3 contain approx 15% CD3+ cells **(B)**, approx 5% CD14+ macrophages **(C)**, and 70% CD56+ natural killer cells **(D)**.

1. Prewarm 20 mL of 0.2% trypsin in 0.02% EDTA to 37°C.
2. Clean decidual tissue is washed and finely chopped.
3. Add the minced tissue to the trypsin and digest at 37°C with mixing for 12 min (*see* **Note 3**).
4. The digestion is stopped by the addition of 20 mL of RPMI 20% FCS. The suspension is then filtered through sterile gauze.
5. Cells are pelleted by centrifugation at 450*g* for 5 min and then resuspended in 20 mL RPMI 10% FCS. The cell suspension is then separated into two 10-mL

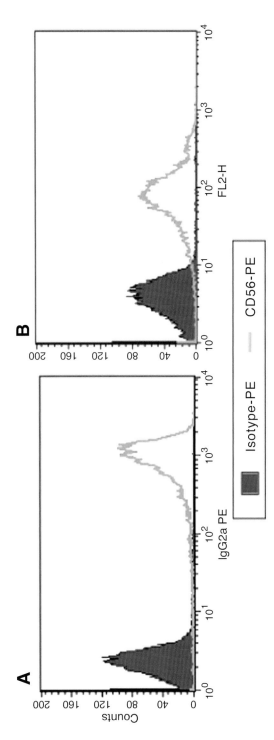

Fig. 3. Fluorescence-activated cell sorting analysis of natural killer (NK) cells purified using CD56-microbeads and magnet-assisted cell separation (MACS). (**A**) Decidual NK cells are 98% pure. The majority of these cells are CD56bright. (**B**) A similar preparation of blood NK cells shows that the majority of blood NK cells are CD56dim.

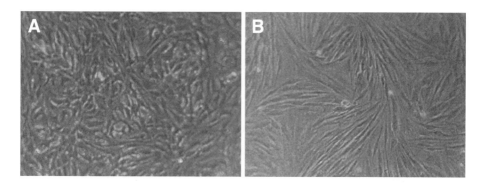

Fig. 4. Culture of decidual stromal cells. (**A**) Stromal cells after overnight culture. The stromal cells are plump and secretory, an appearance which can be maintained by the addition of exogenous estrogen and progesterone. (**B**) After one passage and 7 ds in culture without the addition of exogenous factors, the stromal cells have a fibroblastic appearance.

      aliquots and each of these is layered onto 10 mL Lymphoprep. The layers are then centrifuged at 710*g* for 20 min with no brake.

6. The white cellular interface is collected, diluted in a large excess of RPMI 10% FCS, and then centrifuged at 700*g* for 5 min. The cells are finally resuspended in 16 mL RPMI 10% FCS and cultured in a 75-cm^2 flask overnight.

7. The next morning the supernatant is removed and the adherent layer is washed with RPMI 10% FCS to remove any nonadherent cells. 20 mL of fresh RPMI 10% FCS is then added. In our experience, the cells remain viable for two passages and between 7 and 14 d in culture (**Fig. 4**). When the cells become round and flattened, they cease to proliferate and eventually become nonadherent.

3.7. Isolation of Decidual Glandular Epithelial Cells

1. The first part of this isolation is the same as for decidual leukocytes (*see* **Subheading 3.3.**, steps 1–3).

2. After the digested tissue has been allowed to sediment, a drop of the supernatant is taken and examined under a phase-contrast microscope in order to identify intact glandular structures rather than single cells. If these are not present, the digestion is continued for a further 20 min and then the process is repeated. Carry on until numerous glandular structures are observed. We find that this takes approx 2 h.

3. Pass the supernatant through a 100-µm cell filter (*see* **Note 23**). The tissue remaining on the filter will mostly be partially-digested glands. Wash the filter gently with RPMI and then turn the filter over and back wash the glands into a dish or tube.

4. Centrifuge at 400*g* for 5 min. Resuspend the cell pellet in 3 mL of RPMI 20% FCS for culture in a 35 mm dish (*see* **Note 24**).

4. Notes

1. The manufacturer recommends degassing the buffer to prevent the formation of air bubbles, which may block the column.
2. The decision whether to pool samples will depend on the nature of the experiments to be undertaken. Single samples are ideal for studies of immune recognition as different individuals will express different HLA and immune receptor phenotypes, which can be defined by keeping aside a piece of tissue for reverse-transcription (RT)-polymerase chain reaction (PCR) analysis. However, pooled samples are useful for the analysis of the general features of a certain cell population and also will provide larger numbers of cells. Typically, we find that from 1 g of decidua, we can obtain $3–5 \times 10^6$ decidual leukocytes and $1–3 \times 10^6$ purified decidual NK cells. The yield of trophoblast cells is very variable and less predictable. This may be related to different ages of samples or batches of trypsin. Typically, we obtain 4×10^6 trophoblast cells per sample.
3. In our experience, each batch of trypsin gives different results and may require a variation of a minute either way in the digestion time. When tissues are available, it is advantageous to empirically determine the best timing when each new batch of trypsin is made. In the hope of avoiding this empiricism we have, in the past, attempted to use commercially available, ready-made, pure trypsin solutions. For reasons we do not understand, these do not work.
4. Lymphoprep is a ready-made solution that is most often used for the purification of peripheral blood mononuclear cells by density gradient centrifugation (there are similar products which can be used such as Ficoll from Amersham Biosciences, Buckinghamshire, UK). It contains a chemical that aggregates red blood cells, which causes them to sediment faster than the white blood cell fraction. This technique can also be used to separate other cells from red blood cells. For those unfamiliar with this technique, there is a knack. The heterogeneous cell suspension is very gently overlaid onto the Lymphoprep solution so that there is no mixing of the layers. There are several ways to approach this: one is to place the Lymphoprep in the tube and then, holding the tube at a 45° angle, very slowly pipet the cell suspension down the side of the tube with the pipet tip fairly close to the Lymphoprep. This addition should start drop-wise and then gradually build up, keeping the flow steady. The tubes should be handled very carefully thereafter to prevent mingling of the layers and also the tubes should be balanced so that the centrifugation is as smooth as possible. After centrifugation, there should be four visible layers in the tube: red blood cells in a pellet at the bottom, Lymphoprep clear solution, a thin white cloudy layer (the interface), and a top layer of media supernatant. Holding the tube to eye level, use a Pasteur pipet to remove the cells from the interface. It is important to avoid removing too much Lymphoprep because this can prevent the recovered cells from pelleting. If this has happened, cell recovery may be improved by further dilution of the aspirated solution at the washing step.
5. In freshly purified trophoblast, before overnight culture on fibronectin there are approx 20% HLA-negative cells, which are, therefore, of the villous phenotype.

More information on the identification of trophoblast and other cell types at the fetal–maternal interface can be found in **refs. *4* and *8*.**

6. The isolation takes approx 2.5 h from scraping to plating of the trophoblast on fibronectin.

7. It is not yet known whether this increase in HLA-G+ cells is due to preferential sticking of HLA-G+ cells to the matrix or due to a switching of phenotype.

8. We usually use these cells within 3 d, but they can be plated on fibronectin for a further 4–6 d.

9. Fine mincing should take at least 10 min using two scalpels. We have found that placing a damp paper towel under the dish prevents it from slipping and makes chopping easier. At the required consistency for a 1-h digest, the tissue should appear granular but homogenous with no visible lumps. For an overnight digest, one-half of the amount of chopping is required: small pieces of tissue (approx 2 mm^3) will still be visible.

10. DNAse I is added to digest DNA extruded by dying cells which might otherwise stick to surrounding live cells and reduce their recovery. This is particularly important if one plans to use the MACS technique later on, because sticky clumps of cells can block the column.

11. If there is concern that enzymic digestion may affect the phenotype of the isolated cells, then the collagenase procedure described in **Subheading 3.3., steps 2–3** can be replaced with mechanical disaggregation. The chopped tissue is forced through a 20-cm diameter, 53-μm metal sieve (Endecotts Ltd., London, UK) with a large rubber bung (both sterile). RPMI is added as required to wash the tissue through and also from the bottom of the sieve. The suspension is then filtered as in **Subheading 3.3., step 4**, and the rest of the protocol is the same.

12. For practical purposes, it may be useful to digest the tissue overnight so that the cells can be extracted the next morning. Overnight digestion of the whole tissue does not obviously adversely affect the viability of the recovered cells compared with the 1-h digest. In this case, the tissue is chopped into small pieces but not as finely as for a 1-h digest. Ten grams of tissue is digested in 20 mL of RPMI 10% with 0.6 mg/mL collagenase. The digestion is performed on a roller for 18 h at room temperature.

13. This solution is used to remove dead cells from the preparation. The dead cells take on azide and are sedimented to the bottom of the Lymphoprep. The azide is washed off after this step and, in our experience, is not detrimental to cell functions. However, the azide can be left out.

14. Anti-CD19 or anti-CD20 antibodies can be used in fluorescence-activated cell sorting (FACS) analysis to test for contamination of the sample by maternal blood. From a combination of immunohistology and FACS analysis we would expect that only 1–2% of the purified decidual leukocytes would be B-cells.

15. One of the problems that can occur with this method is that the column blocks, which is why it is best to only add a small amount of cells at a time. If the column blocks, it should be washed and flushed to elute the cells. The procedure is then re-started using a new column. Blockage can also be avoided by increasing the

dilution of the cells before they are applied to the column, although this does make the procedure longer.

16. Removing the plunger and reflushing the column is not recommended, because this generates much cellular debris, which may adversely affect later analysis. The recovered cells can be stored on ice and recombined later. It is also important to prevent the column from running dry.

17. The presence of CD56 MicroBeads on the CD56 antigen does not prevent labeling with Becton Dickinson CD56-PE antibody for FACS analysis. However, they will interfere with indirect labelling with mouse antibodies, because the secondary anti-mouse antibody can bind to the CD56 antibody on the beads. We have found that the MicroBeads are lost after a few days in culture.

18. Some investigators may be concerned that the positive selection procedure may alter the decidual NK cell phenotype. However, CD56 is of unknown function, and cross-linking this receptor has never been shown to have an effect on known functions of NK cells. Indeed, anti-CD56 is regularly used as a negative control antibody in NK cell functional assays. MicroBead cocktails are also available for the isolation of decidual NK cells by negative selection, although these are more costly than the CD56 MicroBeads.

19. This method can easily be adapted for the recovery of other leukocytes such as CD14+ macrophages or CD3+ T-cells using different sets of MicroBeads.

20. The MACS procedure generally takes about 90 min. Tissue sorting to purified decidual NK cells will probably take 3–4 h.

21. Purified decidual NK cells do not survive long in culture, so they should be used immediately. In our experience, only 30% of purified decidual NK cells will be viable after overnight culture in RPMI 10% FCS. Decidual NK cells can be made to proliferate by culturing with a combination of 50 ng/mL SCF and 5 ng/mL interleukin (IL)-15 (Both R&D Systems, Oxford, UK). We have then cultured these cells over a period of 4 d.

22. The cells that pass through the filter will mostly be stromal cells. These cells can be pelleted by centrifugation at 450g for 5 min and then resuspended in 10 mL RPMI 20%. The suspension is then layered onto an equal volume of Lymphoprep and then the layers are centrifuged at 710g for 20 min. The white interface is recovered and then washed with a large excess of RPMI 20%. Recovered cells are cultured in RPMI 20%.

23. Those wishing to remove leukocytes from these cultures could consider using CD45-conjugated Dynabeads.

24. These cells are not grown in vitro for longer than 1 wk. There are always a small number of residual stromal cells that eventually proliferate and over grow the glands.

Acknowledgments

We would like to acknowledge the support and enthusiasm of Professor Y. W. Loke, who has been instrumental in the design and refinement of the techniques contained in this chapter.

References

1. Boyd, J. D. and Hamilton, W. J. (1970) *The Human Placenta*. W. Heffer and Sons, Cambridge, UK.
2. Kam, E. P., Gardner, L., Loke, Y. W., and King, A. (1999) The role of trophoblast in the physiological change in decidual spiral arteries. *Hum. Reprod.* **14,** 2131–2138.
3. Burrows, T. D., King, A., and Loke, Y. W. (1996) Trophoblast migration during human placental implantation. *Hum. Reprod. Update* **2,** 307–321.
4. Loke, Y. W. and King, A. (1995) *Human Implantation: Cell Biology and Immunology.* Cambridge University Press, Cambridge.
5. King, A. (2000) Uterine leukocytes and decidualization. *Hum. Reprod. Update* **6,** 28–36.
6. Trundley, A. and Moffett, A. (2004) Human uterine leukocytes and pregnancy. *Tissue Antigens* **63,** 1–12.
7. Moffett-King, A. (2002) Natural killer cells and pregnancy. *Nat. Rev. Immunol.* **2,** 656–663.
8. King, A., Thomas, L., and Bischof, P. (2000) Cell culture models of trophoblast II: trophoblast cell lines—a workshop report. *Placenta* **21(Suppl A),** S113–S119.

8

In Vitro Models for Studying Human Uterine and Placental Macrophages

Ramsey H. McIntire, Margaret G. Petroff, Teresa A. Phillips, and Joan S. Hunt

Summary

Human monocytes and macrophages, which are also called mononuclear phagocytes, represent a major arm of the innate immune system. These cells not only protect against infection but are also central to tissue remodeling and production of chemokines, cytokines, and growth factors. Tissue macrophages reside in the human placenta and uterine decidua throughout pregnancy, where they comprise part of the host defense network and facilitate placental and extraembryonic development. The purpose of this chapter is to describe methods for establishing useful models of human uteroplacental macrophages: (1) differentiated U937 myelomonocytic cells, (2) peripheral blood monocytes, (3) peripheral blood monocyte-derived macrophages, (4) decidual macrophages, and (5) placental macrophages.

Key Words: Myelomonocytic cell lines; peripheral blood monocyte; decidual macrophage; placental macrophage.

1. Introduction

Human monocytes and macrophages are mononuclear phagocytic cells that comprise a major arm of the innate immune system. During prenatal development, granulocyte-monocyte progenitor cells originate in the fetal yolk sac. These cells migrate and take up residence in the mesenchyme of the placental villi as placental macrophages. In first-trimester placentas, these are termed Hofbauer cells (**Fig. 1**). Subsequently, in both the fetus and in adults, pluripotent myeloid stem cells in the bone marrow differentiate into several types of progenitor cells, including the granulocyte-monocyte progenitor. This progenitor differentiates into a promonocyte, which departs the bone marrow and enters the blood stream, where it differentiates into a mature monocyte. After circulating for approx 8 h, the monocyte then enters various organs and tissues, where tissue-specific factors induce final differentiation into a tissue mac-

From: *Methods in Molecular Medicine, Vol. 122: Placenta and Trophoblast: Methods and Protocols, Vol. 2*
Edited by: M. J. Soares and J. S. Hunt © Humana Press Inc., Totowa, NJ

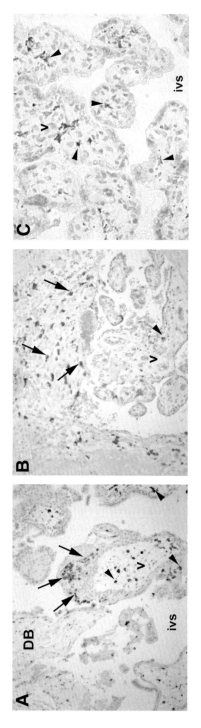

Fig. 1. Immunohistological localization of maternal and fetal macrophages in placentas. (A) Anti-CD68 staining of 12-wk placenta showing a placental villus (v) with adherent fibrin containing macrophages that are presumably maternal in origin (arrows). Fetal macrophages inside the villus are marked with arrowheads. (B) Anti-CD68 staining of term placenta showing maternal macrophages (arrows) in the basal plate, which is adjacent to a placental villus (v). A fetal macrophage (arrowhead) is located inside the villus. (C) Anti-CD14 staining of term placenta showing fetal macrophages (arrowheads) in the stroma of placental villi (v). Original magnifications: A,B ×200; C ×400.

rophage. Tissue macrophages in the placental mesenchyme and in the uterine decidua (**Fig. 1**) are poised to participate in host defense as well as to influence the processes of implantation, placental growth, vascular transformation, trophoblast survival and differentiation, and parturition *(1,2)*.

Tissue macrophages are highly heterogeneous cells in both phenotype and function. They are essential to tissue homeostasis and processes such as wound healing and tissue remodeling because of their remarkable ability to phagocytose and digest tissue and dead cells *(2–4)*. These cells also control cell and tissue function through production of an abundant and diverse group of molecules that include growth factors, chemokines, cytokines, proteolytic enzymes, and adhesion molecules. Importantly, tissue macrophages are powerful cells central to both innate immunity and the development of acquired immune responses *(5–7)*. In response to infectious pathogens, macrophages are potent cellular promoters of inflammation through their production of nitric oxide, reactive oxygen species, proteolytic enzymes, and inflammatory cytokines. Conversely, macrophages have the ability to control immune responses by secreting antiinflammatory cytokines such as interleukin (IL)-10 and transforming growth factor (TGF)-β1. Regarding acquired immunity, macrophages can be induced to express Human Leukocyte Antigen (HLA) class II molecules, which facilitate presentation of breakdown products from phagocytosed material along with co-stimulatory molecules such as B7 (CD80, CD86) to T lymphocytes.

In the human uterus, implantation and pregnancy bring about major changes to the resident leukocyte population in the decidua such that antigen-specific lymphocytes are virtually undetectable. Uterine natural killer (uNK) cells are present in greater numbers during the first and second trimesters whereas macrophage populations remain stable *(8–10)*, comprising 10 to 15% of the total cells in the decidua and 18 to 25% of the decidual leukocyte population *(8–13)*. Possibly because of the continued presence of macrophage differentiation factors such as macrophage colony stimulating factor (M-CSF) *(14–17)* and activation factors such as interferon (IFN)-γ *(18–21)* in the pregnant uterus, human decidual macrophages are potentially immunologically active. This is evidenced by their display of HLA class II and the adhesion molecule CD11c, as well as their ability to produce potent modulators of inflammation such as cytokines, prostaglandins, proteolytic enzymes, and chemotactic peptides *(13,22)*. Decidual macrophages respond to endogenous factors emanating from the placenta that influence maternal immune responses to the fetus as well as to exogenous factors emanating from microorganisms during infections.

This chapter reports methods for the isolation and culture of placental and decidual macrophages as well as other monocyte/macrophage models. These latter models include peripheral blood monocytes, in vitro-generated, monocyte-derived macrophages, and myelomonocytic cell lines, all of which are useful tools because of the relative ease of their isolation and culture. Importantly, the in vitro models are "naïve" to pregnancy-associated factors to which maternal and fetal macrophages are exposed in vivo, such as placental and decidual hormones. Myelomonocytic cell lines are particularly convenient as a result of their unlimited cell yields and uniformity, which is not the case with cells in tissues and blood taken from patients and donors. This chapter will describe the isolation, characterization, and culture of (1) differentiated U937 myelomonocytic cells, (2) peripheral blood monocytes, (3) monocyte-derived macrophages, (4) decidual macrophages, and (5) placental macrophages.

2. Materials

2.1. U937 Cells (American Type Culture Collection [ATCC], Manassas, VA, Cat. No. CRL-1593.2)

2.1.1. Media for Growth, Differentiation, and Activation

1. Growth medium: RPMI-1640 (Mediatech, Herndon, VA) containing 10% heat-inactivated fetal bovine serum (FBS; Atlanta Biologicals, Norcross, GA), 100 U/mL penicillin and 100 µg/mL streptomycin (Invitrogen-Gibco, Carlsbad, CA), 2 mM L-glutamine (Mediatech), 1 mM sodium pyruvate (Mediatech), and 50 µM 2-mercaptoethanol (2-ME; Sigma, St. Louis, MO).
2. Differentiation Medium: growth medium plus 160 nM phorbol myristate acetate (PMA; Sigma).
3. Activation medium: growth medium plus 100 U/mL recombinant human IFN-γ (R&D Systems, Minneapolis, MN).

2.1.2. Morphology, Viability, Characterization, and Proliferation Assays

1. Sterile tissue culture plates (*see* **Note 1**).
2. CellStripper™ cell dissociation solution (Mediatech).
3. Glass slides and Shandon Cytospin® (Thermo Electron Corp., Woburn, MA).
4. Diff-Quik® Stain Set (Dade Behring Inc., Newark, DE).
5. Trypan blue dye (Mediatech).
6. Fixation solutions, blocking solutions, antibodies, detection reagents, and equipment for flow cytometric or immunocytochemical analysis.
7. ^{3}H-thymidine (ICN Biomedicals Inc., Irvine, CA), cell harvester (Brandel, Gaithersburg, MD), and γ scintillation counter. Contact your institute for appropriate storage, use, and disposal protocols for radioactive materials.

2.2. Peripheral Blood Monocytes

2.2.1. Isolation and Purification

1. Histopaque 1077 (Sigma, cat. no. H8889).
2. Low-speed, swinging bucket, temperature-controlled centrifuge.
3. Sterile polypropylene conical tubes (15 mL and 50 mL) (*see* **Note 1**).
4. Serum-free macrophage medium (Invitrogen-Gibco, cat. no. 12065-074) con-

taining 100 U/mL penicillin and 100 μg/mL streptomycin (Invitrogen-Gibco), and 2 m*M* L-glutamine (Mediatech).

5. Serum-containing macrophage medium (Invitrogen-Gibco, cat. no. 12065-074) containing 10% heat-inactivated FBS (Atlanta Biologicals), 100 U/mL penicillin and 100 μg/mL streptomycin (Invitrogen-Gibco), and 2 m*M* L-glutamine (Mediatech).

6. Cell separation buffer (phosphate-buffered saline [PBS] without calcium or magnesium] containing 0.5% bovine serum albumin [BSA; low endotoxin, Sigma] and 2 m*M* ethylenediamine tetraacetic acid [EDTA; Invitrogen-Gibco], and filter sterilized [0.22 μm]).

7. Preseparation filters (Miltenyi Biotec Inc., Auburn, CA, cat. no. 130-041-407).

8. CD14 MicroBeads (Miltenyi, cat. no. 130-050-201).

9. Separation column-MS (Miltenyi, cat. no. 130-042-201).

10. MiniMACS separation unit (magnet, Miltenyi, cat. no. 421-02).

11. Magnet-assisted cell separation (MACS) Multi-Stand (Miltenyi, cat. no. 130-042-303).

2.2.2. Culture (Optional Media)

1. Sterile tissue culture plates (*see* **Note 1**).
2. Serum-free macrophage medium (without antibiotics).
3. Serum-containing macrophage medium (as outlined previously).
4. RPMI-1640 (Mediatech) plus 10% heat-inactivated FBS (Atlanta Biologicals), 100 U/mL penicillin and 100 μg/mL streptomycin (Invitrogen-Gibco), and 2 m*M* L-glutamine (Mediatech).

2.2.3. Morphology, Viability, Characterization, and Proliferation Assays

See **Subheading 2.1.2.**

2.3. Monocyte-Derived Macrophages

2.3.1. Differentiation and Activation

1. Differentiation: Medium (*see* **Subheading 2.2.2.**) plus 150 IU/mL recombinant human M-CSF (R&D Systems).
2. Activation: Medium (*see* **Subheading 2.2.2.**) plus 100 U/mL recombinant human IFN-γ (R&D Systems).

2.3.2. Morphology, Viability, Characterization, and Proliferation Assays

See **Subheading 2.1.2.**

2.4. Decidual Macrophages

2.4.1. Tissue Dissection and Isolation

1. Preweighed, sterile 200-mL beaker containing 50 mL PBS (without calcium or magnesium).
2. 1-L glass beakers for waste.

3. 100-mL glass beaker or 150-mm tissue culture dish for mincing.
4. 500-mL Erlenmayer flask(s).
5. Sterile large forceps.
6. Sterile sharp scissors.
7. Sterile scalpel.
8. Sterile, 100-μm metal sieve.
9. Sterile funnel.
10. Cotton surgical gauze.
11. Histopaque 1077 (Sigma).
12. Low-speed, swinging-bucket, temperature-controlled centrifuge.
13. Sterile polypropylene conical tubes (15 mL and 50 mL) (*see* **Note 1**).
14. 70-μm and 100-μm sterile nylon cell filters (Falcon).
15. Digestion solution: Hank's balanced salt solution (HBSS, Mediatech) containing 20 mM N-(2-hydroxyethyl)piperazine-N'-(2-hemisodium salt) (HEPES, Sigma), 100 U/mL penicillin and 100 μg/mL streptomycin (Invitrogen-Gibco), 30 mM sodium bicarbonate (Mediatech), 10 mg/mL BSA (low endotoxin, Sigma), 200 U/mL collagenase (Type IV, Sigma), 1 mg/mL hyaluronidase (Type 1-S, Sigma), 150 μg/mL DNase I (Type IV, Sigma) (*see* **Note 2**).
16. RPMI-1640 (Mediatech) containing 10% heat-inactivated FBS (Atlanta Biologicals), 100 U/mL penicillin and 100 μg/mL streptomycin (Invitrogen-Gibco), 2 mM L-glutamine (Mediatech), and 25 mM HEPES (Sigma).

2.4.2. Culture (Optional Media)

1. RPMI-1640 (Mediatech) containing 10% heat-inactivated FBS (Atlanta Biologicals), 100 U/mL penicillin and 100 μg/mL streptomycin (Invitrogen-Gibco), 2 mM L-glutamine (Mediatech).
2. Serum-free macrophage medium (without antibiotics).

2.4.3. Morphology, Viability, Characterization, and Proliferation Assays

See **Subheading 2.1.2.**

2.5. Term Placental Macrophages

2.5.1. Tissue Dissection and Isolation

1. *See* **Subheading 2.4.1.**
2. 100-μm sterile nylon cell filters (Falcon).
3. Digestion solution: Medium 199 (Sigma) containing 100 U/mL penicillin and 100 μg/mL streptomycin (Invitrogen-Gibco), 10 mg/mL BSA (Sigma, low endotoxin), 200 U/mL collagenase (Type IV, Sigma), 150 μg/mL Dnase I (Type IV, Sigma) (*see* **Note 2**).
4. M199: Medium 199 (Sigma) containing 10% heat-inactivated FBS (Atlanta Biologicals), 100 U/mL penicillin and 100 μg/mL streptomycin (Invitrogen-Gibco), 2 mM L-glutamine (Mediatech), and 25 mM HEPES (Sigma).

5. HBSS (Mediatech).
6. Anti-human epidermal growth factor receptor (EGF-R) mouse monoclonal antibody, immunoglobulin (Ig)G_{2a}, at 200 µg/mL (Santa Cruz Biotechnology, Santa Cruz, CA, cat. no. SC-120).
7. Goat anti-mouse IgG MicroBeads (Miltenyi, cat. no. 484-01).
8. Cell separation buffer (PBS without calcium or magnesium) containing 0.5% BSA (Sigma, low endotoxin) and 2 mM EDTA (Invitrogen-Gibco), and sterile filtered (0.22 µm).
9. Preseparation filters (Miltenyi, cat. no. 130-041-407).
10. Separation column-MS (Miltenyi, cat. no. 130-042-201).
11. 23- to 27-gauge needle to be attached to separation column.
12. MiniMACS separation unit (magnet, Miltenyi, cat. no. 421-02).
13. MACS Multi-Stand (Miltenyi, cat. no. 130-042-303).

2.5.2. Culture

M199. Medium 199 (Sigma) containing 10% heat-inactivated FBS (Atlanta Biologicals), 100 U/mL penicillin and 100 µg/mL streptomycin (Invitrogen-Gibco), 2 mM L-glutamine (Mediatech).

2.5.3. Morphology, Viability, Characterization, and Proliferation Assays

See **Subheading 2.1.2.**

3. Methods

The methods below describe (1) the differentiation, activation, and characterization of U937 human myelomonocytic cells;, (2) the isolation and purification of peripheral blood monocytes; (3) the differentiation, activation, and characterization of human peripheral blood monocyte-derived macrophages; (4) the isolation and characterization of decidual macrophages from term amniochorion membranes; and (5) the isolation and characterization of placental macrophages from term placental villi.

3.1. U937 Myelomonocytic Cells

U937 cells are a myelomonocytic cell line derived from a human histiocytic lymphoma. The U937 tumor cell line is one of several human monocyte cell lines that are highly proliferative in the undifferentiated state and resemble immature cells of the myelomonocytic lineage. In order to study macrophage-like functions, these cells must first be differentiated. The methods described below employ PMA, a phorbol ester, as the differentiation factor. In addition, because the goal of this chapter is to describe potential models for the decidual macrophage, which is exposed to IFN-γ and is known to be activated in vivo, IFN-γ is used to activate the cells (*see* **Notes 1** and **3**).

3.1.1. PMA Differentiation and IFN-γ Activation

1. Cells are cultured at 37°C and 5% CO_2.
2. To induce differentiation, seed cells at a density of approx 50,000 cells/cm^2 in U937 PMA-differentiation medium for 24 h.
3. To induce activation, remove culture supernatant and treat cells with U937 activation medium for 48 h.

3.1.2. Morphology (**Fig. 2**)

1. Harvest undifferentiated (nonadherent) cells and centrifuge onto glass slides using a Shandon Cytospin centrifuge.
2. PMA-treated and PMA/IFN-γ-treated cells, which are adherent, can be harvested from culture dishes by incubation in CellStripper cell dissociation solution (Mediatech) for 30 min on ice followed by gentle scraping before centrifuging onto glass slides.
3. After drying overnight at room temperature, the glass slides are stained using the Diff-Quik Stain Set following the manufacturer's instructions.
4. Alternatively, cells can be stained in the culture wells by aspirating the supernatants, adding and aspirating the Diff-Quik reagents one at a time, and rinsing several times with water.

3.1.3. Viability by Trypan Blue Dye exclusion (**Fig. 3**)

Viability during PMA differentiation and IFN-γ activation can be done in the wells by staining with trypan blue dye (*see* **Note 4**).

3.1.4. Proliferative Activity by ^{3}H-Thymidine Incorporation (**Fig. 3**)

1. The proliferative activity of undifferentiated U937 cells is fairly high, with a doubling time of approx 24 h. One characteristic of differentiated U937 cells is a loss of proliferative activity without a loss of viability. Cell proliferation can be measured by ^{3}H-thymidine incorporation (*see* **Note 4**). Seed U937 cells in the differentiation and/or activation medium in triplicate wells of 96-well tissue culture plates.
2. Eighteen hours prior to harvesting, add 1 μCi ^{3}H-thymidine to each well.
3. At the end of the culture period, harvest the samples onto filters using a cell harvester and determine cpm in a scintillation counter.

3.2. Peripheral Blood Monocytes

Monocytes are one of the subsets of the bone marrow-derived cells that circulate in peripheral blood. To acquire the monocytes, first isolate peripheral blood mononuclear cells (PBMC), which includes both monocytes and lymphocytes, by density gradient centrifugation. This removes contaminating polymorphonuclear cells (neutrophils, granulocytes), red blood cells, and dead cells. The monocytes are then purified by CD14-positive selection and magnetic bead separation (*see* **Note 1**).

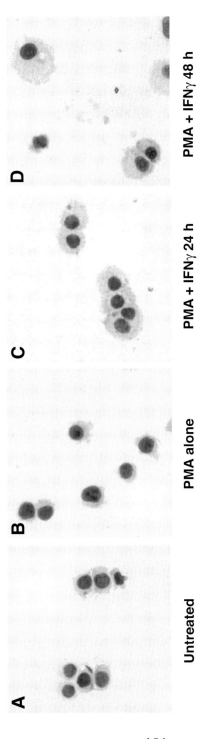

Fig. 2. Morphology of U937 myelomonocytic cells during phorbol myristate acetate (PMA) differentiation and interferon (IFN)-γ activation. (**A**) Untreated U937 cells are small, nonadherent cells. (**B**) In the presence of PMA, the cells adhere to plastic tissue culture dishes but do not demonstrate other readily apparent morphological changes. (**C**) With the further addition of IFN-γ, cell size increases, nuclear density decreases, the nuclear: cytoplasmic ratio decreases, cytoplasmic vacuoles are formed, and cell membrane blebbing is evident by 24 h. (**D**) These changes are more dramatic after 48 h in the presence of IFN-γ. Original magnifications ×400.

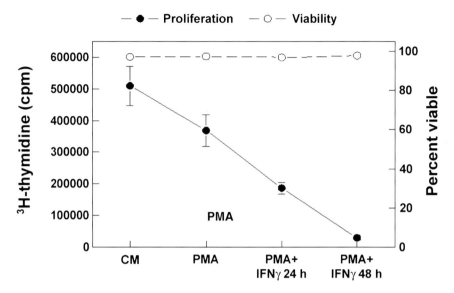

Fig. 3. Proliferative activity and viability of U937 myelomonocytic cells during phorbol myristate acetate (PMA) differentiation and interferon (IFN)-γ activation. Untreated U937 cells are highly proliferative, as indicated by ^{3}H-thymidine uptake of >500,000 cpm. Treatment with PMA alone reduces proliferative activity (closed circles), and subsequent treatment with IFN-γ further decreases proliferative activity. The reduction in proliferative activity is not accompanied by a loss of viability (open circles).

3.2.1. Peripheral Blood Mononuclear Cell Isolation

1. Collect the desired volume of whole blood in heparin-containing tubes and mix thoroughly by gentle inversion to prevent blood from clotting. In calculating the volume to be collected, expect approx 1×10^6 PBMC per 1 mL of whole blood. From PBMC, the expected yield of purified monocytes is approx 10% of PBMC, or 1×10^5 monocytes per 1 mL of whole blood.
2. Transfer whole blood to sterile, 50-mL conical polypropylene tubes and dilute 1:2 using serum-free macrophage medium.
3. Gently layer diluted blood (no more than 15 mL) onto 15 mL Histopaque in a 50-mL conical tube at room temperature, being careful not to mix. Centrifuge for 40 min at 400*g* at room temperature with the brake off (*see* **Note 5**).
4. Carefully aspirate and discard the topmost layer above the interface to approximately the 20-mL mark. Then collect the interface cells (7 mL) from approximately the 20-mL mark to the 13-mL mark.
5. Transfer the interface cells (these are the PBMC) into fresh 50-mL tubes and dilute 1:4 using serum-containing macrophage medium.

6. Wash by centrifugation at $200g$ for 15 min, combine the pellets, transfer to a 15-mL conical tube, and wash twice more at $200g$ for 10 min in serum-containing macrophage medium.

7. Resuspend the cell pellet in appropriate medium for the experiments to be done, determine cell yield by counting using a hemocytometer or automated cell counter, and determine viability (normally 90 to 95%) by trypan blue dye exclusion.

3.2.2. Magnetic Purification of Monocytes (Fig. 4) (See also manufacturer's instructions)

1. Set centrifuge to 4°C and chill cell separation buffer (*see* **Subheading 2.2.1.**) on ice.

2. Centrifuge the PBMC (in the 15-mL conical tube) at $200g$ for 10 min. Resuspend cells in ice-cold cell separation buffer (80 µL per 1×10^7 cells).

3. Add CD14 MicroBeads (20 µL per 1×10^7 cells) and mix by pipetting. Incubate for 15 min at 6 to 12°C (*see* **Note 6**).

4. Wash cells by adding 10 to 20 times the labeling volume of cell separation buffer and centrifuge at $300g$ for 10 min. Aspirate supernatant and resuspend cells in ice-cold cell separation buffer ($1 \text{ mL}/10^8$ cells).

5. Set up Miltenyi separation apparatus (Multi-Stand, magnet, separation column, preseparation filter). Prewet the preseparation filter and the separation column with 500 µL cell separation buffer, allowing the buffer to drain into a new 15-mL tube labeled "negative."

6. Apply 500 µL of the cell suspension (no more than 5×10^7 cells/column) to each preseparation filter. Allow the cells to pass through the pre-separation filter and the separation column into the 15 mL "negative" tube.

7. As a result of surface tension, some of the cell suspension will remain on the preseparation filter. Aspirate the remaining cell suspension through the preseparation filter by using a 200-µL pipet positioned underneath the filter membrane, and pipet onto the separation column.

8. Rinse the 15-mL tube in which the cells are labeled (**steps 2–4**) with another 500 µL of cell separation buffer and pass through the preseparation filter and column.

9. After the rinse volume from **step 8** (500 µL) has passed through the separation column, wash the preseparation filter with 500 µL cell separation buffer (wash No.1) and again pipet the buffer from the bottom of the pre-separation filter (as in **step 7**) onto the separation column. Discard the preseparation filter.

10. Allow the full volume (500 µL) of wash No. 1 from **step 9** to pass through the separation column, and follow with five 500-µL washes, allowing each complete volume to drain into the "negative" collection tube before adding another wash volume.

11. Remove the separation column (containing CD14$^+$-bound cells) from the magnet by pulling the column straight out (not up, because this will shear the cells). Place the separation column containing CD14$^+$ cells over a new 15-mL collection tube labeled "positive," add 1 mL cell separation buffer to the separation column, and flush the bound cells through using the plunger (provided with separation column).

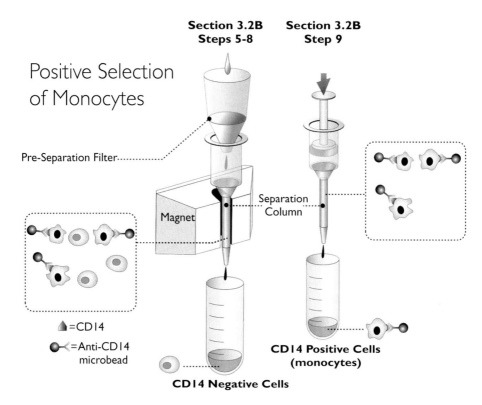

Fig. 4. Positive selection of peripheral blood monocytes using magnetic separation. Peripheral blood mononuclear cells are labeled with anti-CD14 MicroBeads, resulting in direct magnetic bead labeling of CD14$^+$ monocytes. After applying the labeled cell suspension to the preseparation filter and the separation column, the magnet will cause CD14$^+$ monocytes to remain bound to the separation column. Any cells not bound by the anti-CD14 MicroBeads will fall through the separation column into the "negative" tube. After washing several times to ensure all CD14$^-$ cells have passed through the separation column, the column is removed from the magnet, placed over a new "positive" tube, and the plunger is used to flush the CD14$^+$ cells through the column into the "positive" tube.

12. Determine cell yield by counting using a hemocytometer or an automated cell counter, and determine viability (normally 90 to 95%) by trypan blue dye exclusion. Cells can be kept in cell separation buffer on ice during counting.
13. Centrifuge the cells at 200g for 5–10 min, and resuspend in appropriate medium at the desired cell density for culture or analysis.

3.2.3. Purity of Cell Preparation

1. Purity of monocytes can be determined by flow cytometry using a directly-conjugated antibody to CD14 or other monocyte markers (*see* **Note 7**).
2. Alternatively, purity of monocytes can be determined by immunocytochemistry of cells centrifuged onto glass slides using a directly-conjugated antibody (*see* **Note 7**).
3. Expected purity after magnetic purification is 90% CD14$^+$ cells.

3.2.4. Culture (*Fig. 5*)

1. Cells are cultured at 37°C and 5% CO_2.
2. Seed monocytes at a density of approx 600,000 cells/cm^2 in the appropriate medium for the experiment. Cells will maintain 85 to 95% viability for 2 to 3 d.
3. Cell adherence to culture dishes and the length of time that cells can be maintained in vitro increases in serum-containing medium.

3.3. Peripheral Blood Monocyte-Derived Macrophages

Because decidual macrophages are continually exposed in vivo to M-CSF, a monocyte proliferation and differentiation factor, the methods below describe M-CSF differentiation of peripheral blood monocytes. In addition, because IFN-γ, a macrophage activation factor, is also present in the decidua throughout human pregnancy, IFN-γ is used as the activation factor (*see* **Note 8**).

3.3.1. M-CSF Differentiation and IFN-γ Activation

1. Cells are cultured at 37°C and 5% CO_2.
2. Seed purified monocytes in M-CSF-differentiation medium at a density of approx 250,000 cells/cm2 for 5 days. This density is less than monocyte culture because the cells will proliferate in the presence of M-CSF, which can lead to overcrowding.
3. To induce activation, remove culture supernatant and treat cells with IFN-γ-activation medium for 48 h.

3.3.2. Morphology and Characterization (*Fig. 5*)

1. Cells, which are adherent, can be harvested from culture dishes by incubation in CellStripper cell dissociation solution (Mediatech) for 30 min on ice followed by gentle scraping in order to label the cells for flow cytometric characterization.
2. For characterization by immunocytochemistry, centrifuge the cells onto glass slides (*see* **Note 7**).
3. For morphology characterization, after drying overnight at room temperature, cells on the glass slides can be stained using the Diff-Quik Stain Set following the manufacturer's instructions. Alternatively, cells can be stained in the culture wells by aspirating the supernatants, adding and aspirating the Diff-Quik reagents one at a time, and rinsing several times with water.

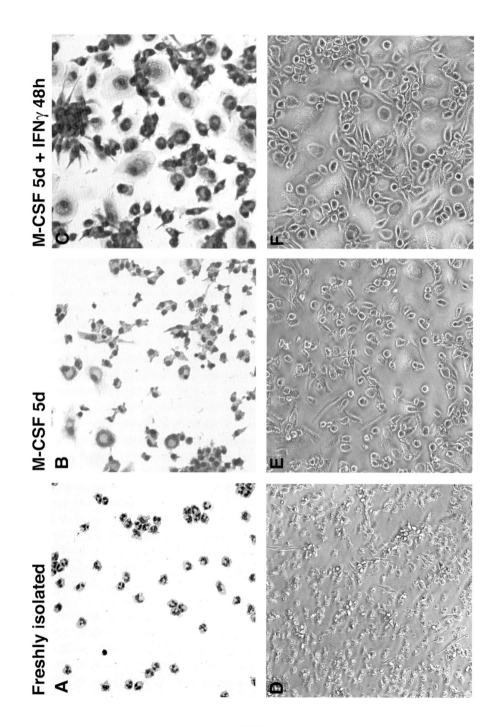

Freshly isolated   M-CSF 5d   M-CSF 5d + IFNγ 48h

A   B   C

D   E   F

3.4. Decidual Macrophages

During human pregnancy, maternal macrophages can be found throughout the specialized uterine endometrium (decidua), and are abundant in the decidua basalis as well as the region of juxtaposition between the chorionic trophoblast layer and the thin layer of decidua capsularis adherent to the extraplacental membranes at term (**Fig. 1**). The methods that follow, adapted from Vince and coworkers *(9)* and Narahara and Johnston *(12)*, describe the dissection of decidual tissue by scraping the decidua capsularis away from the chorionic layer of term extraplacental membranes. This is followed by mincing, enzymatic digestion, and, finally, gradient centrifugation (*see* **Note 1**).

3.4.1. Tissue Dissection, Digestion, and Gradient Centrifugation

1. Add BSA and enzymes to the Digestion Solution (*see* **Subheading 2.4.**) and filter-sterilize.
2. Obtain a fresh, term placenta from a vaginal delivery or a cesarean section (*see* **Note 9**). Place specimen on a sterile surface and cut membranes away from placenta. Place the membranes with the amnion membrane (smooth side) down and the decidua capsularis (red, "lacy" side) up. Remove any blood clots from decidual surface using forceps.
3. Scrape decidual layer away from chorionic layer using a scalpel, and place tissue (approx 10 g) in a preweighed 200-mL beaker of PBS or sterile saline. Re-weigh the beaker and note the amount of tissue collected.
4. Rinse the tissue in the beaker by swirling with PBS or sterile saline, allow the tissue to settle, pour off excess PBS, and repeat two to three times to remove blood.

Fig. 5. (*opposite page*) Bright-field and phase-contrast microscopy demonstrate morphological changes of cultured peripheral blood monocytes and monocyte-derived macrophages during macrophage colony-stimulating factor (M-CSF) differentiation and IFN-γ activation. In the upper panels, cells were centrifuged onto glass slides using a Shandon Cytospin centrifuge, stained with Diff-Quik®, and examined by light microscopy. In the lower panels, cells growing in culture dishes were examined by phase contrast microscopy. (**A,D**) Freshly isolated peripheral monocytes show classic monocyte nuclear morphology (kidney- or horseshoe-shaped nuclei) in preparations where cells were centrifuged onto glass slides. In live cultures, the cells are heterogeneous in size and shape and adhere to culture dishes. (**B,E**) After 5 d in the presence of M-CSF, cells remain heterogeneous in size and shape, but morphological changes and increases in cell size are evident. (**C,F**) Subsequent treatment with IFN-γ for 48 h induces dramatic increases in cell size as well as the number of cellular extensions (pseudopods). Original magnifications: **A,B,C,E,** and **F** ×200; **D** ×100.

5. Transfer tissue to a 100-mL beaker or 150-mm tissue culture dish. Using very sharp scissors, mince tissue into small pieces of approx 1 mm³.
6. Rinse the minced tissue with PBS, and pour through a 100-µm metal sieve, collecting eluate in a waste container. Repeat until the eluate runs clear (is free of blood).
7. Scrape the tissue from the sieve into a 500-mL Erlenmayer digestion flask, rinse the mincing beaker several times with fresh digestion solution, and transfer into the 500-mL digestion flask. The total volume of digestion solution should be 10 mL per gram of tissue collected. Use one 500-mL flask for each 10 to 15 g of collected tissue (100 to 150 mL digestion solution).
8. Place covered digestion flask in 37°C water bath and shake gently for 1 h (*see* **Note 10**).
9. If visible clumps of tissue are present after digestion, filter the cell digest from the 500-mL digestion flask through sterile cotton gauze (unfolded to two layers thickness) draped over a funnel into a 250-mL flask. No tissue should pass through, and DNA slurry should not be a problem.
10. Pass the cell suspension from the 250-mL flask through a 100-µm nylon cell filter, and then through a 70-µm nylon cell filter into 50-mL conical tubes to remove smaller undigested fragments and clumps.
11. Centrifuge filtrate at 250*g* for 10 min to collect dissociated cells. Resuspend with RPMI medium containing 10% FBS, pooling the pellets into 15-mL vol (15 mL per 5 g tissue), and repeat wash.
12. Layer 15 mL cells onto 15 mL room temperature Histopaque gradient in a 50-mL conical tube, being careful not to mix layers. Centrifuge 400*g* for 40 min at room temperature with the brake off (*see* **Note 5**). It is recommended to use one Histopaque gradient for each 5 g of tissue.
13. Aspirate and discard the topmost layer above the interface, and then collect the interface cells.
14. Transfer the interface cells into fresh 50-mL tubes and dilute 1:4 using RPMI medium containing 10% FBS. Centrifuge at 200*g* for 10 min, aspirate supernatants, and wash combined cells twice more in 10- to 20-mL vol.
15. Resuspend the cell pellet in culture medium, determine cell yield by counting using a hemocytometer or an automated cell counter, and determine viability by trypan blue dye exclusion. Expected cell yield is approx 3×10^6 cells per 10 g tissue, but individual samples can vary with yields ranging from 1 to 5×10^6 cells per 10 g tissue. Viability should be approx 85 to 90%, but individual samples range from less than 80% to 95% viability.

3.4.2. Purity of Cell Preparation (*Fig. 6*)

1. Purity of decidual macrophages can be determined by flow cytometry using antibodies to macrophage markers (e.g., CD14, CD68, HLA-DR, HLA-DQ) (*see* **Note 7**).
2. Alternatively, purity of macrophages can be determined by immunocytochemistry on cells centrifuged onto glass slides as shown in **Fig. 6** (*see* **Note 7**).

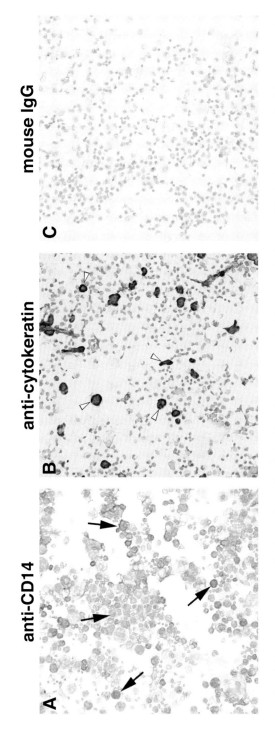

Fig. 6. Immunocytochemical staining of cells isolated from term decidua capsularis. Freshly isolated term decidual macrophages were centrifuged onto glass slides using a Shandon Cytospin. (**A**) Staining with anti-CD14 shows that the macrophages (arrows) are heterogeneous in size, shape, and staining intensity. (**B**) Chorion membrane cytotrophoblast cells (open arrowheads) are identified by staining with anti-cytokeratin. (**C**) An isotype-specific control monoclonal antibody does not bind to any cells. Original magnifications ×200.

3. Expected purity after tissue digestion and gradient centrifugation is 80 to 90% CD14[+] cells, although individual variation is likely. The major cellular contaminants are chorionic cytotrophoblasts, which stain positively using an anti-cytokeratin antibody as shown in **Fig. 6** (*see* **Note 10**).

3.4.3. Culture

1. Cells are cultured at 37°C and 5% CO_2.
2. Seed macrophages at a density of approx 600,000 cells/cm^2 in either RPMI medium containing 10% FBS or serum-free macrophage medium. Cells will maintain viability for 5 to 7 d in serum-containing medium.

3.5. Placental Macrophages

Placental macrophages, which are termed Hofbauer cells in first-trimester tissue, are fetal macrophages that reside in the mesenchyme of placental villi (**Fig. 1**). The methods that follow, adapted from Hunt and coworkers *(23)*, describe the dissection of term placental villous tissue followed by mincing, enzymatic digestion, gradient centrifugation, and magnetic purification by negative selection using an anti-EGF-R antibody to remove trophoblast cells *(24,25)*.

3.5.1. Tissue Dissection, Digestion, and Gradient Centrifugation

1. Add BSA and enzymes to the digestion solution (*see* **Subheading 2.5.**) and filter-sterilize.
2. Obtain a fresh placenta from a vaginal delivery or a cesarean section (*see* **Note 9**). Place specimen on a sterile surface with the umbilical cord facing down and the basal plate facing up. Remove any blood clots from the surface using forceps.
3. Cut decidual surface (basal plate) away from the villous placenta and discard. Harvest sections of placental villi, and place tissue (approx 30 g) in a preweighed 200-mL beaker of PBS or sterile saline. Re-weigh the beaker and note the amount of tissue collected.
4. Rinse the tissue in the beaker by swirling with PBS or sterile saline, allow the tissue to settle, pour off excess PBS, and repeat two to three times to remove as much blood as possible.
5. Transfer tissue to a 100-mL beaker or 150-mm culture dish. Using very sharp scissors, mince tissue into small pieces of approx 1 mm^3.
6. Rinse the minced tissue with PBS, and pour through a 100-μm metal sieve, collecting eluate in a waste container. Repeat until the eluate runs clear (is free of blood).
7. Scrape the tissue from the sieve into a 500-mL digestion flask, rinse the mincing dish several times with fresh digestion solution, and transfer into the 500-mL digestion flask. Add 200 mL warm digestion solution to the tissue. Place covered digestion flask in a 37°C water bath and shake gently for 1 h (*see* **Note 10**).
8. If visible clumps of tissue are present after digestion, filter the cell digest from the 500-mL digestion flask through sterile cotton gauze (unfolded to two layers

of thickness) draped over a funnel into a 250-mL flask. No tissue should pass through, and DNA slurry should not be a problem.

9. Transfer filtered supernatant from the 250-mL flask to sterile 50-mL tubes containing 5 mL FBS. Centrifuge at 250g for 10 min and resuspend in M199 (approx 20 to 25 mL in each of two tubes).

10. Filter the cell suspension through a 100-μm nylon cell filter into two 50-mL conical tubes. Centrifuge at 250g for 10 min and resuspend in M199 (30 mL per tube).

11. Layer 15 mL cells onto 15 mL room temperature Histopaque gradient in four 50-mL conical tubes being careful not to mix layers. Centrifuge at 400g for 30 min at room temperature with the brake off (*see* **Note 5**).

12. Aspirate and discard the topmost layer above the mononuclear cell layer, and then collect the interface cells.

13. Transfer the interface cells into four fresh 50-mL tubes and add 40 mL M199 to each. Centrifuge at 250g for 10 min, aspirate supernatants, resuspend and combine cell pellets in M199, and repeat the wash.

14. Resuspend the cell pellet in M199, determine cell yield by counting using a hemocytometer or an automated cell counter, and determine viability by trypan blue dye exclusion. Expected cell yield is approx 3×10^6 cells per 30 g tissue with viability of approx 80%, but individual samples can vary.

3.5.2. Magnetic Purification by Negative Selection (*Fig. 7*)

1. Set centrifuge to 4°C and place cell separation buffer on ice.

2. Transfer cells to a 15-mL conical tube and spin at 200g for 10 min. Resuspend cells in ice-cold cell separation buffer (80 μL per 1×10^7 cells).

3. Add the mouse anti-EGF-R antibody, which will bind the EGF-R on trophoblast cells (20 μL of the 200 μg/mL stock per 1×10^7 cells), and mix by pipetting. Incubate for 10 min at 6 to 12°C.

4. Wash cells by adding 10 to 20 times the labeling volume of cell separation buffer and centrifuge at 300g for 10 min. Aspirate supernatant and resuspend cells in ice-cold cell separation buffer (80 μL/1×10^7 cells).

5. Add the goat anti-mouse MicroBeads, which will bind the mouse anti-EGF-R antibodies, (20 μL/1×10^7 cells) and mix by pipetting. Incubate for 15 min at 6 to 12°C (*see* **Note 6**).

6. Wash cells by adding 10 to 20 times the labeling volume of cell separation buffer and centrifuge at 300g for 10 min. Aspirate supernatant and resuspend cells in ice-cold cell separation buffer (0.5 mL/10^8 cells).

7. Set up Miltenyi separation apparatus (Multi-Stand, magnet, separation column, preseparation filter). Prewet the preseparation filter and the separation column with 500 μL cell separation buffer, allowing the buffer to drain into a 15-mL tube.

8. Attach the needle to the end of the separation column. Because this protocol utilizes negative selection of desired cells (macrophages), using the needle slows the rate of flow through the separation column, allowing appropriate time for the EGF-R$^+$ cells (trophoblast cells) to bind the column.

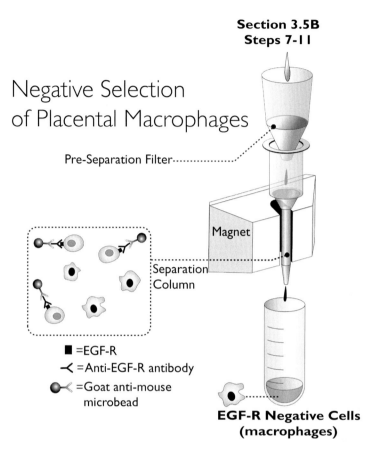

Negative Selection
of Placental Macrophages

Pre-Separation Filter

Magnet

Separation
Column

■ =EGF-R
‹ =Anti-EGF-R antibody
●‹ =Goat anti-mouse
       microbead

**EGF-R Negative Cells
(macrophages)**

Fig. 7. Selection of placental macrophages from villous cell suspension by magnetic separation. The placental cell suspension is labeled with a mouse anti-epidermal growth factor receptor (EFG-R) antibody followed by a goat anti-mouse MicroBead, resulting in magnetic labeling of EGF-R$^+$ trophoblast cells. After applying the labeled cell suspension to the preseparation filter and the separation column, the magnet will cause the EGF-R$^+$ cells to remain bound to the separation column, allowing EGF-R$^-$ cells to fall through the separation column into the "macrophage" tube.

9. Place a fresh 15-mL tube labeled "macrophages" below the column, and apply 500 µL of the cell suspension (no more than 5×10^7 cells/column) to each preseparation filter.
10. As a result of surface tension, some of the cell suspension will remain on the preseparation filter. Aspirate the remaining cell suspension through the preseparation filter by using a 200-µL pipet positioned underneath the filter membrane, and pipet onto the separation column.

11. Rinse the 15-mL tube in which the cells were labeled (**steps 2–6**) with another 500 µL cell separation buffer and pass through the preseparation filter and the separation column.

12. After the rinse volume from **step 11** (500 µL) has passed through the separation column, wash the preseparation filter with 500 µL cell separation buffer (wash No. 1) and again pipet the buffer from the bottom of the preseparation filter (as in **step 10**) onto the separation column. Discard the preseparation filter.

13. Allow the full volume of wash No. 1 from **step 12** (500 µL) to pass through the separation column, and follow with two more 500-µL washes, allowing the complete volume to drain into "macrophage" collection tube before adding another wash volume. Because of the occasional cell clumps and air bubbles between the separation column and the needle, it may be necessary to apply gentle, rocking pressure to the top of the column using the plunger (provided with separation column) to keep the column flowing. It is important not to insert the plunger into the separation column, because this will shear the cells.

14. Determine cell yield by counting using a hemocytometer or an automated cell counter, and determine viability (normally 80 to 90%) by trypan blue dye exclusion. Cells can be kept in cell separation buffer on ice during counting. Expected yield is approx 1×10^6 macrophages, but individual samples can vary.

15. Centrifuge cells at $200g$ for 5 to 10 min, and resuspend in M199 at the desired cell density for culture or analysis.

3.5.3. Purity of Cell Preparation

1. Purity of placental macrophages can be determined by flow cytometry or immunocytochemistry on cells centrifuged onto glass slides. Fetal macrophages are less mature than maternal macrophages and do not express many common macrophage markers. For example, first-trimester Hofbauer cells are CD14$^+$, HLA-DR-, and HLA-DQ-, whereas term placental macrophages are CD14^{lo}, intracellular CD68$^+$ *(24)*, HLA-DR$^+$, and HLA-DQ$^-$ (*see* **Note 7**).

2. Alternatively, the percentage of contaminating cells (mainly trophoblast cells) can be determined by staining purified cells with a labeled anti-mouse secondary antibody. This will result in positive labeling of any cells bound by the anti-EGF-R antibody (*see* **Note 7**).

3.5.4. Culture

1. Cells are cultured at 37°C and 5% CO_2.
2. Seed macrophages at a density of approx 600,000 cells/cm^2 in M199. Cells will maintain viability for 5 to 7 d in serum-containing medium.

4. Notes

1. When working with human blood or tissue, personal protective equipment (gloves, lab coat, eye protection) is required, even when the sample donor is thought to be "healthy." Contact your institute for appropriate biohazardous waste

disposal protocols. As with any cell culture procedure, all cell and tissue manipulation should be performed using sterile equipment and aseptic techniques inside a sterile, laminar flow hood if possible. In addition, all solutions used should be tissue-culture grade, low-endotoxin certified. If any solutions are made in the laboratory, they should be autoclaved and sterile-filtered (0.22 µm) before use. All culture dishes or plates should be sterile tissue culture grade. Sterile conical tubes should be polypropylene, because monocytes/macrophages stick more easily to polystyrene during the isolation protocols, which will result in decreased cell yield.

2. Monocyte and macrophage responses are strongly influenced by bacterial products including endotoxins. Therefore, BSA and all enzymes used in the tissue digestion solution should be cell culture grade (low endotoxin). In addition, for optimal enzymatic activity, all enzymes should be added to the digestion solution and the solution should be sterile-filtered (0.22 µm) just before use. Do not autoclave the digestion solution after the addition of the enzymes.

3. The use of PMA-differentiation and IFN-γ-activation with the U937 cell line as a macrophage model is common practice *(26–34)*. However, other human monocyte cell lines to consider include THP-1 cells (ATCC, cat. no. TIB-202) and HL-60 cells (ATCC, cat. no. CCL-240) *(35–38)*. Alternative methods for differentiation can also be employed, including vitamin D3, tumor necrosis factor (TNF), retinoic acid, butyrate, hypoxanthine, dimethylsulfoxide (DMSO), and actinomycin D.

4. MTT assays are also widely used to measure cell number or cell viability. However, when treating monocytes or macrophages with differentiation or activation factors such as PMA and IFN-γ, significant cellular changes occur, resulting in increased mitochondrial activity. Because the MTT substrate reaction reflects mitochondrial activity, this method may give incorrect results when comparing cell number or viability between nonactivated and activated monocytes or macrophages. For this reason, we employ in-well trypan blue dye exclusion to measure cell viability and ^{3}H-thymidine incorporation to measure proliferative activity.

5. It is important that the gradient centrifugation procedure is performed at room temperature, as temperature affects the gradient density. Do not exceed 15 mL Histopaque per 50 mL-conical tube, and do not layer more cell suspension volume than Histopaque volume, as surface area and gradient depth are important factors in cell yield and purity.

6. Incubations with MicroBeads should be at 6 to 12°C (in the refrigerator) as working on ice increases the incubation time. Additionally, higher temperatures and longer incubation times may lead to unspecific cell labeling. For peripheral monocyte purification, this could also lead to internalization of the CD14 MicroBeads and labeling of cells with low CD14 expression (granulocytes). Because MicroBeads bind unspecifically to dead cells, density gradient centrifugation should always be done before labeling. The maximum cell concentration is 10^8 cells/500 µL buffer and 5×10^7 cells per magnetic column.

7. Because the anti-CD14-MicroBead and the anti-EGF-R are mouse monoclonal antibodies with intact Fc regions, any flow cytometric or immuncytochemical labeling of magnetically separated cells must be performed using a directly conjugated primary antibody. If not, an anti-mouse secondary antibody will bind to the primary antibody of interest as well as the CD14-MicroBeads or the anti-EGF-R antibody, resulting in false-positive staining. Additionally, in order to avoid nonspecific labeling and high background signals when labeling monocytes or macrophages with antibodies for flow cytometry or immunocytochemistry, it is very important to block Fc receptors with 40% heat-inactivated human serum for 30 min prior to antibody labeling.

8. In addition to M-CSF-differentiation *(39,40)*, other macrophage differentiation factors such as granulocyte/macrophage colony stimulating factor (GM-CSF) and IL-13 can be used *(41–43)*. In addition to IFN-γ activation, there are other methods of macrophage activation, which include treatment with bacterial products such as lipopolysaccharide (LPS) *(44)*. However, these models for macrophage activation pertain to states of infection, which are associated with preterm delivery rather than normal pregnancy.

9. The placenta must be obtained within 30 min of delivery, placed in a sterile container, and kept at room temperature until the tissue is dissected and processed. Importantly, no preservatives should be added to the tissue, as this will kill the cells. As mentioned in **Note 2**, macrophage responses are strongly influenced by bacterial products. For this reason, placentas obtained by cesarean section are preferred over vaginal deliveries because the vaginal mucosa contains many commensal bacteria, which contaminate the specimen as it passes through the birth canal.

10. Macrophages in the decidua and placental mesenchyme are more loosely associated with the extracellular matrix than the trophoblast cells, which are tightly associated with each other and the basal lamina. Therefore, to reduce the potential for trophoblast cell contamination of macrophage preparations, do not increase the time of enzyme digestion or add fresh enzymes during the digestion procedure.

Acknowledgments

The authors thank the many students and technicians who have contributed to the development of these protocols. This work is supported by grants from the National Institutes of Health to J. S. H. (HD24212; U54 HD33994 Project IV; PO1 HD39878 Project III) and the University of Kansas Biomedical Research Training Grant to R. H. M.

References

1. Hunt, J. S. (1989) Cytokine networks in the uteroplacental unit: macrophages as pivotal regulatory cells. *J. Reprod. Immunol.* **16,** 1–17.
2. Mor, G. and Abrahams, V. M. (2003) Potential role of macrophages as immunoregulators of pregnancy. *Reprod. Biol. Endocrinol.* **1,** 119.

3. Leibovich, S. J. and Ross, R. (1975) The role of the macrophage in wound repair. A study with hydrocortisone and antimacrophage serum. *Am. J. Pathol.* **78,** 71–100.
4. Clarke, R. A. F. (1996) *The Molecular and Cellular Biology of Wound Repair* (Clarke, R. A. F., ed.). Kluwer Academic/Plenum, New York: pp. 3–50.
5. Janeway, C. A. (1992) The immune system evolved to discriminate infectious non-self from noninfectious self. *Immunol. Today* **13,** 11–16.
6. Fearon, D. T., and Locksley, R. M. (1996) The instructive role of innate immunity in the acquired immune response. *Science* **272,** 50–54.
7. Gordon, S. (1998) The role of macrophages in immune regulation. *Res. Immunol.* **149,** 685–688.
8. Starkey, P. M., Sargent, I. L., and Redman, C. W. (1988) Cell populations in human early pregnancy decidua: characterization and isolation of large granular lymphocytes by flow cytometry. *Immunology* **65,** 129–134.
9. Vince, G. S., Starkey, P. M., Jackson, M. C., Sargent, I. L., and Redman, C. W. (1990) Flow cytometric characterisation of cell populations in human pregnancy decidua and isolation of decidual macrophages. *J. Immunol. Methods* **132,** 181–189.
10. Hunt, J. S., Petroff, M. G., and Burnett, T. G. (2000) Uterine leukocytes: key players in pregnancy. *Semin. Cell Dev. Biol.* **11,** 127–137.
11. Bulmer, J. N., Pace, D., and Ritson, A. (1988) Immunoregulatory cells in human decidua: morphology, immunohistochemistry and function. *Reprod. Nutr. Develop.* **28,** 1599–1614.
12. Narahara, H. and Johnston, J. M. (1993) Effects of endotoxins and cytokines on the secretion of platelet-activating factor-acetylhydrolase by human decidual macrophages. *Am. J. Obstet. Gynecol.* **169,** 531–537.
13. Hunt, J. S. and Robertson, S. A. (1996) Uterine macrophages and environmental programming for pregnancy success. *J. Reprod. Immunol.* **32,** 1–25.
14. Pollard, J. W., Bartocci, A., Arceci, R., Orlofsky, A., Ladner, M. B., and Stanley, E. R. (1987) Apparent role of the macrophage growth factor, CSF-1, in placental development. *Nature* **330,** 484–486.
15. Yong, K., Salooja, N., Donahue, R. E., Hegde, U., and Linch, D. C. (1992) Human macrophage colony-stimulating factor levels are elevated in pregnancy and in immune thrombocytopenia. *Blood* **80,** 2897–2902.
16. Saito, S., Motoyoshi, K., Ichijo, M., Saito, M., and Takaku, F. (1992) High serum human macrophage colony-stimulating factor level during pregnancy. *Int. J. Hematol.* **55,** 219–225.
17. Praloran, V., Coupey, L., Donnard, M., Berrada, L., and Naud, M. F. (1994) Elevation of serum M-CSF concentrations during pregnancy and ovarian hyperstimulation. *Br. J. Haematol.* **86,** 675–677.
18. Hunt, J. S., Miller, L., and Platt, J. S. (1998) Hormonal regulation of uterine macrophages. *Dev. Immunol.* **6,** 105–110.
19. Ashkar, A. A. and Croy, B. A. (1999) Interferon-gamma contributes to the normalcy of murine pregnancy. *Biol. Reprod.* **61,** 493–502.
20. Veith, G. L. and Rice, G. E. (1999) Interferon gamma expression during human pregnancy and in association with labour. *Gynecol. Obstet. Invest.* **48,** 163–167.

21. Bowen, J. M., Chamley, L., Mitchell, M. D., and Keelan, J. A. (2002) Cytokines of the placenta and extra-placental membranes: biosynthesis, secretion and roles in establishment of pregnancy in women. *Placenta* **23,** 239–256.

22. Mellor, A. L. and Munn, D. H. (2000) Immunology at the maternal-fetal interface: lessons for T cell tolerance and suppression. *Annu. Rev. Immunol.* **18,** 367–391.

23. Hunt, J. S., King, C. R., Jr., and Wood, G. W. (1984) Evaluation of human chorionic trophoblast cells and placental macrophages as stimulators of maternal lymphocyte proliferation in vitro. *J. Reprod. Immunol.* **6,** 377–391.

24. Wetzka, B., Clark, D. E., Charnock-Jones, D. S., Zahradnik, H. P., and Smith, S. K. (1997) Isolation of macrophages (Hofbauer cells) from human term placenta and their prostaglandin E2 and thromboxane production. *Hum. Reprod.* **12,** 847–852.

25. Phillips, T. A., Ni, J., and Hunt, J. S. (2001) Death-inducing tumour necrosis factor (TNF) superfamily ligands and receptors are transcribed in human placentae, cytotrophoblasts, placental macrophages and placental cell lines. *Placenta* **22,** 663–672.

26. Sundstrom, C., and Nilsson, K. (1976) Establishment and characterization of a human histiocytic lymphoma cell line (U937). *Int. J. Cancer* **17,** 565–577.

27. Ishizuka, T., Hirata, I., Adachi, M., et al. (1995) Effects of interferon-gamma on cell differentiation and cytokine production of a human monoblast cell line, U937. *Inflammation* **19,** 627–636.

28. Caron, E., Liautard, J. P., and Kohler, S. (1994) Differentiated U937 cells exhibit increased bactericidal activity upon LPS activation and discriminate between virulent and avirulent Listeria and Brucella species. *J. Leukoc. Biol.* **56,** 174–181.

29. Vrana, J. A., Saunders, A. M., Chellappan, S. P., and Grant, S. (1998) Divergent effects of bryostatin 1 and phorbol myristate acetate on cell cycle arrest and maturation in human myelomonocytic leukemia cells (U937). *Differentiation* **63,** 33–42.

30. Dey, A., Kim, L., and Li, W. (1999) Gamma interferon induces expression of Mad1 gene in macrophage, which inhibits colony-stimulating factor-1-dependent mitogenesis. *J. Cell. Biochem.* **72,** 232–241.

31. Hida, A., Kawakami, A., Nakashima, T., et al. (2000) Nuclear factor-kappaB and caspases co-operatively regulate the activation and apoptosis of human macrophages. *Immunology* **99,** 553–560.

32. Chabot, S., Charlet, D., Wilson, T. L., and Yong, V. W. (2001) Cytokine production consequent to T cell—microglia interaction: the PMA/IFN gamma-treated U937 cells display similarities to human microglia. *J. Neurosci. Methods* **105,** 111–120.

33. Bosisio, D., Polentarutti, N., Sironi, M., et al. (2002) Stimulation of toll-like receptor 4 expression in human mononuclear phagocytes by interferon-gamma: a molecular basis for priming and synergism with bacterial lipopolysaccharide. *Blood* **99,** 3427–3431.

34. Naldini, A., Carney, D. H., Pucci, A., and Carraro, F. (2002) Human alpha-thrombin stimulates proliferation of interferon-gamma differentiated, growth-arrested U937 cells, overcoming differentiation-related changes in expression of p21CIP1/WAF1 and cyclin D1. *J. Cell. Physiol.* **191,** 290–297.

35. Drexler, H. G. and Minowada, J. (1998) History and classification of human leukemia-lymphoma cell lines. *Leukemia Lymphoma* **31,** 305–316.

36. Tsuchiya, S. (1980) Establishment and characterization of a human acute monocytic leukemia cell line (THP-1). *Int. J. Cancer* **26,** 171–176.

37. Gallagher, R. (1979) Characterization of the continuous, differentiating myeloid cell line (HL-60) from a patient with acute promyelocytic leukemia. *Blood* **54,** 713–733.

38. Collins, S. J. (1987) The HL-60 promyelocytic leukemia cell line: proliferation, differentiation, and cellular oncogene expression. *Blood* **70,** 1233–1244.

39. Becker, S., Warren, M. K., and Haskill, S. (1987) Colony-stimulating factor-induced monocyte survival and differentiation into macrophages in serum-free cultures *J. Immunol.* **139,** 3703–3709.

40. Munn, D. H. and Armstrong, E. (1993) Cytokine regulation of human monocyte differentiation in vitro: the tumor-cytotoxic phenotype induced by macrophage colony-stimulating factor is developmentally regulated by gamma-interferon. *Cancer Res.* **53,** 2603–2613.

41. Allavena, P., Piemonti, L., Longoni, D., et al. (1998) IL-10 prevents the differentiation of monocytes to dendritic cells but promotes their maturation to macrophages. *Eur. J. Immunol.* **28,** 359–369.

42. Hashimoto, S., Suzuki, T., Dong, H. Y., Yamazaki, N., and Matsushima, K. (1999) Serial analysis of gene expression in human monocytes and macrophages. *Blood* **94,** 837–844.

43. Finnin, M., Hamilton, J. A., and Moss, S. T. (1999) Characterization of a CSF-induced proliferating subpopulation of human peripheral blood monocytes by surface marker expression and cytokine production. *J. Leukoc. Biol.* **66,** 953–960.

44. Dobrovolskaia, M. A. and Vogel, S. N. (2002) Toll receptors, CD14, and macrophage activation and deactivation by LPS. *Microbes Infect.* **4,** 903–914.

9

Macrophage–Trophoblast Interactions

Gil Mor, Shawn L. Straszewski-Chavez, and Vikki M. Abrahams

Summary

During implantation and pregnancy, the invading trophoblast population is within close contact to maternal immune cells, particularly macrophages. During this period, a low level of trophoblast cell death occurs as part of the normal process of tissue renewal. Macrophage engulfment of apoptotic trophoblast cells prevents the release of potentially pro-immunogenic intracellular contents and prevents a maternal immune response. Furthermore, the uptake of apoptotic cells suppresses macrophages from secreting pro-inflammatory cytokines and promotes the release of anti-inflammatory cytokines, thus creating a microenvironment that will promote trophoblast survival and a successful pregnancy. The present chapter will describe some of the approaches used to study the interaction between macrophages and trophoblast cells.

Key Words: Macrophage; trophoblast; pregnancy; placenta; apoptosis; co-culture; cytokines; conditioned media; caspase; XIAP.

1. Introduction

The removal of cellular debris, generated as a result of apoptosis, is a challenging task that must be performed in order to maintain cellular homeostasis. Different morphological changes accompany the induction of the apoptotic program. Cells first become round and detach from their neighbors. Then, condensation of both the nucleus and cytoplasm occurs without major modification to the other intracellular organelles. Following condensation, nuclear fragmentation and membrane blebbing is observed, resulting in the formation of apoptotic bodies with intact membranes. These morphological changes are a translation of the biochemical modifications, mediated by the activation of the caspase cascade, that are occurring inside of the cell.

Another important cellular change that occurs during apoptosis is the redistribution of membranal proteins, which will allow macrophages to recognize apoptotic cells and direct the phagocytic process. Several receptors have been

From: *Methods in Molecular Medicine, Vol. 122: Placenta and Trophoblast: Methods and Protocols, Vol. 2*
Edited by: M. J. Soares and J. S. Hunt © Humana Press Inc., Totowa, NJ

implicated in the recognition and engulfment of apoptotic cells *(1,2)*, suggesting that the process of phagocytosis is well regulated and functionally relevant.

Implantation and trophoblast invasion is characterized by a progressive, continuous induction of apoptosis in the maternal tissue surrounding the fetus *(3)*. During this period, numerous macrophages are present at the implantation site and this was originally thought to represent an immune response occurring against the invading trophoblast. However, we propose that this may not be the case. We suggest that macrophage engulfment of apoptotic cells prevents the release of potentially pro-inflammatory and pro-immunogenic intracellular contents that occurs during secondary necrosis *(4)*. Because of the allogenic nature of the placenta, this process may be essential for the well being of the fetus. Trophoblast cells are carriers of proteins, which are antigenically foreign to the maternal immune system and if released, as result of cell death, may initiate or accelerate immunological responses with lethal consequences for the fetus. Therefore, the appropriate removal of dying trophoblast cells prior to the release of these intracellular components is critical for the prevention of fetal rejection.

1.1. Macrophages and Apoptosis

Histological analysis of normal placental beds, as well as in preeclampsia, shows the presence of a large number of macrophages, which are in the majority of cases, localized to the vicinity of apoptotic cells. Indeed, macrophages are one of the major cell types in both the maternal and fetal compartments of the uteroplacental unit *(5)*. In humans, during the first weeks of implantation, macrophages are found in high numbers in the maternal decidua and in tissues close in proximity to the placenta *(6)*. Similarly, in rodents, macrophages accumulate at or near the implantation site *(7)*. The dense macrophage infiltration at the maternal–fetal interface suggests that these cells are also involved in specific pregnancy-associated functions, and not only to perform their usual immunological tasks *(8)*. Hunt and co-workers have implied that maternal macrophages assist in the tissue remodeling necessary to accommodate expansion of extraembryonic tissue *(9)*. However, macrophages are not merely scavengers of dying cells, but also actively orchestrate apoptosis of unwanted cells during tissue remodeling *(2)*. Macrophages synthesize and secrete cytokines and growth factors, which govern the local cellular and tissue interactions *(6,9)*. Numerous findings propose that the capacity for macrophages to influence cell death is regulated by the extent of uptake of apoptotic cells *(2)*. For example, the cytolysis of tumor cells by activated macrophages is inhibited by the ingestion of apoptotic but not necrotic cells *(10)*. Similarly, during embryo implantation, uterine epithelial cells surrounding the blastocyst undergo apoptosis and may form an anti-inflammatory environment by increasing Th-2 type cytokines.

This may explain the surprising cohabitation of macrophages and trophoblast cells at the implantation site. The type of cytokines produced by a macrophage depends on its activation state *(11)*. We propose that in *normal pregnancy*, the uptake of apoptotic cells suppresses these activated macrophages from secreting pro-inflammatory cytokines such as tumor necrosis factor (TNF)-α and interferon (IFN)-γ *(12,13)* and promotes the release of anti-inflammatory and immunosuppressive cytokines *(12)*. However, we postulate that in pregnancies complicated with intrauterine growth restriction (IUGR) or preeclampsia, activated macrophages secrete pro-inflammatory cytokines such as TNF-α and IFN-γ and induce apoptosis in the extravillous trophoblast. This hypothesis is supported by a report of Pijnenborg et al. *(14)*, who found a higher incidence of cell clusters secreting TNF-α, probably macrophages, in the placental bed of patients with severe forms of preeclampsia.

Macrophages are also located near the spiral arteries during trophoblast invasion and transformation. Our own and previous studies of placental bed specimens demonstrate changes in the distribution of macrophages during pathological conditions such as preeclampsia *(15)*. Whereas in normal pregnancies, macrophages are located in the stroma surrounding the transformed spiral arteries and extravillous trophoblast, in preeclampsia, macrophages are located within and around the spiral arteries separating them from the trophoblast cells *(16)*. Their distribution resembles a barrier between the invading trophoblast and the spiral arteries. We propose a differential role for uterine macrophages during trophoblast invasion/differentiation, according to their stage of activation. In normal pregnancies, macrophages function as support cells by facilitating trophoblast invasion through the placental bed. In pathological conditions, macrophages function as a barrier for trophoblast invasion and differentiation by inducing trophoblast apoptosis (**Fig. 1** and **ref. 12**). Therefore, this raised the question, "what determines this dual role."

1.2. Consequences of Apoptotic Cell Clearance

Recent studies indicate that the removal of apoptotic bodies is neither a neutral nor a passive process, but rather an active physiological event that may influence not only immune responses, but also the proliferation and differentiation of surrounding cells *(2)*. Voll et al. *(13)* found that monocyte secretion of the pro-inflammatory cytokine TNF-α was inhibited, whereas production of the anti-inflammatory cytokines, transforming growth factor (TGF)-β and interleukin (IL)-10 was increased following co-culture of monocytes with apoptotic lymphocytes. Furthermore, in vivo studies have clearly demonstrated that the TGF-β released by macrophages ingesting apoptotic cells has anti-inflammatory effects in inflamed peritoneum and lungs *(17)*. Therefore, we propose that the clearance of apoptotic cells by decidual macrophages protects

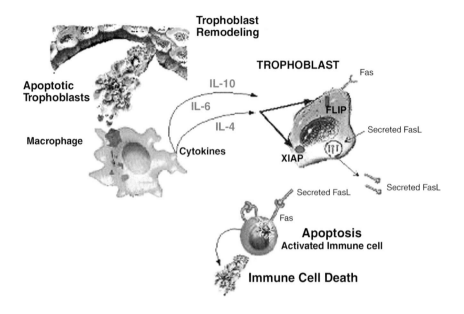

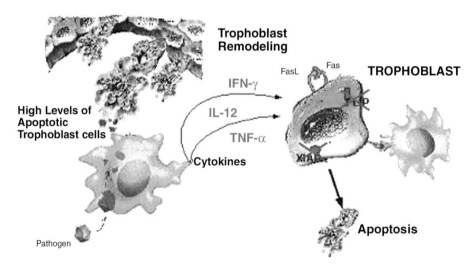

Fig. 1 (*see* companion CD for color version). Apoptotic cell clearance by macroph-ages. (**A**) Clearance of low levels of apoptotic cells by macrophages induces their production of anti-inflammatory cytokines, which in turn promote trophoblast cell survival. (**B**) Elevated levels of apoptosis and consequential inefficient clearance of apoptotic cells will result in a pro-inflammatory microenvironment, which will pro-mote further trophoblast cell death.

the trophoblast by: (1) macrophages phagocytosing apoptotic trophoblast cells will prevent the release of intracellular proteins of paternal origin, which could trigger an immune response; (2) decidual macrophages will influence the local microenvironment following phagocytosis of apoptotic trophoblast cells, and this in turn will have an effect on trophoblast susceptibility to pro-apoptotic signals.

In the following section we describe the main techniques used in our laboratory for the previously described studies.

2. Materials

2.1. Equipment

1. 100- × 20-mm Petri dishes (BD Biosciences, Bedford, MA).
2. 50-mL conical tubes (BD Biosciences).
3. 15-mL conical tubes (BD Biosciences).
4. Sterile scissors, forceps and scalpel.
5. Sieve (40 μm).
6. 25-cm^2/75-cm^2 flasks (BD Biosciences).

2.2. Reagents

1. Hanks' balanced salt solution (HBSS) without calcium and magnesium (Invitrogen, Carlsbad, CA).
2. 2.5 % trypsin–ethylenediamine tetraaceti acid (EDTA) (Invitrogen).
3. Minimum essential medium (MEM) with D-val prepared using custom kit (ICN Biomedicals, Inc., Irvine, CA).
4. Human serum (HS; Gemini Bio-Products, Woodland, CA).
5. Lymphocyte Seperation Media (ICN Biomedicals, Inc).
6. Dulbecco's modified Eagle's medium (DMEM) (Invitrogen).
7. Fetal bovine serum (FBS; Hyclone, Logan, UT).
8. Sterile double-distilled water (ddH$_2$O).
9. Fat-free powdered milk.
10. RPMI (Invitrogen) containing 10% FBS (HyClone).
11. OptiMEM (Invitrogen).
12. Phorbol 12-myristate 13-acetate (PMA, Sigma Chemical Company, St. Louis, MO).
13. Camptothecin (Sigma).
14. Propridium iodide (Sigma).
15. Hoechst 33342 dye (Molecular Probes, Eugene, OR).
16. Lysis buffer: phosphate-buffered saline (PBS) containing 0.01% NP40 and 0.001% sodium dodecyl sulfate (SDS).
17. Phenylmethylsulfonylfluoride (PMSF; Sigma).
18. Protease inhibitor cocktail (PIC; Roche Applied Science, Indianapolis, IN).
19. Bicinchoninic acid (BCA) assay (Pierce Chemical Company, Rockford, IL).
20. Caspase-Glo 3/7 substrate (Promega, Madison, WI).

21. PKH26 and PKH67 dyes (Sigma).
22. Lower Gel: 6 mL Tris (pH 8.8), 9.5 mL polyacrylamide (for 12% gels), 200 μL 50% glycerol, 8.3 mL ddH$_2$O, 240 μL fresh 10% ammonium persulphate, 12 μL *N,N,N',N'*-tetramethylethylenediamine (TEMED).
23. 6.5 mL ddH$_2$O, 2.5 mL upper Tris (pH 6.8), 1 mL polyacrylamide, 45 μL fresh 10% ammonium persulphate, 22.5 μL TEMED.

3. Methods

The methods described below outline (a) preparation and cell culture of macrophages, (b) the isolation and culture of primary trophoblasts, (c) the preparation of apoptotic trophoblast cells, (d) the co-culturing of apoptotic cells with macrophages and (e), evaluating the effect apoptotic cell clearance by macrophages on trophoblast cell survival in vitro.

3.1. Macrophage Culture

Macrophages are obtained by differentiating monocytes in vitro. To avoid the need to isolate peripheral blood monocytes for each experiment, the monocyte cell line, THP-1, is used. Differentiation of monocytes into macrophages can be performed by culturing THP-1 cells with PMA (**Fig. 2**) (*see* **Note 1**).

1. In six-well tissue culture plates, seed 1×10^6 cells in 3 mL RPMI/10% FBS containing 10 ng/mL PMA.
2. Culture at 37°C in 5% CO$_2$ for 72 h (*see* **Note 2**).
3. Differentiation can be determined by checking cell morphology by light microscopy

3.2. Preparation of First-Trimester Trophoblast Cell Cultures

3.2.1. Before Starting

1. Sterilize scissors, forceps and scalpel.
2. Thaw 2.5% trypsin-EDTA.
3. Turn-on shaker to 37°C.
4. All steps must be performed under sterile conditions in the hood.

3.2.2. Tissue Collection

1. Tissue specimens should be collected in *cold*, sterile PBS.
2. Transfer tissue to a 50-mL conical tube if not already in one.
3. Wash the tissue in *cold* HBSS (*see* **Note 3**) until solution is clear to remove excess blood.
4. Transfer tissue to a Petri dish and cover with HBSS.
5. Remove any blood clots with forceps.
6. Scrape trophoblast cells from the membranes using a scalpel.
7. Remove any leftover membranes using forceps.
8. Transfer the tissue back to the 50-mL conical tube and wash with HBSS.

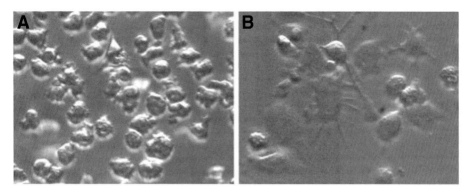

Fig. 2. THP-1 cells cultured for 72 h with or without phorbol 12-myristate 13-acetate (PMA) **(A)** Undifferentiated THP-1 cells **(B)** PMA differentiated THP-1 cells

9. Allow trophoblast cells to sediment and then carefully remove the supernatant by vacuum pipet.
10. Repeat the two previous steps until the solution is clear.
11. Carefully remove the supernatant by vacuum pipet and mince the tissue into little pieces using scissors.

3.2.3. Typsinization

1. Measure the volume of the tissue and add an equal volume of 2.5% trypsin-EDTA.
2. Incubate the tissue at 37°C for 10 min with shaking.
3. After the incubation, add *prewarmed* DMEM + 10 % FBS so that the serum reaches a final concentration of 2%. The serum will stop the trypsinization process.
4. Add DMEM + 10% FBS to the tissue until the final volume is between 30 mL and 40 mL depending on the amount of tissue.
5. Vortex the mixture for 20 s and then allow the tissue to sediment.
6. Collect the supernatant using a transfer pipet and transfer to a new 50-mL conical tube.
7. Repeat the three previous steps except add DMEM + 10% FBS until the final volume is between 25 and 35 mL and then between 20 and 30 mL.
8. Centrifuge the supernatant at 800g for 10 min.

3.2.4. Filtering

1. Remove the supernatant by vacuum pipet and resuspend the pellet in 10 mL of DMEM + 10% FBS.
2. Equilibrate the sieve with sterile ddH$_2$O.
3. Filter the resuspension through the sieve to remove pieces of tissue and collect the filtrate in a Petri dish.

4. If you have more than one sample, wash the sieve with sterile ddH$_2$O to remove the leftover tissue before filtering the next sample.
5. Centrifuge the filtrate at 800g for 10 min.

3.2.5. Gradient

1. Remove the supernatant by vacuum pipet and resuspend the pellet in 10 mL of DMEM + 10% FBS.
2. Add 5 mL of the lymphocyte separation media to a 15-mL conical tube.
3. Carefully layer the resuspended cells over the separation media.
4. Centrifuge at 1000g for 30 min with the brake off.
5. Collect the white band of cells with a transfer pipet and transfer to a 15-mL conical tube.
6. Wash the cells with 10 mL DMEM + 10% FBS and centrifuge at 800g for 10 min.

3.2.6. Culture

1. Remove the supernatant by vacuum pipette and resuspend the pellet in 5–10 mL of MEM with D-val + 10% HS depending on the size of the pellet (see **Note 4**).
2. Plate the cells in either a 25-cm^2 or a 75-cm^2 flask depending on the size of the pellet.
3. Remove any unattached cells the following day and add fresh MEM with D-val + 10% HS.

3.2.7. Characterization

Trophoblast cells should be cytokeratin 7$^+$/vimentin-/CD45-.

3.3. Preparation of Apoptotic Trophoblast Cells

The SVneo transformed first trimester human extravillous trophoblast cell line, HTR8 (**18**), hereafter referred to as H8, was a gift from Dr. Charles Graham (Queen's University, Kingston, ON, Canada).

3.3.1. Treatment of Trophoblast Cells With Camptothecin

1. Resuspend trophoblast cells in RPMI/10% FBS and seed 2×10^6 cells in 100 mm tissue culture Petri dishes. At this time also plate 2×10^5 of trophoblast cells in a tissue culture chamber slide (see **Note 5**).
2. Culture at 37°C for 18–24 h, after which time cells should be 70–80% confluent.
3. Remove media from the cells and replace with OptiMEM containing 4 μM camptothecin.
4. Culture at 37°C for 24 h.

3.3.2. Evaluation of Trophoblast Cell Apoptosis

1. Check cells in chamber slide by microscopy. A large number should be unattached.
2. Without removing the unattached cells, to the culture media add 1 μL propridium iodide at 1 μg/mL and 1 μL Hoechst 33342 dye at 5 μg/mL.

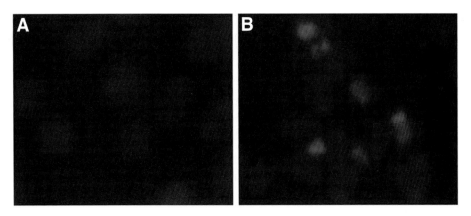

Fig. 3 (*see* companion CD for color version). Trophoblast cells stained with Hoechst 33342 dye. **(A)** Untreated trophoblasts **(B)** Trophoblast cells undergoing apoptosis.

3. Incubate cells at room temperature in the dark for 15 min.
4. Evaluate the number of apoptotic cells by fluorescence microscopy (*see* **Note 6**). Viable cells will be negative for propidium iodide and positive for Hoechst 33342 dye (**Fig. 3A**). Apoptotic cells will stain positive for both propidium iodide and Hoechst 33342 dye and the Hoechst staining of the nucleus will be condensed and intense (**Fig. 3B**).

3.3.3. Collection of Apoptotic Trophoblast Cells

1. Harvest apoptotic trophoblast cells by passing a cell scraper gently over the dish once and collecting all cells, transferring them into a 15-mL tube.
2. Centrifuge cells at 800g and room temperature for 10 min and aspirate off the supernatant.
3. Resuspend cells in 10 mL OptiMEM containing 10 ng/mL PMA

3.4. Macrophage and Apoptotic Trophoblast Co-Culture In Vitro

3.4.1. Co-Culture Experiment for Monitoring Macrophage Phagocytosis of Apoptotic Cells (*Fig. 4*)

1. In tissue culture chamber slides, prepare 2×10^5 macrophages (*see* **Subheading 3.1.**).
2. Prepare apoptotic trophoblast cells (*see* **Section 3.2.**).
3. Wash macrophages three times with PBS and then to cells add 200 µL of PKH26 red fluorescent cell linker dye at 0.04 µM.
4. Incubate at room temperature for 5 min and then add 200 µL of RPMI/10% FBS.
5. Wash cells three times with 1 mL of RPMI/10% FBS.
6. Add 1 mL OptiMEM/10 ng/mL PMA to macrophages and place at 37° while **steps 7–11** are performed.
7. Wash apoptotic trophoblast cells with PBS.

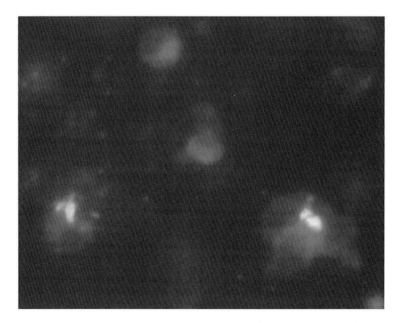

Fig. 4 (*see* companion CD for color version). Phorbol 12-myristate 13-acetate (PMA)-differentiated THP-1 cells (dark) phagocytosing apoptotic trophoblast cells (clear).

8. Resuspend apoptotic trophoblast cells in 1 mL PKH67 green fluorescent cell linker dye at 0.02 μ*M*.
9. Incubate at room temperature for 5 min and add 1 mL of RPMI/10% FBS.
10. Wash apoptotic cells three times with 1 mL of RPMI/10% FBS.
11. Resuspend apoptotic cells in OptiMEM containing 10 ng/mL PMA.
12. Remove media from THP-1 cells and add 1×10^6 apoptotic trophoblast cells (1:5 ratio).
13. Incubate at 37°C for 3 h and visualize by fluorescent confocal microscopy.

3.4.2. Co-Culture Experiment for Collection of Macrophage Conditioned Media

1. Resuspend apoptotic trophoblast cells in OptiMEM containing 10 ng/mL PMA.
2. Remove media from macrophages and replace with either 1 mL apoptotic trophoblasts (*see* **Note 7**) or 1 mL OptiMEM containing 10 ng/mL PMA (no treatment control). Also set up macrophage free treatments.
3. Culture at 37°C for 24 h.
4. Collect culture supernatants and remove cells by centrifuging at 1000*g* and 4°C for 10 min.
5. Collect cell-free conditioned media and store at –40°C.

3.5. Treatment of Trophoblast Cells
With Macrophage-Conditioned Media

1. In 60-mm tissue culture Petri dishes seed 8×10^5 of H8 cells in RPMI/10% FBS.
2. Culture cells at 37°C for 18–24 h until cells are 70% confluent.
3. Remove media and replace with 2 mL OptiMEM and culture for 18 h.
4. Remove media and replace with 1 mL of fresh OptiMEM.
5. Add 1 mL of treatments: OptiMEM as a no treatment control, camptothecin (8 μM) as a positive control or macrophage conditioned media.
6. Culture at 37°C for 48 h.
7. Prepare trophoblast cell lysates (*see* **Subheading 3.6.1.**)

3.6. Evaluation of the Effect of Macrophage-Conditioned Media on Trophoblast Cell Survival

3.6.1. Preparation of Trophoblast Cell Lysate

1. Using a cell scraper, detach all adherent cells.
2. Transfer all cells to a 15-mL tube and add 5 mL of cold PBS.
3. Centrifuge cells at 800g and 4°C for 10 min and remove the supernatant.
4. Resuspend cell pellet in 100 µL of lysis buffer containing 2 µL PMSF and 2 µL PIC.
5. Incubate on ice for 20 min and then centrifuge at 10,000g and 4°C for 15 min.
6. Collect the supernatant into a fresh Eppendorf tube and add 2 µL PMSF and 2 µL PIC.
7. Test protein concentration using the BCA assay and store at –40°C.

3.6.2. Western Blot Analysis for Caspase and XIAP Activation

The effect of macrophage conditioned media on trophoblast cell survival can be determined by evaluating the activation status of XIAP, an inhibitor of apoptosis and the activation of caspase-3, the effector caspase critical for apoptosis, by using Western blot analysis (**Fig. 5**).

3.6.2.1. GEL PREPARATION (*SEE* **NOTE 8**)

1. Prepare the lower gel:
2. Load 7 mL for each gel immediately and slowly layer 500 µL ddH$_2$O on top of each gel.
3. Allow the gel to polymerize for about 30 min.
4. Prepare the upper gel.
5. Remove water from lower gels and immediately add upper gel.
6. Position combs and allow upper gel to polymerize for about 30 min.

3.6.2.2. SAMPLE PREPARATION

1. Adjust the protein concentration of all samples to 25 µg in 20 µL using dH$_2$O and to this add 10 µL of 3X sample buffer.
2. Boil samples for 5 min and then centrifuge for a few seconds.
3. Place on ice.

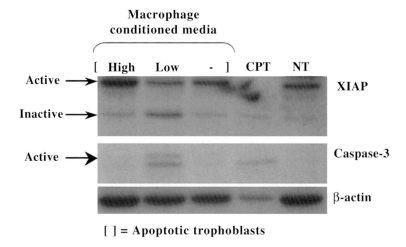

Macrophage conditioned media

[ ] = Apoptotic trophoblasts

Fig. 5. Conditioned media collected from macrophages co-cultured with high levels of apoptotic cells results in the inactivation of XIAP and activation of caspase-3 in trophoblast cells. Only the active form of XIAP is expressed by trophoblast cells treated with conditioned media collected from macrophages that were co-cultured with low levels of apoptotic cells

3.6.2.3. RUNNING GELS

1. Place gels in gel box and fill the inner and outer chamber with 1X running buffer.
2. Remove combs (*see* **Note 9**) and load 25 µL of sample to each lane.
3. Run gels at 100 V.
4. Meanwhile, cut PDVF membranes (9 × 6 cm) and filter paper (10 × 7 cm) and prepare fresh transfer buffer. Keep the buffer at –20°C until needed.

3.6.2.4. TRANSFER

1. Wash membranes for a few seconds in methanol to remove coating and then wash with dH$_2$O for 5 min.
2. Place membranes and sponges in transfer buffer.
3. Remove the gels from the glass plates and carefully transfer them into a container with transfer buffer.
4. For the transfer, prepare a sandwich as follows: sponge–filter paper–gel–membrane–filter paper–sponge (*see* **Note 10**).
5. Place in transfer box and fill with transfer buffer and run at 32 V overnight.

3.6.2.5. IMMUNOBLOTTING

1. Following transfer, stain membranes in Ponceau red to visualize proteins.
2. Wash membranes with dH$_2$O and then block in 5% milk/PBS-Tween for 1 h at room temperature.

3. Wash membranes three times for 10 min with PBS-Tween.
4. Incubate membranes overnight in primary antibody made up in 1% milk/PBS-Tween at 4°C with constant motion.
5. Wash membranes three times for 10 min with PBS-Tween.
6. Incubate membranes for 1 h at room temperature with secondary antibody made up in 1% milk/PBS-Tween.

3.6.2.6. DEVELOPING

1. Wash membranes three times for 10 min with PBS-Tween and three times for 10 min in dH$_2$O.
2. Remove fluid from membrane and add enhanced chemiluminescence (ECL), making sure that the membrane is fully covered.
3. Incubate for 1 min.
4. Place membranes between transparent sheets and ensure that all air bubbles are pushed away from the membrane.
5. Expose to film and develop.

3.6.3. Measuring Caspase Activity

Although Western blot analysis is a powerful tool for evaluating the activation of the apoptotic pathway, caspase activation does not necessarily equate to caspase activity. Furthermore, Western blot analysis is, at best, semi-quantitative. Therefore, to confirm Western blot results and to quantify caspase activation, the luciferacse-based luminescent Caspase-Glow assay can be used to measure caspase-3 activity.

1. Adjust cell lysate protein concentrations to 10 µg/50 µL using dH$_2$O and transfer 50 µL to polyprolylene tubes for luminometer.
2. Add 50 µL Caspase-Glow 3/7 substrate and mix gently (*see* **Note 11**).
3. Incubate at room temperature in the dark for 1 h.
4. Measure luminescence of each sample using a single sample luminometer.

4. Notes

1. If the PMA is removed once the monocytes have differentiated into macrophages, cells will undergo apoptosis. Therefore, PMA should be present throughout the experiment.
2. During the 72-h incubation, the media will most likely become yellow. As this occurs remove the media and replace with fresh RPMI/10% FBS containing 10 ng/mL PMA.
3. HBSS must be without calcium and magnesium, which inhibit trypsin.
4. Trophoblast cells are cultured in MEM with D-valine because fibroblasts can only grow in L-valine.
5. The trophoblast cells seeded in the chamber slides will allow the extent of cell death to be determined prior to collecting the apoptotic trophoblast cells.
6. Unattached cells will be apoptotic. However, cells still attached are not necessarily viable. The propidium iodide/Hoechst staining should reveal the majority of

attached cells to be undergoing apoptosis. If this is not the case, then continue to culture the trophoblast cells with camptothecin for longer.

7. The ratio of macrophages: trophoblasts will depend on whether the experiment warrants high or low levels of apoptotic cells. For example, a 1:5 ratio would represent high levels of apoptotic cells.

8. The concentrations indicated are for preparing two mini gels. Add the 10% ammonium persulphate and TEMED last just before loading.

9. It is important to fill up the chamber with buffer prior of removing the combs in order to prevent the collapse of the wells.

10. It is important to remove any air bubbles between each layer because these will interfere with the transfer of proteins from the gel to the membrane.

11. Do not vortex the Caspase-Glow 3/7 substrate, because this will affect its activity.

References

1. Fadok, V. A. and Chimini, G. (2001) The phagocytosis of apoptotic cells. *Semin. Immunol.* **13,** 365–372.

2. Savill, J. and Fadok, V. (2000) Corpse clearance defines the meaning of cell death. *Nature* **407,** 784–788.

3. Piacentini, M. and Autuori, F. (1994) Immunohistochemical localization of tissue transglutaminase and Bcl-2 in rat uterine tissues during embryo implantation and post-partum involution. *Differentiation* **57,** 51–61.

4. Savill, J., Dransfield, I., Gregory, C., and Haslett, C. (2002) A blast from the past: clearance of apoptotic cells regulates immune responses. *Nat. Rev. Immunol.* **2,** 965–975.

5. De, M. and Wood, G. W. (1990) Influence of oestrogen and progesterone on macrophage distribution in the mouse uterus. *J. Endocrinol.* **126,** 417–424.

6. Miller, L. and Hunt, J. (1996) Sex steroids hormones and macrophage function. *Life Sciences* **59,** 1–14.

7. Tachi, C. and Tachi, S. (1986) Macrophages and implantation. *Ann. NY Acad. Sci.* **476,** 158–182.

8. Ben-Hur, H., Gurevich, P., Berman, V., Tchanyshev, R., Gurevich, E., and Zusman, I. (2001) The secretory immune system as part of the placental barrier in the second trimester of pregnancy in humans. *In Vivo* **15,** 429–435.

9. Hunt, J. (1989) Cytokine networks in the uteroplacental unit: Macrophages as pivotal regulatory cells. *J. Reprod. Immunol.* **16,** 1–17.

10. Reiter, I., Krammer, B., and Schwamberger, G. (1999) Differential effect of apoptotic versus necrotic tumor cells on macrophage antitumor activities. *J. Immunol.* **163,** 1730–1732.

11. Cavaillon, J.M. (1994) Cytokines and macrophages. *Biomed. Pharmacother.* **48,** 445–453.

12. Abrahams, V. M., Kim, Y. M., Straszewski, S. L., Romero, R., and Mor, G. (2004) Macrophages and apoptotic cell clearance during pregnancy. *Am. J. Reprod. Immunol.* **51,** 275–282.

13. Voll, R. E., Herrmann, M., Roth, E. A., Stach, C., Kalden, J. R., and Girkontaite, I. (1997) Immunosuppressive effects of apoptotic cells. *Nature* **390,** 350–351.
14. Pijnenborg, R., McLaughlin, P. J., Vercruysse, L., et al. (1998) Immunolocalization of tumour necrosis factor-alpha (TNF-alpha) in the placental bed of normotensive and hypertensive human pregnancies. *Placenta* **19,** 231–239.
15. Reister, F., Frank, H. G., Kingdom, J. C., et al. (2001) Macrophage-induced apoptosis limits endovascular trophoblast invasion in the uterine wall of preeclamptic women. *Lab. Invest.* **81,** 1143–1152.
16. Mor, G. and Abrahams, V. (2003) Potential role of macrophages as immunoregulators of pregnancy. *Reprod. Biol. Endocrinol.* **1,** 119 (http://www.rbej.com/content/1/1/119).
17. Huynh, M. L., Fadok, V. A., and Henson, P. M. (2002) Phosphatidylserine-dependent ingestion of apoptotic cells promotes TGF-beta1 secretion and the resolution of inflammation. *J. Clin. Invest.* **109,** 41–50.
18. Graham, C. H., Hawley, T. S., Hawley, R. G., et al. (1993) Establishment and characterization of first trimester human trophoblast cells with extended lifespan. *Exp. Cell. Res.* **206,** 204–211.

10

Methods for Evaluating Histocompatibility Antigen Gene Expression in the Baboon

Daudi K. Langat, Asgerally T. Fazleabas, and Joan S. Hunt

Summary

A wide variety of techniques has been developed for qualitative and quantitative analysis of gene expression in human cells and tissues. Two commonly used methods are reverse-transcription (RT)-polymerase chain reaction (PCR) to analyze the transcribed messenger RNAs (mRNA) and immunohistochemistry to detect the translated proteins. These techniques can be modified and adapted for use in analyzing gene expression in animal models. In particular, as a result of the close phylogenetic relationship between humans and nonhuman primates, human reagents, especially antibodies, cross-react with nonhuman primate tissues. However, the results are not always satisfactory as some antibodies may cross-react with irrelevant antigens in these tissues. In this chapter, we describe the use of RT-PCR and immunohistochemical techniques to analyze expression of Paan-AG, a novel class Ib major histocompatibility complex antigen in the olive baboon (*Papio anubis*) placenta. We used Paan-AG-specific primers to amplify Paan-AG transcripts from baboon placenta, and generated Paan-AG isoform-specific polyclonal antibodies for use in immunohistochemistry.

Key Words: Baboon; MHC; placenta; nonhuman primate; RT-PCR; immunohistochemistry.

1. Introduction

Nonhuman primates are important models to study human disease or biology because they share a high degree of similarity with humans. They have been widely used in studies of human infectious diseases, neurological disorders, vaccine development, and transplantation biology *(1)*. For an experimental animal to be a good model, the genetic make-up needs to be studied in detail. In this respect, the major histocompatibility complex (MHC) has received much attention, mainly because of its central role in modulating the immune system. The MHC loci in different species of non-human primates have been described *(2–5)*. They show a high degree of similarity with their human counterparts as shown by their clustering by locus and/or lineage and by the sharing of similar peptide-binding profiles *(5–7)*.

From: *Methods in Molecular Medicine, Vol. 122: Placenta and Trophoblast: Methods and Protocols, Vol. 2*
Edited by: M. J. Soares and J. S. Hunt © Humana Press Inc., Totowa, NJ

The most common techniques used in MHC studies are reverse-transcription (RT)-polymerase chain reaction (PCR) to analyze the messages, and immunohistochemistry to analyze protein expression. Oligonucleotide primers that are used to amplify human MHC loci using PCR have been successfully used to amplify their nonhuman primate homologs *(8–10)*. However, although antibodies that are used in human studies cross-react with nonhuman primate tissues, the results are not always satisfactory. Our preliminary studies showed that some antibodies, such as 87G, a human leukocyte antigen (HLA)-G- specific monoclonal antibody, cross-reacted nonspecifically with multiple baboon tissues (Langat, D. K., Morales, P. J., Fazleabas, A. T., Hunt, J. S., unpublished data).

We and others have utilized RT-PCR and immunohistochemistry to identify MHC class I molecules expressed in baboon placenta *(8,11)*. In this chapter, we describe the techniques we used to characterize *Paan-AG*, a novel baboon class Ib gene that possesses characteristics of the human class Ib gene, *HLA-G*, and is expressed in the baboon placenta *(11)*. We used Paan-AG specific primers to amplify Paan-AG messages and generated Paan-AG isoform-specific polyclonal antibodies for immunohistochemical studies to determine the pattern of protein expression of this gene in baboon tissues *(11)*. In addition, strategies for amplifying other baboon class I genes are discussed.

2. Materials

2.1. RNA Isolation, Reverse Transcription, and Polymerase Chain Reaction

1. Trizol Reagent (Invitrogen, Carlsbad, CA, cat. no. 15596-018), store at 4°C.
2. Total RNA samples, stored at –80°C.
3. RT-PCR reagents, stored at –20°C:
   a. Moloney-murine leukemia virus reverse transcriptase (MMLV-RTase), 200 U/ μL (Invitrogen, cat. no. 28025-013).
   b. 5X First Strand buffer (Invitrogen, cat. no. Y00146, comes with MMLV-RT enzyme).
   c. 0.1 *M* Dithiothreitol (Invitrogen, cat. no. Y00147, comes with MMLV-RT enzyme).
   d. RNase inhibitor (RNasin, Promega, cat. no. N2511, 40 U/μL).
   e. Oligo d(T)$_{12–18}$, (0.5 μg/μL) (Invitrogen, cat. no. 18418-012).
   f. Deoxynucleotide triphosphate (dNTP) mix, 10 m*M* (Invitrogen, cat. no. 18427-013).
   g. *Taq* DNA polymerase (Invitrogen, cat. no. 10342-020).
   h. 10X PCR buffer minus Mg (Invitrogen, cat. no. Y02028, comes with *Taq* enzyme).
   i. 50 m*M* MgCl$_2$ (Invitrogen, cat. no. Y02016, comes with *Taq* enzyme).

4. MicroAmp 200-µL thin-walled PCR tubes (PE Applied Biosystems, Foster City, CA, cat. no. N801-0540).
5. Autoclaved water containing 0.1% diethyl pyrocarbonate (DEPC-H_2O) for diluting RNA samples, and sterile water for PCR (e.g. Sterile water for irrigation, Baxter Healthcare Corp., Deerfield, IL).
6. Deoxyribonuclease I (DNAse I) reagents, available as a kit (cat. no. AMP-DI, Sigma, St. Louis, MO) containing the following):
   a. Amplification grade DNAse I (cat. no. 5307, 1 U/µL).
   b. 10X Reaction buffer (cat. no. R6273, 200 mM Tris-HCl, pH 8.3, 20 mM $MgCl_2$).
   c. Stop solution: 50 mM ethylenediamine tetraacetic acid (EDTA) (cat. no. S4809).
7. Primers for PCR, custom-synthesized (*see* **Notes 1** and **2**). Reconstitute the lyophilized samples to 100 µM stocks in 10 mM Tris-HCl, pH 8.0. Make 20-µM working dilutions (100 µL each) with sterile water and store at –20°C.
8. Reagents for agarose gel analysis of DNA products: Agarose:Nusieve (3:1) (Amresco Inc., Solon, OH, cat. no. E776); 50X Tris-Acetate-EDTA (TAE) buffer; DNA molecular weight marker (Invitrogen, cat. no. 15615-016); 6X tracking dye/loading buffer; ethidium bromide, 10 mg/mL (Sigma, cat. no. E-1510).
9. Thermocycler.
10. Electrophoresis unit.
11. Ultraviolet (UV) transilluminator.
12. Polaroid camera.

2.2. Extraction and Sequencing of the PCR Products

1. QIAquick Gel Extraction Kit (Qiagen Inc., Valencia, CA, cat. no. 28704).
2. 3 M Sodium acetate, pH 5.2.
3. GenElute LPA Reagent (5 mg/mL, Sigma, cat. no. 5-6575).
4. Ethanol (100%, 70%).
5. ABI 377 Prism™ Sequencer (PE Applied Biosystems).
6. ABI Prism dRhodamine Terminator Cycle-Sequencing Ready Reaction Kit (PE Applied Biosystems, cat. no. 403044).

2.3. Antibody Production and Purification

1. Appropriate animal host (chickens, goat, etc.).
2. Peptides for use as immunogens. We used 10 amino acid peptides corresponding to unique portions of Paan-AG1, Paan-AG2, and soluble Paan-AG1 (*see* **Fig. 1** for the sequence and location of each peptide). Each peptide was linked to Keyhole Limpet Hemocyanin to increase immunogenicity.
3. EGGstract® immunoglobulin (Ig)Y Purification System kit (Promega Corp., Madison, WI, cat. no. G1531), used to isolate IgY antibodies from egg yolk.
4. UltraLink™ EDC/Diaminodipropylamine Immobilization Kit (Pierce, Rockford, IL, cat. no. 53154), used for affinity purification of antibodies.

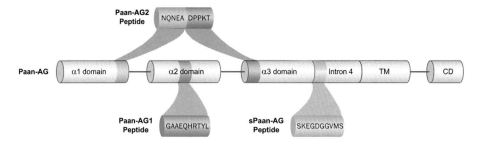

Fig. 1. Location and sequence of the peptides used to generate anti-Paan-AG antibodies (anti-Paan-AG1, anti-Paan-AG2 and anti-sPaan-AG1) on the full-length Paan-AG protein. α1, α2, α3, external domains; TM, transmembrane region; CD, cytoplasmic domain.

2.4. Enzyme-Linked Immunosorbent Assay

1. SureBlue™ TMB 1-Component Microwell Peroxidase Substrate (0.02% hydrogen peroxide, with 0.4 g/L 3,3',5,5'-tetramethylbenzidine chromogen (Kirkegaard & Perry Laboratories, Gaithersburg, MD, cat. no. 52-00-00).
2. Enzyme-linked immunosorbent assay (ELISA) plates (Costar®, Corning Inc., Corning, NY).
3. Non-fat dry milk, blotting grade (Bio-Rad, Hercules, CA, cat. no. 170-6404).
4. Negative control antibodies: chicken IgY (Promega Corp., cat. no. G1161) and goat IgG (Sigma, cat. no. I5256).
5. Horseradish peroxidase (HRP)-conjugated secondary antibodies: HRP-anti-chicken IgY (Promega Corp., cat. no. G135A,), HRP-anti-goat IgG (Jackson ImmunoResearch Lab Inc., West Groove, PA, cat. no. 305-035-045).
6. 1 *M* Phosphoric acid (H_3PO_4).
7. ELISA reader, with a 450-nm filter.
8. Buffers: phosphate-buffered saline (PBS), pH 7.4 (for dilutions), and Tris-buffered saline, pH 8.0, containing 0.05% Tween-20 (TBS-T, wash buffer).

2.5. Immunohistochemistry

1. 4% Paraformaldehyde in 70 m*M* phosphate buffer (*see* **Note 3**).
2. Histo-Processor (e.g., Fisher Histo-Processor, Fisher Scientific, Pittsburgh, PA).
3. Microtome (e.g., 820 Spencer Microtome, American Optical, Buffalo, NY).
4. Microscope slides (e.g., Superfrost®/Plus microscope slides, Fisher Scientific, Pittsburgh, PA).
5. Ethanol (50%, 70%, 90%, 95%, 100%).
6. Histo-Clear (National Diagnostics, Atlanta, GA, cat. no. HS-200).
7. Blocking Reagent: 10% normal horse serum (Sigma, cat. no. H0146) or normal rabbit serum (Sigma, R9133).
8. Wash buffer: PBS, pH 7.4, containing 0.3% Tween-20.

9. Negative control antibodies: chicken IgY (Promega Corp., cat. no. G1161) and goat IgG (Sigma, cat. no. I5256).
10. Biotin-labeled secondary antibodies: rabbit anti-chicken IgY (Promega Corp., cat. no. G2891), horse anti-goat IgG (Vector Laboratories, Burlingame, CA, cat. no. BA9500).
11. Streptoavidin-labeled peroxidase enzyme (Zymed Laboratories Inc., San Francisco, CA, cat. no. 50-242).
12. Aminoethyl cabarzole substrate kit (Zymed Labs Inc., cat. no. 00-2007).
13. Mayer's hematoxylin (Sigma, cat. no. 51275).
14. Crystal Mount (Biomeda Corp., Foster City, CA).
15. Permount (Fisher Scientific).

3. Methods

3.1. RNA Isolation, Reverse Transcription, and Polymerase Chain Reaction

1. Obtain fresh placental tissue, cut into small pieces (<0.5 cm^3) and immediately perform RNA extraction. Alternatively, wrap the tissues in sterile aluminium foil and immerse in liquid nitrogen for 10 min, then store the tissue at $-80°C$.
2. Isolate total RNA from placental tissue using Trizol® Reagent, following manufacturer's protocols, then measure the RNA concentration using a spectrophotometer at a wavelength of 260 nm. One A_{260} unit is equal to 40 µg of RNA. Store the RNA at $-70°C$ until required for PCR.
3. Thaw RNA sample on ice. Heat at $55–60°C$ for 10 min, then place immediately on ice.
4. Add to an RNAse-free PCR tube on ice: 1 µg RNA sample in 8 µL sterile water, 1 µL 10X reaction buffer and 1 µL amplification grade DNase I, 1 U/µL. Prepare duplicate tubes for reactions with and without reverse transcriptase. Incubate this for 15 min at room temperature.
5. Add 1 µL of stop solution to bind calcium and magnesium and to inactivate the DNase I, followed by heating at $70°C$ for 10 min to denature both DNase and the RNA. Chill on ice.
6. Prepare RT reaction cocktail containing the following: 8 µL 5X First Strand buffer, 4 µL dithiothreitol, 2 µL dNTP, 2 µL RNase inhibitor, 2 µL Oligo d(T)$_{12–18}$ and 2 µL MMLV RTase, made up to 29 µL with sterile water, per sample. Also make a cocktail without RTase to be used as a control for each RNA preparation sample
7. Add 29 µL reaction cocktail to each tube in **step 5**.
8. Mix well; spin briefly in a microcentrifuge ($16,000g$ for 1 min) to settle contents.
9. Incubate 10 min at $25°C$, 1 h at $37°C$, 5 min at $99°C$ and 5 min at $5°C$ (use thermocycler in all incubations) (*see* **Note 4**).
10. Proceed immediately with PCR reaction, or store the RT reaction products at $-80°C$ (can be stored for short-term at $-20°C$).
11. Prepare a PCR cocktail by mixing the following reagents (amounts indicated are per sample) as follows: 5 µL 10X PCR buffer, 1 µL dNTP, 1 µL MgCl$_2$, 0.5 µL

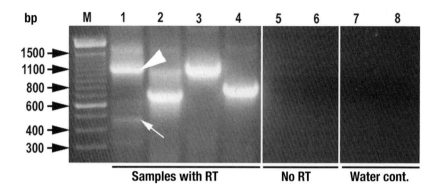

Fig. 2. A typical polymerase chain reaction (PCR) experiment to amplify mRNAs from total RNA, with the required controls included. Paan-AG transcripts were amplified from cDNA synthesized from baboon term placenta RNA using primers that amplify all the alternatively spliced transcripts of Paan-AG (bG7-26F and bG1078-1099R, **lane 1**). The arrowhead shows the full-length transcript (Paan-AG1), whereas the small arrow indicates the location of Paan-AG3. The other alternatively spliced transcripts are faint. The rest of the lanes (**lanes 2–8**) represent positive and negative controls for this experiment. **Lanes 2, 6,** and **8** represent amplification of placenta cDNA with actin primers, using placental cDNA (**lane 2**) or "mock-reverse transcribed cDNA" (reverse transcription without transcriptase enzyme, **lane 6**) as template, and substituting template with water (**lane 8**). **Lanes 3, 4, 5,** and **7** shows PCR with bG7-26/bG1078-1099 primers, using plasmid DNA containing either sPaan-AG1 (**lane 3**) or Paan-AG2 (**lane 4**) as positive control templates, and using "mock-reverse transcribed cDNA" (**lane 5**) and substituting template with water (**lane 7**) as negative controls (*see* **Note 4** for further information).

each of the forward and reverse primers (stock is 20 μ*M*), 37.6 μL sterile water and 0.4 μL *Taq* polymerase. Add 4 μL of cDNA and 46 μL of the PCR cocktail to a PCR tube. Include appropriate positive and negative controls (*see* **Note 5**).

12. Mix well; centrifuge briefly in a microcentrifuge (16,000*g* for 1 min) to settle contents.

13. Incubate in the thermocycler: 94°C for 1 min, followed by 30 cycles of denaturation at 94°C for 45 s, annealing at the appropriate temperature (*see* **Notes 6** and **7**) for 30 s and extension at 72°C for 2 min, and a final extension at 72°C for 10 min, then cool the PCR products to 4°C.

14. Mix the whole 50 μL each PCR reaction with 10 μL 6X dye-gel loading buffer and load all 60 μL per well of a 3% agarose gel, containing 0.1 μg/mL ethidium bromide. Load 10 μL of DNA molecular weight marker in one of the wells, and perform the electrophoresis for 1–2 h at 100 volts (**Fig. 2**).

3.2. Extraction and Sequencing of the PCR Products

1. Cut off each of the amplified product bands and extract it from the agarose gel using the QIAquick Gel Extraction kit, following the manufacturer's instructions (*see* **Note 8**).
2. To concentrate the eluted DNA, precipitate the DNA as follows: Add 0.1 vol of 3 M sodium acetate, pH 5.2, to each sample, and vortex.
3. Add 2 µL of GenElute LPA reagent to each tube and vortex (*see* **Note 9**).
4. Add 2.5 vol of 100% ethanol to precipitate the DNA, vortex and centrifuge for 10 min at maximum speed (16,000g) in a microcentrifuge at 4°C.
5. Remove supernatant, air-dry the pellet for 5–10 min, and then wash by adding 1 mL of 70% ethanol followed by centrifugation for 10 min at 4°C.
6. Remove supernatant, air-dry the pellet and redissolve in 20 µL sterile water, then determine the concentration with a spectrophotometer at 260 nm. One A_{260} unit is equal to 50 µg of DNA. The sample is now ready for sequencing (*see* **Note 10**).
7. Sequence the samples using the PCR primers or clone them into an appropriate plasmid and sequence using plasmid-specific primers *(11)*. For a 10-µL reaction, add 2 µL of Terminator-Ready Mix, 3.2 pmol of primer, 500 ng of sample plasmid DNA (if cloned) or 30–90 ng PCR product, and water (to a total of 10 µL) to a 200-µL PCR tube.
8. Mix the reagents by vortexing, then centrifuge briefly (16,000g, 1 min) and place in a thermocycler. Perform the sequence reaction for 25 cycles using the following conditions: denaturation at 96°C for 10 s, annealing at 50°C for 5 s, and extension at 60°C for 4 min.
9. Transfer the sequence reactions to a 1.5-mL chilled Eppendorf tube and add 2 µL of 3 M sodium acetate, pH 5.2 and 50 µL of 95% ethanol.
10. Place the samples on ice for 10 min to precipitate the extension products, then centrifuge for 30 min at maximum speed (16,000g) in a microcentrifuge at 4°C.
11. Wash the pellet with 250 µL of 70% ethanol and centrifuge for 10 min at 16,000g in a microcentrifuge at 4°C.
12. Discard the supernatant and air-dry the pellets for 10 min at room temperature, then resuspend in 4 µL gel-loading buffer (deionized formamide, containing 25 mM EDTA, pH 8.0, and 50 mg/mL blue dextran), vortex briefly and centrifuge for 1 min at 16,000g to settle the contents.
13. Heat the samples to 97°C for 2 min to denature the DNA, then chill in ice. Load 2 µL of each sample onto a 4.75% 0.2-mm vertical slab polyacrylamide sequencing gel (48 cm long) and perform the electrophoresis overnight in an ABI 377 sequencer. Analyze the sequence data using appropriate software (e.g., EditSeq and MegALIGN, DNAStar Inc., Madison, WI).

3.3. Antibody Production and Purification

The immunization protocols that we use to obtain antibodies in chickens and goats are similar. They differ only in the number of booster injections given and the method of collecting the antibodies (from eggs and serum in chicken and from serum in goat). The protocol below describes antibody production in the chicken, with information pertaining to the goat in parentheses.

1. Collect 2 mL pre-immune serum from 2 chickens (5 mL from goat), followed by an intra-muscular injection with 0.5 mg KLH-peptide (subcutaneous injection of 2 mg peptide in goat, **Fig. 1**) emulsified in Freund's complete adjuvant (FCA; day 1).
2. Boost the immunization after 1 wk by an intra-muscular injection of 0.5 mg of KLH-peptide emulsified in Freund's incomplete adjuvant (FIA) (1 mg of KLH-peptide in FIA in the goat at 3-wk intervals, for a total of four boosters. The first booster subcutaneous, the rest intramuscular).
3. Collect 2 mL immune serum (5 mL for goat) 1 wk after each booster injection, for antibody titer determination.
4. Collect eggs daily from day 21 for 1 wk.
5. Give a second booster injection on day 42, and collect eggs for 1 wk from day 48 (production bleeds for the goat obtained on days 73, 94, and 115).
6. On day 55, euthanize the chicken and perform a terminal bleed (terminal bleed obtained from goat at day 118).
7. Extract the total IgY antibodies from the egg yolk using the EGGstract IgY Purification System kit, following manufacturer's recommendations.
8. Isolate peptide-specific antibodies from the total IgY antibody isolate (or from goat serum) by affinity purification with peptide-coated antibody purification columns such as the UltraLink™ EDC/Diaminodipropylamine Immobilization Kit (Pierce).
9. Test the specificity of the purified antibodies by ELISA, described later.

3.4. Enzyme-Linked Immunosorbent Assay

1. Coat 96-well ELISA plates with 10 µg/mL of recombinant HLA-G5, HLA-G6, the peptide used to generate the antibody (positive control) and the glutathione-S-transferase (GST) fusion protein used in the generation of recombinant HLA-G5 and HLA-G6 (negative control, 50 µL per well) overnight at 4°C (*see* **Note 11**).
2. Block nonspecific binding for 1 h at room temperature using 5% fat-free skim milk in PBS, pH 7.2 (200 µL per well).
3. Wash four times with 200 µL per well using TBS-T, pH 8.0.
4. Dilute the eluted antibody to obtain concentrations varying between 1 µg/mL and 20 µg/mL, using blocking buffer. Dilute the negative control antibodies (chicken IgY or goat IgG) similarly. Add 50 µL of the diluted antibody or controls to each well and incubate for 30 min at 37°C.
5. Wash the plates as described above, and then add 50 µL of the appropriate secondary antibody diluted 1:1000, and incubate for 30 min at 37°C.
6. Wash as described above, and then incubate the plates with 100 µL of substrate for 15 min at room temperature.
7. Stop the reaction by adding 50 µL per well of 1 M H_3PO_4.
8. Read the optical density of each well at a wavelength of 450 nm using an ELISA reader, and analyze the results (**Fig. 3**).

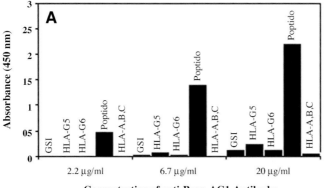

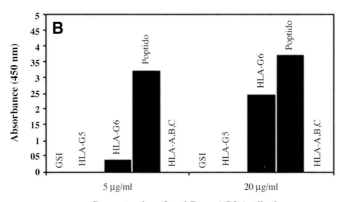

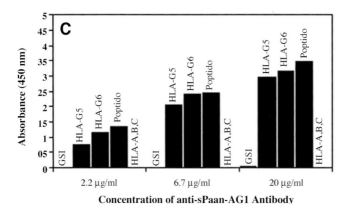

Fig. 3. Summary of the reactivities of **(A)** anti-Paan-AG1, **(B)** anti-Paan-AG2 and **(C)** anti-sPaan-AG1 antibodies with recombinant soluble Human Leukocyte Antigen (HLA)-G proteins using an enzyme-linked immunosorbent assay (ELISA). The ELISA plates were coated with 10 μg/mL of glutathione-*S*-transferase (GST) protein and HLA-A,B,C (class Ia) protein mixture as negative controls, the peptide used for immunization as a positive control, or recombinant HLA-G5 or HLA-G6 proteins.

3.5. Immunohistochemistry

1. Fix the placental and other tissues (<0.5 cm^3) overnight in 4% paraformaldehyde at 4°C.
2. Dehydrate the tissues in increasing concentrations of ethanol (50%, 70%, 90%, 95%) for 30 min each, then in absolute ethanol (100%) repeated twice for 30 min each time.
3. Immerse the tissues in Histo-Clear (with two changes) for 30 min each, and then embed in paraffin wax for 1 h using a Histo-Processor (*see* **Note 12**).
4. Cut 5-μm sections using a Microtome, float the sections on warm water (at 40°C), place on precleaned microscope slides and bake overnight at 40°C (or for 1 h at 60°C) in an oven. Store the sections at 4°C until required.
5. Warm the tissue sections to room temperature and immerse in Histo-Clear (with three changes) for 5 min each.
6. Rehydrate the tissue sections by immersing in decreasing concentrations of ethanol (100% ethanol repeated twice, 95%, 80%, 70%, 50%) for 5 min each, then in distilled water for 2 min (*see* **Notes 12** and **13**).
7. Block nonspecific binding for 1 h at room temperature in a moist chamber, using 10% normal serum (*see* **Note 14**).
8. Add the experimental, negative and positive control antibodies diluted in blocking buffer (enough to cover the sections) and incubate for 1 h in a humid chamber at 37°C (*see* **Notes 15** and **16**).
9. Wash the sections three times for 5 min each in wash buffer.
10. Block endogenous peroxidase activity using 0.5% hydrogen peroxide in methanol, for 25 min at room temperature, and then wash as described previously.
11. Incubate the slides with the appropriate biotin-labeled secondary antibody for 30 min.
12. Wash as described previously.
13. Add 100 μL of streptoavidin-labeled peroxidase enzyme and incubate for 10 min.
14. Add 100 μL of substrate and incubate for 5–10 min, until the red color develops sufficiently.
15. Wash the sections three times for 5 min each with distilled water, counter-stain with hematoxylin for 20 s, rinse with tap water and fix overnight at room temperature with Crystal Mount. Add a drop of Permount, place a coverslip and air-dry for 1 h, then examine under a microscope (**Fig. 4**).

4. Notes

1. There are three strategies that may be used to amplify class I MHC by PCR in nonhuman primates where the sequence of the template is unknown:
   a. Use of pan class I primers that anneal to conserved regions in MHC class I, and are expected to amplify all MHC cDNAs *(12)*. These primers anneal to Exon 2 (forward) and exon 5 (reverse), and their sequences are shown in **Table 1**. The PCR products can then be cloned and sequenced. The sequences obtained can then be used as templates to design species-specific primers (*see* **Note 2**).

Anti-cytokeratin   **Anti-sPaan-AG1**

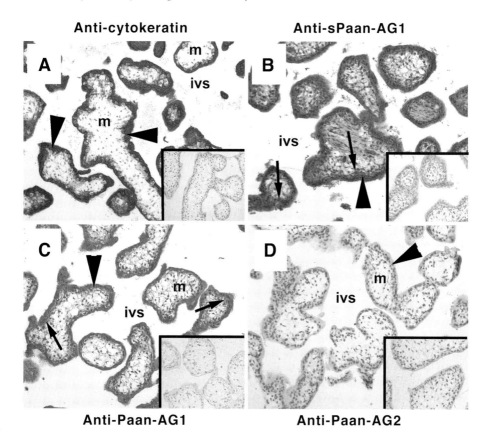

Anti-Paan-AG1   **Anti-Paan-AG2**

Fig. 4. Immunohistochemical localization of soluble and membrane-anchored Paan-AG glycoproteins in first trimester (day 54) baboon placenta. **(A)** Placental villi stained with anti-cytokeratin antibody used as a marker to identify trophoblast cells (arrowheads). **(B–D)** Soluble **(B)** and membrane-anchored **(C)** Paan-AG1 proteins were highly expressed by villous syncytiotrophoblast (arrowheads). The villous cytotrophoblast cells were also labeled but not as strongly as the syncytiotrophoblast (arrows), whereas anti-Paan-AG2 antibody did not label the villi **(D)**. Inset in each picture is the negative control section, stained with isotype control antibodies to confirm specificity of the staining of the test antibodies. m, mesenchymal stroma; ivs, intervillous space. Magnification ×200.

b. Use of locus-specific primers. These primers anneal to the 5' and 3' untranslated regions of class I MHC that flank the coding regions, and selectively amplify all alleles of each locus in HLA *(13)*. These primers have been used to amplify full-length *MHC-A* and *MHC-B* genes from the olive (*Paan-A* and *Paan-B*) and yellow baboons (*Pacy-A* and *Pacy-B*), respectively *(9,10)* (*see* **Table 1** for sequence of the primers).

Table 1
List of Polymerase Chain Reaction Primers Used to Amplify Major Histocompatibility Complex Class I Genes From Baboon Tissues

Name	Sequence	Comment
1.3H3[a]	5'-GCA AGC TTA TGG TGG TCA TGG CGC CCC GAA CC-3'	Exon 1, forward
4.2R1[a]	5'-GCG AAT TCT TTG TCT CTC AAA TTT CAG GA-3'	3'UT, reverse
bG7-26 (F)[b]	5'-CCC TCC TCC TGG TGC TCT CA-3'	Paan-AG-specific, Exon 1, forward
bG1078-1099 (R)[b]	5'-ACA CAA GGC AGC TGT CTC ACA C-3'	Paan-AG-specific, Exon 8, reverse
β-Actin (F)[b]	5'-CAC CCC GTG CTG CTG ACC GAG GCC-3'	forward
β-Actin(R)[b]	5'-CCA CAC GGA GTA CTT GCG CTC AGG-3'	reverse
Pan Class I (F)[c]	5'-TCC CAC TCC ATG AGG TAT TTC-3'	Exon 2, forward
Pan Class I (R)[c]	5'-TCC AGA AGG CAC CAC AG-3'	Exon 5, reverse
HLA5UTA[d]	5'-GCG CGT CGA CCC CAG ACG CCG AGG ATG GCC-3'	HLA-A-specific, 5'UT, forward
HLA3UTA[d]	5'-CCG CAA GCT TTT GGG GAG GGA GCA CAG GTC AGC GTG GGA AG-3'	HLA-A-specific, 5'UT, reverse
HLA5UT[d]	5'-GGG CGT CGA CGG ACT CAG AAT CTC CCC AGA CGC CGA G-3'	HLA specific, 5'UT, forward
HLA3UTB[d]	5'-CCG CAA GCT TCT GGG GAG GAA ACA CAG GTC AGC ATG GGA AC-3'	HLA-B-specific, 3'UT, reverse
HLA3UTC[d]	5'-CCG CAA GCT TTC GGG GAG GGA ACA CAG GTC AGT GTG GGG AC-3'	HLA-C-specific, 3'UT, reverse

HLA, Human Leukocyte Antigen.
[a]Primer sequence from **ref. 8**.
[b]Primer sequence from **ref. 11**.
[c]Primer sequence from **ref. 12**.
[d]Primer sequence from **ref. 13**.

c. Use of multiple sets of primers that amplify HLA loci in humans. Because of the similarity between human and nonhuman primate MHC genes, there is a high probability that human MHC primers would amplify the non-human primate homologous genes. This strategy was initially used to amplify Paan-AG messages from baboon placenta using the HLA-G specific primers 1.3H3 and 4.2R1 *(8)*.

2. In designing PCR primers, the following points should be noted: (a) primers should be 20–25 bases long, (b) the melting temperature of the pair of primers should be matched or differ by only a few degrees, (c) if the sequence of the template is known, the primer sequence at the 3' end of each primer should exactly match the template, (d) the primers should not exhibit intramolecular complementarity to avoid hair-pin formation, (e) the primers should not be complementary at their 3' ends to avoid formation of primer dimers, (f) primers should have an average GC content (40–55%) and should not have consecutive runs of guanines (over 3), and (g) the base distribution should be balanced throughout the primer (as opposed to having a disproportionate density of GC at one end and AT on the other end). For further information, consult the laboratory guide of Farrell *(14)*.

3. To make 4% paraformaldehyde in 70 mM phosphate buffer, dissolve 40 g paraformaldehyde in 600 mL distilled water, stir on a hot plate and heat to steaming (not boiling, 70°C). Add a few drops of 1 N NaOH dropwise until solution clears. Dissolve 4.0 g NaH_2PO_4 and 6.5 g Na_2HPO_4 in 80 mL distilled water. Add to the paraformaldehyde solution, pH 7.0 and make up to 1 L. Store at 4°C and use within 2 wk.

4. The conditions may vary according to the source of reverse transcriptase used. The conditions shown are for MMLV-RT from Invitrogen (see product insert for the recommended conditions for other reverse transcriptase enzymes).

5. Include negative and positive controls for each stage of the PCR reaction. Appropriate negative controls include substituting water for sample (for each pair of primers) to confirm the water and reagents were not contaminated, and using the No-RT sample (sample "mock-reverse transcribed" without the reverse transcriptase) to confirm that there is no genomic DNA contamination. Positive controls include using cDNA or plasmid DNA known to contain the template being amplified, and using primers that amplify a ubiquitously expressed gene such as actin, to confirm the presence of cDNA in the reaction. The latter also serves to confirm the absence of genomic DNA contamination in the No-RT sample (**Fig. 3**).

6. The optimal annealing temperature is usually determined empirically. A general rule is to start by annealing at 5°C below the melting temperature (Tm) of the primer pair. For T_m below 68°C, the following formula may be used: $T_m = 2(A+T) + 4(G+C)$. However, there are computer programs that are used to design primers (e.g., PrimerSelect, available from DNAStar Inc.) and these programs usually give the calculated optimal annealing temperature for each primer pair, in addition to determining other optimal primer characteristics.

7. The PCR conditions vary depending on the DNA polymerase enzyme used in the reaction and generally require optimization, especially the salt and primer concentrations. The conditions shown are for *Taq* DNA polymerase (Invitrogen) that was optimized in our laboratory (see product insert for recommended conditions when using other enzymes).

8. Other commercial kits that may be used include Quantum Prep® Freeze 'N' Squeeze DNA Gel Extraction Spin Columns (Bio-Rad Inc., cat. no. 732-6165), GenElute Agarose Spin Columns (Sigma, cat. no. S-6500) and Ultrafree-MC Centrifugation Filter Devices (Millipore Inc., Bedford, MA, cat. no. 42600). They all use proprietary formulation of reagents. However, the basic principle of the method and reagents that can easily be made in the laboratory (instead of purchasing kits, *see* **ref. 15**).

9. GenElute LPA (Linear Polyacrylamide) is an inert neutral carrier for precipitating picogram amounts of nucleic acids with ethanol in the presence of 0.1 *M* salt. The nucleic acid precipitate is visible immediately upon addition of GenElute LPA, eliminating the need for long and low temperature incubation. It allows complete recovery of nucleic acids larger than 20 basepairs and does not interfere with downstream manipulations of the precipitated DNA. A suitable alternative is glycogen (Invitrogen, cat. no. 10814010).

10. At this point, the extracted PCR product may be sequenced directly or cloned into an appropriate vector and sequenced using vector primers. The latter is necessary when the PCR product consists of different sequences that have exactly the same length, hence migrate together in an agarose gel. For example, Paan-AG primary transcript is alternatively spliced (*11*), and two of the spliced transcripts, Paan-AG2 (exon 3 spliced out) and Paan-AG4 (exon 4 spliced out) both have the same length since exon 3 and exon 4 are both 276 bp long. Both transcripts are amplified and migrate together when using primers that bind to exon 1 and exon 8 (e.g., bG7-26 and bG1078-1099, Table 1). They were only distinguished after cloning the 830 bp band and sequencing several clones (*11*).

11. The ELISA protocol described can easily be modified and adapted for analysis of other antibodies or use in other ELISA systems. Optimal conditions must be determined for each ELISA system. In general, the following points are taken into account when optimizing ELISA conditions:

    a. Use 96-well plates that are certified as high protein-binding or designed for ELISA.
    b. Coat the ELISA plates with 5-20 µg/mL protein in a volume of 50–100 µL PBS, pH 7.4, or 0.1 *M* NaHCO$_3$, pH 9.6, per well.
    c. Blocking nonspecific binding maybe performed using a protein that does not cross-react with the antibody being tested. Fat-free skim milk (5%) or bovine serum albumin in PBS give good results.
    d. Washing is critical in ELISA, to reduce non-specific binding. Phosphate-buffered saline or Tris-buffered saline (TBS) containing a mild detergent (such as Tween-20) are good wash buffers. *See* **Ref. 20** for further information on ELISA.

12. Some antibodies do not react with paraffin-embedded tissue. In such cases, embed the fresh tissue in appropriate freezing medium (e.g., Tissue-Freezing Medium™, Triangle Biomedical Sciences, Durham, NC, cat. no. H-TFM) and flash-freeze by immersing in liquid nitrogen. Cut 5- to 7-μm sections of the frozen tissue using a cryostat and place the sections on a glass slide and allow drying for 10 min at room temperature. Fix the tissue with cold acetone for 10 min, air-dry and proceed with **step 7**, or wrap the slides in aluminum foil and store them at –20°C until required.

13. Some fixation procedures result in the epitope being "hidden" such that the antibody cannot bind. In such cases, an extra "antigen-retrieval" step should be included after re-hydration. This includes treatment with trypsin/EDTA (Invitrogen) for 15 min before blocking, or boiling with either BORGdecloaker™ or 10X Reveal (Biocompare Inc., South San Francisco, CA, cat nos. BD1000S and RV1000M)

14. The type of normal serum used to block nonspecific binding sites in a tissue section is determined by the animal species in which the secondary antibody to be used was raised. Thus, in our case, we used normal horse serum to block nonspecific binding in tissues to be stained with the goat antibodies because the secondary antibody we used was horse anti-goat IgG, and for the tissues stained with the primary antibodies from chicken, we used rabbit normal serum and rabbit anti-IgY secondary antibody.

15. Antibodies to different HLA class I loci that have been used in nonhuman primate MHC studies include W6/32, a mouse IgG_{2a} monoclonal antibody that reacts with monomorphic class I heavy chains associated with β_2-microglobulin *(16,17)* and 16G1, a mouse IgG_{2a} monoclonal antibody that reacts with HLA-G5 and HLA-G6, *(18)*. In some cases, specific monoclonal and polyclonal antibodies to nonhuman primate MHC have been generated using peptide immunogens *(11)* or recombinant protein *(19)*.

16. An ideal positive control tissue is one that is known to express the epitope that reacts with the antibody in use. Negative controls include isotype-specific antibodies with specificities to irrelevant antigen but raised in the same species as the experimental antibody, and also using diluent instead of primary antibody, to control for possible cross-reactivity of secondary antibody with tissue (**Fig. 4**).

References

1. Bontrop, R. E. (2001) Non-human primates: essential partners in biomedical research. *Immunol. Rev.* **183,** 5–9.
2. Adams, E. J. and Parham, P. (2001) Species-specific evolution of MHC class I genes in the higher primates. *Immunol. Rev.* **183,** 41–64.
3. Arnaiz-Villena, A., Martinez-Laso, J., Castro, M. J., et al. (2001) The evolution of the MHC-G gene does not support a functional role for the complete protein. *Immunol. Rev.* **183,** 65–75.
4. Doxiadis, G. G., Otting, N., de Groot, N. G., and Bontrop, R. E. (2001) Differential evolutionary MHC class II strategies in humans and rhesus macaques: relevance for biomedical studies. *Immunol. Rev.* **183,** 76–85.

5. Langat, D. K. and Hunt, J. S. (2002) Do nonhuman primates comprise appropriate experimental models for studying the function of human leukocyte antigen-G? *Biol. Reprod.* **67,** 1367–1374.
6. Geluk, A., Elferink, D. G., Slierendregt, B. L., et al. (1993) Evolutionary conservation of major histocompatibility complex-DR/peptide/T cell interactions in primates. *J. Exp. Med.* **177,** 979–987.
7. McKinney, D. M., Erickson, A. L., Walker, C. M., et al. (2000) Identification of five different Patr class I molecules that bind HLA supertype peptides and definition of their peptide binding motifs. *J. Immunol.* **165,** 4414–4422.
8. Boyson, J. E., Iwanaga, K. K., Urvater, J. A., Hughes, A. L., Golos, T. G., and Watkins, D. I. (1999) Evolution of a new non-classical MHC class I locus in two Old World primate species. *Immunogenetics* **49,** 86–98.
9. Prilliman, K., Lawlor, D., Ellxson, M., et al. (1996) Characterization of baboon class I major histocompatibility molecules. *Transplantation* **61,** 989–996.
10. Sidebottom, D. A., Kennedy, R., and Hildebrand, W. H. (2001) Class I MHC expression in the yellow baboon. *J. Immunol.* **166,** 3983–3993.
11. Langat, D. K., Morales, P. J., Fazleabas, A. T., Mwenda, J. M., and Hunt, J. S. (2002) Baboon placentas express soluble and membrane-bound Paan-AG proteins encoded by alternatively spliced transcripts of the class Ib major histocompatibility complex gene, *Paan-AG. Immunogenetics* **54,** 164–173.
12. Paul, P., Rouas-Freiss, N., Moreau, P., et al. (2000) HLA-G, -E, -F preworkshop: tools and protocols for analysis of non-classical class I genes transcription and protein expression. *Hum Immunol.* **61,** 1177–1195.
13. Domena, J. D., Little, A. M., Madrigal, A. J., et al. (1993) Structural heterogeneity in HLA-B70, a high-frequency antigen of black populations. *Tissue Antigens* **42,** 509–517.
14. Farrell, R. E. (1998) *RNA Methodologies: A Laboratory Guide for Isolation and Characterization.* Academic, San Diego, CA.
15. Sambrook, J. and Russell, D. W. (eds.) (2001) *Molecular Cloning: A Laboratory Manual, 3rd Edition.* Cold Spring Harbor Laboratory, Cold Spring Harbor, NY.
16. Stern, P. L., Beresford, N., Friedman, C. I., Stevens, V. C., Risk, J. M., and Johnson, P. M. (1987) Class I-like MHC molecules expressed by baboon placental syncytiotrophoblast. *J. Immunol.* **138,** 1088–1091.
17. Sluvkin, I. I., Boyson, J. E., Watkins, D. I., and Golos, T. G. (1998) The rhesus monkey analogue of human lymphocyte antigen-G is expressed primarily in villous syncytiotrophoblasts. *Biol. Reprod.* **58,** 728–738.
18. Ryan, A. F., Grendell, R. L., Geraghty, D. E., and Golos, T. G. (2002) A soluble isoform of the rhesus monkey nonclassical MHC class I molecule Mamu-AG is expressed in the placenta and the testis. *J. Immunol.* **169,** 673–683.
19. Sluvkin, I. I., Lunn, D. P., Watkins, D. I., and Golos, T. G. (2000) Placental expression of the non-classical MHC class I molecule, Mamu-AG at implantation in the rhesus monkey. *Proc. Natl. Acad. Sci. USA* **97,** 9104–9109.
20. Coligan, J. E., Kruisbeek, A. M., Margulies, D. H., Shevach, E. M., and Strober, W. (1994) *Current Protocols in Immunology.* John Wiley & Sons, Hoboken, NJ.

11

Analysis of the Soluble Isoforms of HLA-G

mRNAs and Proteins

Judith L. Pace, Pedro J. Morales, Teresa A. Phillips, and Joan S. Hunt

Summary

The human major histocompatibility complex (MHC) contains genes encoding the Human Leukocyte Antigens (HLA). Of these antigens, placental immunologists need study only the HLA class I molecules, because HLA class II expression is repressed in the fetal placental cells that are in direct contact with maternal blood and tissues containing maternal immune cells. The class I antigens are subdivided into two general categories. The class Ia antigens are highly polymorphic and are typified by HLA-A, -B, and -C; these are expressed by nearly all somatic cells and stimulate graft rejection when foreign to the host. By contrast, the HLA class Ib antigens, HLA-E, -F, and -G, have restricted expression, few variants, and appear rarely to be immunostimulatory. One class Ia antigen, HLA-C, and the three class Ib antigens are differentially expressed by trophoblast cell subpopulations. In order to understand immune privilege in the pregnant uterus and placenta, it is essential to study the unique structural and functional features of these four genes and their glycoprotein products. In this chapter, we focus on the first class Ib gene identified in human placentas, *HLA-G*, with emphasis on its two soluble isoforms, HLA-G5 and HLA-G6. We describe methods developed in our laboratory to distinguish mRNAs encoding HLA-G5 and HLA-G6, and antibody-based protocols for identification of the soluble isoforms.

Key Words: Enzyme-linked immunosorbent assay (ELISA); flow cytometry; HLA-G; human; immunoblotting; immunohistochemistry; placenta; reverse transcriptase polymerase chain reaction (RT-PCR); recombinant HLA-G; trophoblast cells.

1. Introduction

In humans, the major histocompatibility complex (MHC)-derived antigens are known as the Human Leukocyte Antigens (HLA) because of their having first been identified on leukocytes. Now, it is well documented that essentially all somatic cells express these antigens to a greater or lesser degree, but that some cells select specific genes from among the many members of this family for expression.

From: *Methods in Molecular Medicine, Vol. 122: Placenta and Trophoblast: Methods and Protocols, Vol. 2*
Edited by: M. J. Soares and J. S. Hunt © Humana Press Inc., Totowa, NJ

Trophoblast cells in human placentas are nearly unique in their failure to express HLA class Ia antigens, HLA-A and HLA-B, which are best known for their capacity to facilitate killing of infected and foreign cells and to mediate graft rejection when foreign to the host *(1)*. Nor do these cells express the HLA class II antigens (HLA-D) that have similar abilities. Although many mechanisms that assist in protection of the semiallogeneic fetus from attack by maternal immune cells are in place, this striking genetic restriction in trophoblast cells surrounding and encasing the fetus may be the single most critical element upon which establishment and maintenance of immune privilege in the pregnant uterus rests. There are no examples in the scientific literature of HLA-A, HLA-B, or HLA-D expression in the placentas of either successful or unsuccessful pregnancies.

In humans, the negative approach of simply restricting expression of immunostimulatory paternal antigens on cells at the maternal–fetal interface is paired with a positive approach: certain subpopulations of trophoblast cells express HLA class Ib antigens, and these are most often inhibitory rather than stimulatory of immune cell function. This is a prominent function of HLA-G antigens.

HLA-G is one of the three expressed HLA class Ib genes (*HLA-E, HLA-F,* and *HLA-G*); the glycoprotein products of all are readily detectable in placentas *(2,3)*. These genes have few alleles in comparison with the class Ia genes, which may be the critical feature that permits expression at the maternal–fetal interface. The class Ia antigens are extremely important to efficient generation of cytotoxic T lymphocytes (CTL) and their subsequent recognition of infected and aberrant cells, recognition of HLA-null tumor cells by natural killer (NK) cells, and, possibly, also to binding of growth factors. The functions of the class Ib antigens remain poorly defined, although HLA-G, the best studied of the class Ib antigens, appears to have an immune suppressive role *(4–6)*. Yet much remains to be learned about this and other functions it may have in implantation and pregnancy.

The *HLA-G* gene is unique among the class I genes in several important respects: (1) the interferon (IFN)/Enhancer A region is flawed by a 13-bp deletion; (2) the cytoplasmic tail is short; (3) the γ-activated site (GAS) element is dysfunctional, (4) the single transcript is alternatively spliced to yield seven transcripts (**Fig. 1**) *(7,8)*. These messages encode four membrane-bound antigens and three soluble antigens. The soluble antigens result from a stop sequence in either intron 4 (HLA-G5, HLA-G6) or intron 2 (HLA-G7), which prevents translation of the transmembrane and cytoplasmic regions. The two soluble antigens, HLA-G5 and HLA-G6, are nearly identical to their membrane counterparts, HLA-G1 and HLA-G2, except that they lack the amino acids downstream from intron 4. HLA-G1/G5 and G2/G6 differ from one another by lack of the α2 domain in the latter set.

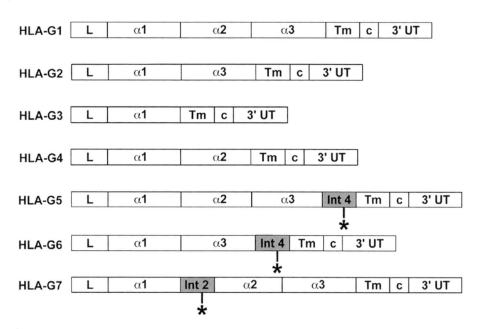

Fig. 1. Schematic representation of messages derived by alternative splicing of the single *HLA-G* primary transcript. The three transcripts encoding soluble proteins are terminated in intron 4 (HLA-G5, HLA-G6) and intron 2 (HLA-G7) by a stop codon (denoted by *), which precludes translation of the balance of the message, including the transmembrane and cytoplasmic domains. L, leader sequence; Int, intron; Tm, transmembrane; c, cytoplasmic; UT, untranslated.

Studies are just now being reported that are directed toward defining isoform-specific functions for the HLA-G proteins. Our interest in learning whether the isoforms had the same or different functions was first stimulated by learning that pregnancy goes forward in women whose HLA-G α2 domain contains a deletion and cannot encode functional HLA-G1 or HLA-G5 glyco-proteins *(9)*. We postulated that other isoforms could compensate for HLA-G1/G5, and this has since been verified by others.

Of all the isoforms, HLA-G1 has received the most attention. The product of this transcript is abundant in migrating extravillous cytotrophoblast (CTB) cells, and is readily detected using monoclonal antibodies (mAb) such as W6/32 that bind HLA class I antigens complexed with light chain, β2-microglobulin (β2m). Although HLA-G1 was originally thought to bind uterine natural killer (uNK) cell receptors and activate inhibitory pathways, this function is now attributed to HLA-E *(10)*. It remains to be determined what the major cellular target of HLA-G1 may be, but recent studies in our laboratory indicate that its soluble counterpart, HLA-G5, binds to both CD8[+] cells *(11)* and to cells of the mononuclear phagocyte lineage *(12)*, and achieves effects that are consistent with immune suppression. Others have reported functions for HLA-G5 that include induction of the Fas/FasL programmed cell death pathway in activated CTL *(13)* and induction of immunosuppressive CD4$^+$ cells *(14)*.

Our recent finding that HLA-G5 and HLA-G6 are differentially expressed in trophoblast subpopulations *(11)* has further stimulated our interest in isoform-specific functions. HLA-G5 transcripts and proteins are readily identified in villous and extravillous trophoblast cells, and proteins are present in both syncytiotrophoblast and maternal blood. By contrast, although HLA-G6 transcripts are present in both villous and extravillous CTB cells, only the extravillous cells contain detectable protein *(11)*. These observations imply different functions, and unpublished DNA microarray data support this novel idea (McIntire, R. and Hunt, J.S., unpublished results).

The class I genes and their glycoprotein products are very similar to one another. As a consequence, studying individual genes requires precise methods. In this chapter, we use our experiences with HLA-G to illustrate how to explore its messages and proteins, and to investigate potential functions, focusing particularly on the two soluble isoforms, HLA-G5 and HLA-G6. The methods include reverse-transcription (RT)-polymerase chain reaction (PCR) with various sets of primers, flow cytometry to identify intracellular antigens, immunoblotting and enzyme-linked immunosorbent assay (ELISA) to identify antigens in cell lysates and supernatant culture media, and immunohistology to locate antigens in tissues.

2. Materials

2.1. Total RNA Extraction, Reverse Transcription and Polymerase Chain Reaction

1. Trizol® Reagent (Invitrogen, Carlsbad, CA, cat. no. 15596-018), stored at 4°C.
2. Total RNA samples, stored at –80°C.
3. Cell lines: JEG-3 (American Type Culture Collection [ATCC], Manassas, VA, cat. no. HTB 36) and S14/8 *(15)*, JAR (cat. no. HTB 144) and L-M(TK⁻) (cat. no. CCL 1.3).
4. Autoclaved, deionized water treated with 0.1% diethyl pyrocarbonate (DEPC-H_2O, *see* **Note 1**) for diluting RNA samples, and sterile, pyrogen-free water for PCR (e.g., sterile water for irrigation, Baxter Healthcare Corp., Deerfield, IL).
5. DNAse I reagents, available as a kit (Sigma-Aldrich, St. Louis, MO, cat. no. AMP-D1) containing the following:
   a. Amplification grade DNAse I (cat. no. 5307, 1 U/µL).
   b. 10X Reaction buffer: 200 mM Tris-HCl, pH 8.3, 20 mM MgCl$_2$ (cat. no. R6273).
   c. Stop solution: 50 mM ethylenediamine tetraacetic acid (EDTA) (cat. no. S4809).

6. RT-PCR reagents, stored at –20°C:
   a. Deoxynucleotide triphosphate (dNTP) mix, 10 mM (Invitrogen, cat. no. 18427-013).
   b. Moloney-murine leukemia virus reverse transcriptase (MMLV-RT), 200 U/µL (Invitrogen, cat. no. 28025-013).
   c. 5X first strand buffer (Invitrogen, cat. no. Y00146, comes with MMLV-RT).
   d. 0.1 M dithiothreitol (DTT) (Invitrogen, cat. no. Y00147, comes with MMLV-RT, enzyme).
   e. RNase inhibitor (RNasin®, Promega, Madison, WI, cat. no. N2511, 40 U/µL).
   f. Oligo d(T)$_{12-18}$, (0.5 µg/µL) (Invitrogen, cat. no. 18418-012).
   g. *Taq* DNA polymerase (Invitrogen, cat. no. 10342-020).
   h. 10X PCR buffer minus Mg^{2+} (Invitrogen, cat. no. Y02028, comes with *Taq* enzyme).
   i. 50 mM $MgCl_2$ (Invitrogen, cat. no. Y02016, comes with *Taq* enzyme).
   j. Custom designed primers, approx 100 µM in 10 mM Tris-HCl, pH 8.0 (*see* **Note 2**).
      Primer pairs for HLA-G5 transcripts (amplicon size 585 bp)
      Gex3b (forward) 5'-GCCTCCTCCGCGGGTATGAAC-3'
      Gi4 (reverse) 5'-GGCCTCACCACCGACCCTGTTA-3'
      Primer pairs for HLA-G6 transcripts (amplicon size 369 bp)
      Gex2-4 (forward) 5'-GCGAGGCCAACCCCCCCAAGA-3'
      Gi4 (reverse) 5'-GGCCTCACCACCGACCCTGTTA-3'
7. 200-µL thin-walled PCR tubes (Midwest Scientific, St. Louis, MO), certified RNase-free/DNase-free.
8. Barrier, presterilized tips (Midwest Scientific), certified free of RNase/DNase, human DNA, PCR inhibitors, and pyrogens.
9. Polypropylene 1.5-mL tubes (Midwest Scientific), RNase-free, DNAase-free.
10. Reagents for agarose gel electrophoresis of DNA products: agarose (3:1), biotechnology grade (Amresco, Solon, OH, cat. no. E776), 50X Tris acetate EDTA (TAE) buffer (*see* **Note 3**), 1 kb DNA ladder (Invitrogen, cat. no. 15615-016), 6X tracking dye/loading buffer, ethidium bromide, 10 mg/mL (Sigma-Aldrich, cat. no. E-1510).
11. Thermocycler.
12. Electrophoresis unit.
13. Ultraviolet (UV) transilluminator.
14. Polaroid camera.

2.2. Intracellular Flow Cytometry

1. Stably transfected HEK293 cells that express either HLA-G5 or HLA-G6 proteins and HEK293 cells transfected with an "empty" expression vector were derived as we have previously described *(11)*. These are designated as 293-HLA-G5, 293-HLA-G6 and 293-Vector, respectively.

2. Culture medium for HEK293 cells: Dulbecco's modified Eagle's medium (Cellgro, Mediatech, Inc., Herndon, VA) supplemented with 10% fetal bovine serum (FBS), 100 U/mL penicillin and 100 µg/mL streptomycin (Invitrogen) and 0.6 mg/mL Geneticin® (Invitrogen).

3. Monensin, Golgi Stop™ (BD Pharmingen, San Diego, CA).

4. Hank's balanced salt solution (HBSS) without Ca^{2+} and Mg^{2+} (Sigma-Aldrich).

5. Trypsin–EDTA solution containing 0.25% trypsin and 0.02% EDTA in HBSS (Sigma-Aldrich) supplemented with 10 mM HEPES (Sigma-Aldrich).

6. Preseparation filters 30-µm mesh size (Milteny Biotec, Auburn, CA).

7. Monoclonal antibody, 16G1 (Daniel Geragthy, Fred Hutchinson Cancer Research Center, Seattle, Washington).

8. Isotype control: mouse immunoglobulin (Ig)G$_1$, κ (BD Pharmingen, Cat. No. 557273).

9. R-Phycoerythrin (PE)-conjugated anti-mouse IgG, F(ab')$_2$ fragment from sheep (Sigma-Aldrich, cat. no. P-8547) (*see* **Note 4**).

10. 10X phosphate-buffered saline (PBS) (for 1 L): 80 g NaCl, 2 g KCl, 14.4 g Na_2HPO_4, and 2.4 g KH_2PO_4.

11. 2X Fixation and Permeabilization reagent: 0.2% saponin (Sigma-Aldrich, cat. no. S-4521), 0.2% bovine serum albumin (BSA) (Sigma-Aldrich, cat. no. A-7906), 0.7–0.8% formaldehyde in 2X PBS, filtered using a 45-µm membrane and stored at 4°C.

12. 1X Permeabilization/wash buffer: 0.1% saponin (Sigma-Aldrich), 0.1% BSA (Sigma-Aldrich), 0.09% sodium azide, in 1X PBS, filtered using a 45-µm membrane and stored at 4°C.

13. Blocking buffer: 20% sheep serum (Sigma-Aldrich, cat. no. S-2263), 20% human serum (Sigma-Aldrich, cat. no. H-4522) in 2X Permeabilization/Wash Buffer, filter (0.22-µm) and store at 4°C.

14. 2% Paraformaldehyde (*see* **Note 5**).

15. Low-speed, swinging-bucket, temperature-controlled centrifuge.

16. Flow cytometer such as FACSCalibur™ and Cellquest™ software (BD Biosciences, San Diego, CA).

2.3. Immunoblots and Immunoprecipitations

1. 293-HLA-G5, 293HLA-G6, and 293-Vector cells (*11*) cultured as described for intracellular staining (*see* **Subheading 2.2.**).

2. Cell solubilization buffer: A basic stock containing 1% NP-40 and 0.1% sodium dodecyl sulfate (SDS) in PBS can be prepared in large volume (e.g., 100 mL) and stored at 4°C. Add the following volumes of protease inhibitor stocks (*see* **Note 6**) immediately before use: 5.74 µL phenylmethylsulfonylfluoride (PMSF), 2.5 µL aprotinin, 2 µL leupeptin and 4 µL EDTA per mL of cell solubilization buffer.

3. SDS reducing Laemli buffer (2X): 20% (v/v) Glycerol, 100 mM Tris-HCl pH 6.8, 10% (v/v) 2-mercaptoethanol, 0.2% (w/v) bromophenol blue 4% (w/v) SDS.

4. SDS-polyacrylamide gel electrophoresis (PAGE) system and transfer apparatus.

5. Nonfat dry milk, blotting Grade (Bio-Rad, Hercules, CA, cat. no. 170-6404).

6. Monoclonal antibody 16G1 (Daniel Geragthy, Fred Hutchinson Cancer Research Center, Seattle, WA).
7. Horseradish peroxidase (HRP)-conjugated secondary antibody: HRP-anti-mouse IgG (Jackson ImmunoResearch Lab. Inc., West Groove, PA, cat. no. 115-035-062).
8. Chemiluminescence substrate, SuperSignal® (Pierce, Rockford, IL) High performance chemiluminiscense film, Hyperfilm™ ECL (Amersham Biosciences, Little Chalfont, Buckinghamshire, England).
9. Broad range protein markers (Bio-Rad, cat. no. 161-0318).
10. SDS-PAGE gradient gels Tris-HCl 4-20% (Bio-Rad, Inc., cat. no. 161-1105).
11. 10X gel running buffer (Bio-Rad, cat. no. 161-0732).
12. 10X transfer buffer (Bio-Rad, cat. no. 161-0734) (*see* **Note 7**).
13. Nitrocellulose membranes (Schleicher & Schuell, Inc., Keene, NH, cat. no. BA-S83).
14. Power supply.
15. Detergent compatible (DC) protein assay (Bio-Rad, cat. no. 500-0112).
16. EZview™ red Protein G affinity Gel (Sigma-Aldrich, cat. no. E-3403).

2.4. ELISA

1. C-shaped Nunc Immuno Plates with MaxiSorp surface (Nalge Nunc Int., Rochester, NY, cat. no. 430341).
2. Purified HLA-G5 and HLA-G6 proteins in 10 m*M* PBS, pH 7.2. (*see* **Note 8**)
3. Purified anti-HLA-G antibodies. Stock solutions were prepared in 10 m*M* PBS, pH 7.2, and diluted appropriately for the type of ELISA (*see* **Note 9**).
   Anti-HLA-G5 (1-2C3) *(11)*
   Anti-HLA-G2/G6 (26-2H11) *(11)*
4. Purified mouse IgG$_1$ (BD Pharmingen, cat. no. 557273)
5. HRP conjugated horse anti-mouse IgG (Vector Laboratories, Burlingame, CA, cat. no. PI-2000); Prepare 1:1000 dilution in blocking solution (*see* **item 10**) just prior to use.
6. Anti-HLA-G5/G6 (9-1F10) (patent pending). The mAb 9-1F10 was derived from the same fusion that produced mAb 1-2C3 *(11)*, but in contrast to 1-2C3, mAb 9-1F10 recognizes both HLA-G5 and HLA-G6 isoforms. The mAb was purified and biotinylated using an EZ-Link™ Sulfo-NHS-Biotinylation Kit (Pierce, cat. no. 21420).
7. ZyMax™ streptavidin-HRP conjugate (Zymed Laboratories, South San Francisco, CA, cat. no. 43-8323). Prepare a 1:10,000 dilution in 10 m*M* PBS, pH 7.2, containing 0.05% Tween-20.
8. Peroxidase substrate: 2-component TMB (KPL, Gaithersburg, MD, cat. no. 50-65-00)
9. Coating solution: 10 m*M* PBS, pH 7.2. Dissolve 9.83 g NaCl and 1.38 g NaH$_2$PO$_4$·H$_2$O in about 950 mL deionized H$_2$O. Adjust to pH 7.2 with 1 *N* NaOH and bring volume to 1000 mL. Filter-sterilize using a 0.22-μm membrane.
10. Blocking solution: 5% nonfat dry milk (BioRad, cat. no. 170-6404) in 10 m*M* PBS, pH 7.2, containing 0.02% Tween-20. Prepare fresh on the day of use.
11. BSA-T diluent: 0.5% BSA in 10 m*M* PBS, pH 7.2 containing 0.05% Tween-20.

12. Wash buffer: 50 mM Tris-buffered saline, pH 8.0, containing 0.05% Tween-20 (TBS-T) Filter-sterilize.
13. Stop reagent: 1 M H_3PO_4.
14. Automatic single- and multi-channel pipetters and tips.
15. Reagent reservoirs (Fisher Scientific, Hampton, NH, cat. no. 13-681-100).
16. Lint-free paper towels.
17. Automatic plate reader with capacity to measure absorbance at 450 nm.

2.5. Immunohistochemistry

1. Refrigerated cryostat (Leica, Model CM1900).
2. Microscope slides (e.g., Superfrost®/Plus microscope slides, Fisher Scientific).
3. Disposable plastic base molds (15 × 15 × 5 mm) (Fisher Scientific).
4. Optimum cutting temperature (OCT) tissue freezing medium (Triangle Biomedical Sciences, Durham, NC).
5. Microscope slides with two 10-μ frozen tissue sections mounted on each.
6. Phosphate buffered saline pH 7.4 (PBS) (10X stock): 80 g NaCl, 2 g KCl, 2 g NaH_2PO_4, 11.4 g Na_2HPO_4, adjust volume to 1000 mL.
7. Acetone (Sigma-Aldrich).
8. Coplin jars (Fisher Scientific).
9. Pap pen (Research Products International Corp, Mount Prospect, IL).
10. Antibody dilution buffer: 100 mL PBS with 0.3% Tween 20, add 1 g bovine serum albumin, adjust pH to 8.0 with Na_2CO_3. Aliquot into 5-mL portions and store at –20°C.
11. Peroxidase blocking reagent (DakoCytomation California Inc., Carpinteria, CA, cat. no. S200130).
12. Horse serum (Sigma-Aldrich).
13. Mouse anti-HLA-G5 (1-2C3) *(11)*.
14. Mouse anti-HLA-G6 (26-2H11) *(11)*.
15. Control mouse IgG$_1$ (BD PharMingen, cat. no. 557273).
16. Secondary antibody: biotinylated horse anti-mouse IgG (Vector Laboratories, cat. no. BA-2000).
17. Human serum (Sigma-Aldrich).
18. Streptoavidin-labeled peroxidase conjugate (Zymed Laboratories, cat. no. 50-242).
19. AEC substrate development kit (Zymed, cat. no. 00-2007).
20. Mayer's hematoxylin (Sigma-Aldrich, cat. no. MHS-32).
21. Crystal Mount (Biomeda Corp., Foster City, CA, Fisher Scientific, cat. no. BMM-02).
22. Humidified chamber (Thermo Shandon, Pittsburgh, PA).
23. Permount® (Fisher Scientific).

3. Methods

3.1. Analysis of HLA-G mRNAs: RT-PCR

RT-PCR is a standard technique that is readily adaptable to evaluation of transcripts encoding the soluble and membrane isoforms of HLA-G. However,

A

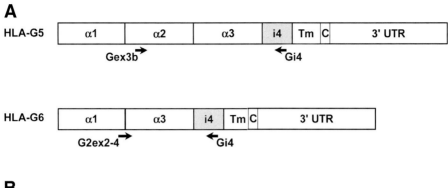

B

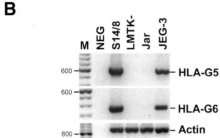

Fig. 2. Analysis of HLA-G5 and -G6 by reverse-transcription (RT)-polymerase chain reaction (PCR). (**A**) Illustration of locations of the pairs of primers used to amplify HLA-G5 and -G6 sequences. The designs were based on majority mismatches with other Human Leukocyte Antigen (HLA) molecules. Note that the primer pairs amplifying HLA-G5 span the α2 domain to intron 4 and the pairs amplifying HLA-G6 span α3 through intron 4. (**B**) Amplifications using these primer pairs show positive signals in the HLA 6.0-transfected S14/8 mouse fibroblasts and no signals in their untransfected LMTK⁻ counterparts. The Jar choriocarcinoma cells are negative, as expected, and the JEG-3 choriocarcinoma cells are positive. HLA-G5 transcripts are found at 585 bp and HLA-G6 transcripts are present at 369 bp. The loading control is β-actin, and is positive in all cells.

the HLA class I gene complex contains somewhere between 19 and 25 genes, most of which are pseudogenes or partial gene fragments. All of these genes have high degrees of sequence similarity to one another. The early scientific literature is rife with errors of identification of HLA class I mRNAs, and only sequencing reveals the authenticity of the amplicon in RT-PCR.

In this section, we describe an RT-PCR procedure for specific identification of HLA-G5 and HLA-G6 transcripts in cells and tissues. The genomic locations of HLA-G5 and HLA-G6 specific primer pairs are shown in **Fig. 2A**. The HLA-G5 and HLA-G6 primers were constructed in accordance with the sequence of the *0101 allele, which is represented by the commonly used HLA 6.0 DNA.

Sequence analysis suggests that the primer pairs will also give accurate data for the other HLA-G alleles.

1. Extract total RNA from cells or tissues of interest using standard procedures (*see* **Note 10**). It is essential to have positive and negative controls for HLA-G expression. Commonly used positive controls include the JEG-3 and S14/8 (*15*) cell lines; with JAR and L-M(TK⁻) cell lines serving as respective negative controls.

2. Digest total RNA samples with DNAse I as described in the AMP-D1 kit (*see* **Note 11**).

3. Set up reverse transcriptase (+RT) reactions using DNAse-treated RNA to generate first strand cDNA (*see* **Note 12**). Also include RNA samples incubated under the same conditions but without reverse transcriptase (–RT) to generate negative control reactions (*see* **Note 13**).

4. Prepare a PCR cocktail with the following volumes per sample, in nuclease-free 1.5-mL tubes:

10X PCR buffer minus Mg^{2+}	5.0 µL
50 mM $MgCl_2$	1.5 µL
10 mM dNTP mix	1.0 µL
5' primer (20 µ*M*)	0.625 µL
3' primer (20 µ*M*)	0.625 µL
Sterile water	36.8 µL
Taq DNA polymerase (5U/µL)	0.4 µL

5. Set up PCR tubes as described below by mixing PCR cocktail containing the primer pairs with +RT and –RT samples. Also prepare a negative control, which contains all reagents except RT samples, for each pair of primers (*see* **Note 14**):

Reagent	+RT samples	–RT samples	Negative control
H_2O	—	—	4 µL
cDNA (+RT reactions)	4 µL	—	—
Mock cDNA (–RT reactions)	—	4 µL	—
PCR cocktail	46 µL	46 µL	46 µL
Final volume	50 µL	50 µL	50 µL

6. Mix well; centrifuge for 2–4 s at 14,000*g* to settle contents.

7. Incubate in a thermocycler under the following conditions: denaturation, 94°C, 45 s; 35 cycles at 94°C, 45 s followed by 65°C, 45 s, followed by 72°C, 2 min. Conclude with extension at 72°C, 10 min. Store at 4°C.

8. Analyze PCR products by standard agarose-ethidium bromide gel electrophoresis (*see* **Note 15**). A product of 585 bp should be obtained for HLA-G5 and 369 bp for HLA-G6 (**Fig. 2B**).

9. Confirm identity of amplified products by DNA sequencing (*see* **Note 16**).

3.2. Analysis of HLA-G5 and HLA-G6 Proteins

Standard methods of analysis can be adapted for specific identification of HLA-G5 and HLA-G6 proteins only if the intrinsic aspects of the antibodies to

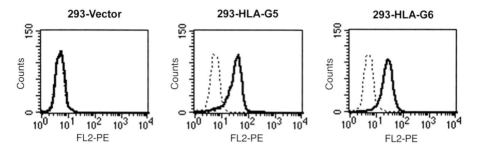

Fig. 3. Detection of intracellular soluble HLA-G by flow cytometry. Human HEK293 cells stably transfected with an empty expression vector (293-Vector), a HLA-G5 expression vector (293-HLA-G5) or a HLA-G6 expression vector (293-HLA-G6) were evaluated for intracellular antigens. The data are presented as overlaid histograms (isotype control, IgG$_1$, dotted lines; mAb 16G1, which binds to both HLA-G5 and HLA-G6, solid lines). Note that 293-G5 and 293-G6 cells were positive for soluble HLA-G as indicated by an increase in fluorescence intensity in cells stained with 16G1 in comparison with the isotype control.

be used are known. The field of HLA-G identification using antibody-based methods is fraught with difficulty because so little has been reported about the specific methods of tissue/cell fixation to be used, the targeted molecules on the HLA-G antigens and the specific isoforms detected by each reagent. Once these important characteristics have been defined and reported, the antibodies can be used to assess expression in vitro in/on isolated cells by flow cytometry and in cell lysates by immunoblotting or ELISA as well as expression in vivo by immunohistology.

Reagents for identifying HLA-G5 and HLA-G6 are now well characterized. The first antibody to be generated against the intron 4 amino acid sequences that are unique to the soluble isoforms was a mouse monoclonal antibody (mAb), 16G1, developed by D. Geraghty. This antibody is extremely versatile. It recognizes HLA-G5 and HLA-G6 antigens *in situ*, even in paraformalde-hyde-fixed placentas (unpublished results), and is effective in identifying HLA-G5 and HLA-G6 by intracellular flow cytometry (*see* **Fig. 3**). 16G1 identifies recombinant HLA-G5 and HLA-G6 in immunoblots and by ELISA as previously reported (*see* Fig. 1B,C in **Ref. 11**).

Distinguishing the two soluble isoforms required the development of new mAb, and this was reported from our laboratory in 2003 *(11)*. The new mAb, anti-HLA-G5 (1-2C3) and anti-HLA-G2/G6 (26-2H11), cannot recognize their proteins in paraformaldehyde-fixed tissues but are highly specific when tested on frozen tissue sections by immunohistology *(11)*. They do not recognize their proteins in immunoblots but are useful in ELISA (**Fig. 4**).

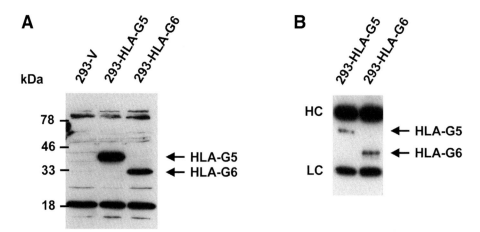

Fig. 4. Electrophoretic characterization of HLA-G5 and -G6 proteins. (**A**) Immunoblots. Cell extracts (30 µg) from human HEK293 cells stably transfected with empty expression vector (293-Vector), HLA-G5 (293-HLA-G5), or HLA-G6 (293-HLA-G6) were separated by using sodium dodecyl sulfate (SDS)-polyacrylamide gel electrophoresis (PAGE), transferred to nitrocellulose membranes and immuno-detected using 16G1, a mAb that identifies both HLA-G5 and HLA-G6 (arrows). (**B**) Immuno-precipitation. Purified HLA-G5 and -G6 were immunoprecipitated with 16G1, subjected to SDS-PAGE, and identified with 16G1 (arrows). IgG heavy chains (HC) and light chains (LC) from anti-mouse immunoglobulin G conjugated to HRP that was used to precipitate HLA-G/16G1 complexes are also visible on the blots.

3.2.1. Analysis of HLA-G5 and HLA-G6 by Intracellular Flow Cytometry

We have established a procedure to detect intracellular HLA-G5 and HLA-G6 in transfected 293-HLA-G5 and 293-HLA-G6 cells by flow cytometry using standard methods that were previously applied for cytokine detection in activated lymphocytes *(16)*. The critical parameters that should be considered when staining intracellular molecules include: (1) conditions for fixation and permeabilization, which can vary among different cell types, (2) time in culture and use of a protein transport inhibitor to limit secretion of the target molecule, and (3) choice of the antibody, as the antigenic determinant to be recognized must be maintained during culture and throughout staining procedures. As described later and shown in **Fig. 3**, mAb 16G1 works well in this procedure. Specificity of staining of HLA-G5 and HLA-G6 using 16G1 is illustrated in two ways. First, 16G1 readily stains 293-HLA-G5 and 293-HLA-G6 cells, but not 293-Vector cells. Second, none of the cells were stained when treated with a control mouse IgG$_1$ immunoglobulin in place of the specific mAb, 16G1.

1. Establish cultures of 293-HLA-G5, 293-HLA-G6, and 293-Vector cells in 75-cm^2 flasks. Incubate the cells until they become approx 70% confluent and add 4 µL of GolgiStop™ to each flask. Continue the culture for 4–6 h (*see* **Note 17**).
2. Harvest the cells from each culture by trypsinization and prepare single cell suspensions for each cell population. For HEK293 cells, aspirate the culture medium and rinse the cell monolayer with 10 mL HBSS. Aspirate the HBSS, add 4 mL of warm trypsin/EDTA solution to each flask and incubate at 37°C for 5 min. Examine the cells under a microscope to confirm that they appear rounded up and released from the growth surface. Add 6 mL fresh, warm culture medium and pipet up and down 10 times (*see* **Note 18**). Centrifuge for 10 min at 200*g*. Discard the culture medium and resuspend the cells in 5 mL fresh culture medium.
3. Count cells and determine viability by trypan blue exclusion. Adjust cell concentration to 10^6 cells/mL of culture medium. For each cell population, pipet 1 mL of the cell supension into each of four 12- × 75-mm polypropylene tubes. These tubes will be processed as sumarized in the table below to evaluate autofluorescence and specific staining by mAb, 16G1

		1° Reagent			2° Reagent
Parameter tested	Sample No.	Perm/wash buffer	IgG1 (1 µg/mL)	16G1 (1 µg/mL)	PE-anti-mouse IgG (1:20)
Autoflourescence	1	+	—	—	—
Secondary antibody	2	+	—	—	+
Isotype control antibody	3	—	+	—	+
Specific antibody	4	—	—	+	+

4. Centrifuge the tubes in a swinging-bucket rotor (200*g* for 20 min at 4°C) to pellet cells. Carefully aspirate the culture medium and thoroughly resuspend cells in 1 mL of fixation and permeabilization reagent. Incubate cells for 1 h on ice.
5. Centrifuge (200*g* for 20 min at 4°C) and wash fixed cells four times with 1 mL of 1X permeabilization/wash buffer.
6. After the final wash, resuspend the cell pellet in 100 µL of blocking buffer and incubate 30 min on ice, in order to block nonspecific binding sites.
7. Add 100 µL blocking buffer containing either no antibody (autoflourescence and secondary antibody controls), or 1 µg/mL of 16G1 or IgG$_1$ isotype control for each cell line. Incubate on ice for 45 min.
8. Add 1 mL of permeabilization/wash buffer and flick tube to mix, then centrifuge as before. Repeat three additional times.
9. Resuspend cells in 100 µL Blocking buffer, alone, or containing a 1:20 dilution of the secondary antibody, PE-conjugated anti-mouse IgG, and incubate on ice and in the dark for 30 min.

10. Wash four times with permeabilization/wash buffer as described in **step 8**. After final wash re-suspend cells in 0.5 mL PBS, add 0.5 mL 2% paraformaldehyde, mix and incubate for at least 30 min at 4°C. Transfer labeled cells to 12- × 75-mm polystyrene tubes.

11. Acquire fluorescence data using a FACSCalibur flow cytometer and CellQuest software. Display data as histograms by plotting fluorescence intensity vs cell number as shown in **Fig. 3**.

3.2.2. Immunoblots and Immunoprecipitation

In this section we demonstrate the utility of mAb 16G1 for detection of HLA-G5 and HLA-G6 by immunoblotting and immunoprecipitation. We have previously used mAb 16G1 to detect our purified recombinant HLA-G5 and HLA-G6 proteins *(11)* and glutathione-*S*-transferase (GST)-fusion proteins of HLA-G5 and HLA-G6 *(17)* by immunoblotting. Here we show that 16G1 detects HLA-G5 and HLA-G6 in whole cell lysates from HEK293 transfected cells (**Fig. 5A**). We also show that 16G1 can immunoprecipitate purified HLA-G5 and HLA-G6 proteins (**Fig. 5B**).

1. Culture HEK293 cells expressing HLA-G5 and HLA-G6 as described *(11)*.

2. Aspirate medium from cells. Wash two times with PBS at room temperature.

3. Place culture dish on ice. Add 500 µL (for a 100-mm dish, 750–1000 µL for a T-75 flask) ice-cold cell solubilization buffer (with freshly added inhibitors) directly to cells. Immediately scrape cells into the buffer and transfer to a 2-mL polypropylene tube.

4. Disrupt cells by three quick cycles of freezing and thawing using liquid nitrogen and a 37°C water bath.

5. Incubate the sample on ice for 30 min. If lysates remain viscous, shear DNA by passing the cell lysate through a 21-gage needle. Centrifuge at 15,000*g* for 10–20 min at 4°C to clarify the solution.

6. Transfer supernatants to clean 1.5-mL tubes and prepare a 25- to 50-µL aliquot (for protein assay) in 0.5-mL tubes. Store all samples at –80°C.

7. Determine protein concentration of lysates using an assay that is compatible with detergents, e.g., BioRad DC (*see* **Note 19**).

8. For immunoblotting experiments, adjust protein concentration of cell extracts to 2–6 mg/mL with solubilization buffer and mix with an equal volume of 2X reducing Laemli SDS-PAGE sample buffer. Heat samples in a boiling water bath for 3 min. Load samples onto gels and proceed with standard SDS-PAGE and immunoblotting (*see* **Note 20**).

9. For immunoprecipitation, samples are kept in cell solubilization buffer and incubated with 16G1 (2 µg) using instructions provided in the EZview kit (*see* **Note 21**). Detect HLA-G5 and HLA-G6 proteins in the precipitated immune complexes by immunoblotting as described in **step 8**.

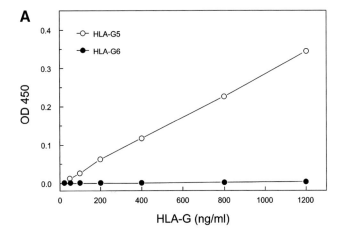

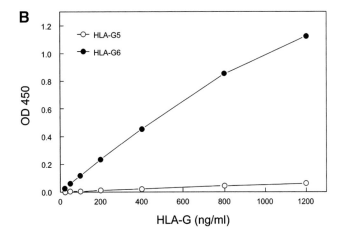

Fig. 5. Detection of HLA-G5 and -G6 by capture enzyme-linked immunosorbent assay (ELISA). Procedures for capture ELISA were performed as described in Methods (*see* **Subheading 3.2.3.**) Wells of microplates were coated with either **(A)** anti-HLA-G5 (1-2C3) or **(B)** anti-HLA-G6 (26-2H11) at concentrations of 5 µg/mL. Varying concentrations (25 to 1200 ng/mL) of purified recombinant HLA-G5 or -G6 proteins were added, and bound HLA-G proteins were detected after sequential treatment with biotinylated 9-1F10 (1 µg/mL), streptavidin-horseradish peroxidase and substrate as previously described. Note that in **(A)**, immobilized anti-HLA-G5 (1-2C3) specifically recognized recombinant HLA-G5 (open circles) in a dose dependent manner, but did not bind to recombinant HLA-G6 (closed circles). In **(B)**, immobilized anti-HLA-G2/G6 (26-2H11) specifically recognized recombinant HLA-G6, but not recombinant HLA-G5. No binding activity was detected when wells were coated with a control mouse immunoglobulin G_1 preparation (not shown).

3.2.3. Enzyme-Linked Immunosorbent Assay

Standard ELISA protocols for detection of HLA-G antibodies and proteins are described as follows. Microwell plates coated with either HLA-G5 or HLA-G6 proteins are used in a so-called *indirect* ELISAs for detection of HLA-G antibodies *(11)*. HLA-G5 and HLA-G6 proteins can also be detected and quantified with *sandwich* or *capture* ELISAs, using immobilized, anti-HLA-G5 (1-2C3) or anti-HLA-G2/G6 (26-2H11) as capture reagents and biotinylated anti-HLA-G5/G6 mAb 9-1F10 for detection. Recommended concentrations and dilutions of reagents for this procedure are given below. However, appropriate titration experiments should be performed for each reagent to assure optimal performance.

3.2.3.1. Indirect ELISA for Detection of HLA-G Antibodies

1. Dilute purified HLA-G5 and HLA-G6 proteins to 5 μg/mL in coating solution, and add 50 μL of the appropriate antigen to each wells of a Nunc microplate according to plate design (*see* **Note 22**).
2. Seal wells with Parafilm™ and incubate overnight (16–18 h) at 4°C.
3. Wash plate three times with 225 μL of TBS-T wash buffer per well for each wash (*see* **Note 23).**
4. Add 225 μL of 5% milk Blocking Solution to each well. Incubate 60 min at room temperature.
5. Remove blocking solution, then add 50 μL of either blocking solution, normal mouse IgG_1 (as controls), anti-HLA-G5 mAb, 1-2C3, or anti-HLA-G2/G6 mAb, 26-2H11 (all IgG reagents diluted to 1 μg/mL in Blocking Solution).
6. Seal the wells with Parafilm and incubate 30 min at 37°C.
7. Wash plates four times with 225 μL of TBS-T wash buffer per well, as before.
8. Add 50 μL HRP-conjugated horse anti-mouse IgG, diluted 1:1000 in blocking solution, to each well.
9. Seal the wells with Parafilm and incubate 30 min at 37°C.
10. Wash four times with 225 μL of TBS-T wash buffer per well, as before.
11. Add 100 μL of TMB substrate to each well. Incubate 5–10 min to allow color development.
12. Add 50 μL stop solution to each well.
13. Read microplate at 450 nm using an automatic plate reader.
14. Data analysis: record absorbance values and compare results from known positive and negative controls. Assay background values, determined from wells treated with blocking buffer in place of the primary antibody, should be low (less than 0.1 absorbance units). Determine assay specificity for a given antigen by comparing results obtained using the mouse control IgG_1 and specific antibody. Absorbance values for control IgG_1 should be similar to assay background.

3.2.3.2. CAPTURE ELISA TO QUANTIFY HLA-G5 AND HLA-G6 PROTEINS

1. Dilute capture mAb, anti-HLA-G5 (1-2C3), anti-HLA-G2/G6 (26-2H11), or mouse IgG$_1$ (as a control) to 5 µg/mL in 10 mM PBS and add 100 µL/well of the appropriate reagent to wells of a Nunc microplate, as in plate design (*see* **Note 22**).
2. Seal plate with Parafil and incubate overnight (16–18 h) at 4°C.
3. Wash four times with 225 µL of TBS-T wash buffer per well for each wash.
4. Add 225 µL of 5% milk blocking solution to all wells and incubate 3 h at room temperature.
5. Dilute HLA-G5 and HLA-G6 proteins in BSA-T diluent to give a range of concentrations from 25 to 1000 ng/mL. Also dilute test samples to assure that ultimate absorbance values are within the linear range of the standards.
6. Add 100 µL of HLA-G standards and test samples to appropriate wells.
7. Seal the plate with Parafilm and incubate overnight (16–18 h) at 4°C.
8. Wash four times with 225 µL of TBS-T wash buffer per well, as before.
9. Add 100 µL of biotinylated-9-1F10, diluted to 1 µg/mL in BSA-T diluent to all wells.
10. Incubate 3 h at room temperature.
11. Wash four times with 225 µL of TBS-T wash buffer per well.
12. Add 100 µL HRP-strepavidin conjugate to each well and incubate 30 min at room temperature.
13. Wash four times with TBS-T wash buffer, as before.
14. Add 100 µL TMB substrate and incubate 15 min at room temperature.
15. Add 50 µL of 1 M H$_3$PO$_4$ to each well to stop the reaction.
16. Read absorbance at 450 nm using an automatic plate reader.
17. Construct a standard curve by plotting HLA-G protein concentration versus absorbance value. Typical standard curves for quantifying HLA-G5 and HLA-G6 are shown in **Fig. 4**.
18. Data analysis: data from capture ELISAs are evaluated in ways similar to those described previously for indirect ELISAs. Controls for the capture antibody and biotinylated detecting antibody should be compared with the respective specific antibodies to determine assay specificity.

3.2.4. Immunohistochemistry

The 16G1 mAb and others are suitable for immunohistochemical localization of soluble forms of HLA-G in human tissues *(11)*, but none can distinguish between HLA-G5 and HLA-G6. Here we describe a specific method for detection of HLA-G5 and HLA-G2/G6 in frozen sections of human placental tissue, using mAbs, anti-HLA-G5 (1-2C3) and anti-HLA-G2/G6 (26-2H11). We have found that staining procedures are also applicable to cytospin preparations of cultured cell lines and isolated trophoblast subpopulations. The results of staining first trimester villi with anti-HLA-G2/G6 (26-2H11) are shown in **Fig. 6**.

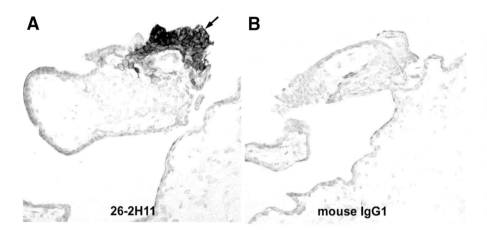

Fig. 6. Identification of HLA-G2/G6 using the mAb 26-2H11 in immunohistology. Tissue sections taken from a gestation-week-13 placenta were immunostained with either **(A)** anti-HLA-G2/G6 or **(B)** isotyped matched mouse immunoglobulin (Ig)G control. Binding was detected by using an anti-mouse IgG-horseradish peroxidase conjugate. Note that in **A**, cytotrophoblast cells distal to the villous express the proteins (arrow) both in the cell membrane and in the cytoplasm, whereas in **B**, no binding was detected.

1. Remove slides containing the frozen sections (*see* **Note 24**) from a –20°C freezer and allow warming to room temperature.
2. Fix for 10 min in acetone chilled to –20°C in a Coplin jar and subsequently air dry.
3. Circle each tissue section using a hydrophobic Pap pen to help localize staining reagents to the tissue section and prevent leakage to adjacent samples, if multiple sections are placed on a slide. Process slides as described below, taking care not to allow the tissue sections to dry out. Staining reagents are usually applied in volumes of approx 100 µL per tissue section.
4. Wash slides two times for 5 min each with PBS in a Coplin jar.
5. Block for endogenous peroxidase with ready to use peroxidase blocking solution, 10 min at room temperature.
6. Wash slides two times by immersing the slides in PBS.
7. Block with 10% horse serum diluted in antibody dilution buffer for 1 h at room temperature in humidified chamber (*see* **Note 25**).
8. Prepare the primary antibody in antibody dilution buffer: 1-2C3 (2.5 µg/mL), 26-2H11 (10 (µg/mL) and negative control IgG$_1$ isotype diluted to same concentration as primary antibody. Add to appropriate tissue sections and incubate one hour at 37°C in a humidified chamber.
9. Wash the slides two times for 5 min in PBS in a Coplin jar.
10. Prepare secondary antibody (biotinylated horse anti-mouse IgG) at 10 µg/mL in antibody dilution buffer plus 5% normal human serum (*see* **Note 26**). Apply to sections and incubate for 30 min at room temperature in a humidified chamber.

11. Wash the slides two times in PBS for 5 min in Coplin jar.
12. Dilute the streptavidin peroxidase conjugate in PBS as directed by the manufacturer. Apply to tissue sections and incubate 10 min in humidified chamber at room temperature.
13. Wash the slides two times in PBS for 5 min.
14. Dilute components of AEC substrate color development kit in distilled water as directed. Apply to tissue sections and incubate up to 15 min at room temperature for color development.
15. To stop the color development reaction wash the slides in distilled water.
16. Counter stain by dipping the slides in Mayer's hematoxylin for 10 s.
17. Wash the slides in tap water until excess hematoxylin is cleared.
18. Remove slides from the Coplin jar and apply one drop of Crystal Mount to each wet tissue section and carefully spread evenly over the entire tissue section.
19. Allow the slides to dry overnight at room temperature.
20. Next day coverslip slides using Permount.
21. Examine tissue sections microscopically to evaluate staining characteristics of the antibodies. Positive staining is indicated by a red color and should not be present in the sections treated with the mouse IgG_1 control.

4. Notes

1. Add 0.1 % DEPC to water, stir vigorously for at least 1 h, then autoclave using a liquid cycle for 15 min.
2. The primers can be custom made by several companies such as Integrated DNA Technologies, Inc. (Coralville, IA). The lyophilized stocks are reconstituted in 10 mM Tris-HCl pH 8.0 to 100 μM. The final concentration is determined by spectrophotometer readings at 260 nm. Working aliquots are prepared by dilution in sterile water to 20 μM, followed by storage –20°C.
3. 50X TAE for 1 L: 242 g of Tris base, 57.1 mL of glacial acetic acid, 100 mL of 0.5 M EDTA (pH 8.0), bring volume to one liter. Filter-sterilize by 0.22-μm filtration. Working solution is 1X, 40 mM Tris-acetate and 1 mM EDTA.
4. Fluorescent conjugates are sensitive to light and temperature. Original stocks of fluorescent conjugates should be protected from light and stored at 4°C. Also, fluorescently labeled cells should be similarly protected during staining procedures by performing incubations on ice and covering the rack of tubes with thick aluminum foil, working in a dimly lit laboratory and finally storing samples in the cold wrapped in thick aluminum foil.
5. 2% paraformaldehyde: weigh the amount needed and add to an appropriate volume of PBS. Place the suspension on a hot plate, under chemical hood and warm the suspension to 70–75°C while stirring until the powder is dissolved. Avoid boiling. Filter the solution through Whatman filter paper and store at 4°C. This solution is stable for a week at 4°C.
6. Stock solutions of protease inhibitors: PMSF, 100 mM, (17.42 mg/mL) dissolved in isopropanol, aliquoted and stored at room temperature. Aprotinin, prepared by dissolving to 4 mg/mL in H_2O, aliquot and store at –20°C. Leupeptin dissolved in H_2O to 5 mg/mL, aliquoted and stored at –20°C. EDTA, 0.5 M.

7. Transfer buffer, for 1 L, add 100 mL of 10X Tris/glycine buffer and 200 mL methanol to water to yield 1 L of solution. Store at 4°C.

8. Recombinant HLA-G5 and HLA-G6 proteins were produced by transfected HEK293 cells and purified as we have previously described *(11)*.

9. Monoclonal antibodies, 1-2C3 and 26-2H11, were produced as previously described *(11)* and purified from hybridoma culture supernatant by affinity chromatography on Protein G-Sepharose using standard methods.

10. The RNA extraction method of choice will depend on the sample available. We normally use TRIzol® reagent for both cells and tissue samples.

11. The RNA obtained by TRIzol extraction is digested with DNAase I (RNAase-free) to degrade any contaminating DNA, thus avoiding false amplification reactions during RT-PCR.

12. In our laboratory, the first strand cDNA synthesized from total RNA is obtained using MMLV-RT from Invitrogen. The final RT reaction sample is diluted fivefold with sterile water and stored in aliquots at –20°C (short term) or –80°C (long term).

13. The –RT reaction samples are used to rule out false amplification of residual genomic DNA and, therefore, confirm efficiency of the DNAse I digestions.

14. There is evidence that HLA-G mRNA levels are variable depending on the allele *(18)*. Therefore when signals are weak, increase the input of diluted cDNA to 10–20 μL, instead of 4 μL, and adjust the volume of water added to the PCR cocktail appropriately to achieve a total PCR reaction volume of 50 μL.

15. We use biotechnology grade agarose and ethidium bromide (20 mg/mL stock). We add ethidium bromide to a final concentration of 0.2 μg/mL after melting the agarose gel (2% agarose 3:1) in 1X TAE.

16. Amplicons obtained are visualized by using a UV transilluminator. The bands are extracted from the gel using QIAquick® gel extraction kit (Qiagen Inc., Valencia, CA) and sequenced using DNA sequencer kit from Applied Biosystems. Note that a pair of high-molecular-weight bands may be observed with the HLA-G5 primers.

17. The amount of GolgiStop™ required and the time of treatment should be determined experimentally for each cell type. Because protein transport inhibitors can become toxic to cells, incubation periods longer than 12 h are not recommended.

18. Cell dissociation: It is important to obtain a suspension of single cells with high viability (>90%). While trypsinization followed by repeated pipetting is sufficient for most applications, some cell lines and primary cell populations tend to aggregate. In these cases, we have been able to reduce the aggregates by passing cells through sterile 30-μm mesh filters immediately after trypsinization .

19. We use the DC protein assay from Bio-Rad Laboratories, Inc., and include Reagent S according to the manufacturer's instructions.

20. Use standard guidelines provided in brochures from Bio-Rad Laboratories for SDS-PAGE and electrotransfer to nitrocelose membranes. For immuno-detection, block membrane with blocking buffer (3% milk in 50 m*M* Tris-buffered saline [TBS], pH 7.4) for 1 h at room temperature. Subsequently, incubate for either 1 h at room temperature or overnight at 4°C with 16G1 mAb diluted to

1 µg/mL with antibody dilution buffer (3% milk in TBS containing 0.05% Tween-20, TBS-T). Wash three times (10 min on rocker) with TBS-T followed by incubation for 1 h at room temperature with HRP-conjugated anti-mouse IgG at 0.04 µg/mL in TBS-T. Wash membrane five times. Detect using HRP chemiluminescence substrate as described by the manufacturer.

21. Use Ezview™ instruction brochure for guidelines in immunoprecipitation.

22. Draw an 8 × 12 grid to represent a 96-well plate. Plan for replicates of three wells for each sample. Denote their position on the plate in a manner that is conducive to using an 8- or 12-channel pipet for adding reagents and washing procedures. Controls should include wells treated with (1) all the reagents except the analyte of interest to determine assay background and (2) control IgG in place of specific antibody or irrelevant protein in place of specific antigen as applicable for the type of assay to determine specificity.

23. Washing procedures: reagents and wash solutions are removed from the plate by flicking the liquid into a sink. The plate is then blotted two or three times onto fresh lint-free paper towels to remove any residual solution from the wells. Add appropriate solutions to the wells immediately after blotting to avoid drying. Avoid bubble formation in the wells whenever possible because they limit washing efficiency and introduce errors if present during absorbance readings. One way to avoid bubbles when adding solutions is to first preload pipet tips with a small volume (5–10 µL) prior to filling the tip. This can be accomplished by pressing the piston of the pipet to the "first stop" and inserting the tips into the solution. Carefully press the piston further and release back to the "first stop" to take up a small amount of solution. Then, fill the tip in the normal manner. Deliver solutions to the side of the wells, but press the piston only to the "first stop." Holding the piston at the "first stop" and return the pipet to the solution. Re-fill the tips normally and continue with reagent additions.

24. There are several methods for tissue fixation but our mAb 1-2C3 and 26-2H11 require tissues embedded in tissue freezing medium such as OCT. Tissue samples no larger than 1 cm^3 are placed in disposable plastic base molds and covered with OCT. The mold containing the tissue is placed on top of dry ice until solid then stored at –80°C. Two 5- to 8-µm thick cryostat sections are usually mounted on the same slide. These can be prepared in advance and stored at –20°C for several days prior to staining. The disadvantage of this method is poor tissue morphology when compared with paraffin embedded tissues.

25. It is necessary to use 10% serum from the animal in which the secondary antibody was raised.

26. When staining tissue that is known to contain large numbers of macrophages increase the percentage of human serum up to 40%.

Acknowledgments

This work was supported by grants from the National Institutes of Health to J. S. H. (HD39878 and HD26429) and to the University of Kansas Center for Reproductive Sciences (HD33994).

References

1. Janeway, C. A., Travers, P., Walport, M., and Capra, J. D. (1999) *Immunobiology.* Garland, New York, NY, pp. 509–516.
2. Ishitani, A., Sageshima, N., Lee, N., et al. (2003) Protein expression and peptide binding suggest unique and interacting functional roles for HLA-E, F, and G in maternal-placental immune recognition. *J. Immunol.* **171**, 1376–1384.
3. McMaster, M. T., Librach, C. L., Zhou, Y., et al. (1995) Human placental HLA-G expression is restricted to differentiated cytotrophoblasts. *J. Immunol.* **154**, 3771–3778.
4. Hunt, J. S. and Hutter, H. (1996) Current theories on protection of the fetal semiallograft, in *HLA and the Maternal-Fetal Relationship* (Hunt, J. S., ed.). Landes, Austin, TX: pp. 27–50.
5. Carosella, E. D., Dausset, J., and Rouas-Freiss, N. (1999) Immunotolerant functions of HLA-G. *Cell Mol. Life Sci.* **55**, 327–333.
6. Hunt, J. S. (2002) Immunogenetics: genetic regulation of immunity in pregnancy, in *Reproductive Medicine: Molecular, Cellular and Genetic Fundamentals* (Fauser, B. C. J. M., ed.). Parthenon, NY: pp. 153–167.
7. Ishitani, A. and Geraghty, D. E. (1992) Alternative splicing of HLA-G transcripts yields proteins with primary structures resembling both class I and class II antigens. *Proc. Natl.Acad. Sci. USA* **89**, 3947–3951.
8. Paul, P., Cabestre, F. A., Ibrahim, E. C., et al. (2000) Identification of HLA-G7 as a new splice variant of the HLA-G mRNA and expression of soluble HLA-G5, -G6, -G7 transcripts in human transfected cells. *Hum. Immunol.* **61**, 1138–1149.
9. Ober, C, Aldrich, C., Rosinsky, B., et al. (1998) HLA-G1 protein expression is not essential for fetal survival. *Placenta* **19**, 127–132.
10. Lee, N., Llano, M., Carretero, M., et al. (1998) HLA-E is a major ligand for the natural killer inhibitory receptor CD94/NKG2A. *Proc. Natl. Acad. Sci. USA* **95**, 5199–5204.
11. Morales, P., Pace, J. L., Platt, J. S., et al. (2003) Placental cell expression of HLA-G2 isoforms is limited to the invasive trophoblast phenotype. *J. Immunol.* **171**, 6215–6224.
12. McIntire, R. H., Morales, P. J., Petroff, M. G., Colonna, M., and Hunt, J. S. (2004) Recombinant HLA-G5 and -G6 drive U937 myelomonocytic cell production of TGF-β1. *J Leukoc Biol.* **76(6)**, 1220–1228..
13. Fournel, S., Aguerre-Girr, M., Huc, X., et al. (2000) Soluble HLA-G1 triggers CD95/CD95 ligand-mediates apoptosis in activated CD8+ cells by interacting with CD8. *J. Immunol.* **164**, 6100–6104.
14. LeMaoult, J., Krawice-Radanne, I., Dausset, J., and Carosella, E. D. (2004) HLA-G1-expressing antigen-presenting cells induce immunosuppressive CD4+ T cells. *Proc. Natl. Acad. Sci. USA* **101**, 7064–7069.
15. Chu, W., Yang, Y., Geraghty, D. E., and Hunt, J. S. (1999) Interferons enhance HLA-G mRNA and protein in transfected mouse fibroblasts. *J. Reprod. Immunol.* **42**, 1–15.

16. Jung, T., Schauer, U., Heusser, C., Neumann, C., and Rieger, S. (1993). Detection of intracellular cytokines by flow cytometry. *J. Immunol. Methods* **159,** 197–207.
17. Hunt, J. S., Pace, J. L., Morales, P. J., and Ober, C. (2003). Immunogenicity of the soluble isoforms of HLA-G. *Mol. Hum. Reprod.* **9,** 729–735.
18. Hviid, T. V. F, Hylenius, S., Rørbye, C., and Nielsen, L. G. (2003). *HLA-G* allelic variants are associated with differences in the *HLA-G* mRNA isoform profile and *HLA-G* mRNA levels. *Immunogenetics* **55,** 63–79.

IV

ANALYSIS OF PLACENTAL FUNCTION
Transport and Endocrinology

12

In Vivo Techniques for Studying Fetoplacental Nutrient Uptake, Metabolism, and Transport

Timothy R. H. Regnault and William W. Hay, Jr.

Summary

This chapter presents experimental methods to measure in vivo uteroplacental nutrient substrate uptake, transfer to the fetus, and metabolism by the uteroplacental unit. The fundamental method involves application of the Fick principle, which requires determination of uterine and umbilical blood flow rates and measurement of nutrient substrate arterial and venous concentrations in the uterine and umbilical circulations. Surgical approaches to placing catheters into these circulations are described. Details are provided to illustrate key concepts for net rates of uteroplacental glucose and amino acid uptake, transfer to the fetus, and net uteroplacental uptake.

Key Words: Placenta; uteroplacental; pregnancy; animal; surgery; vessels; uterine; fetus; umbilical; uterine; blood flow; uptake; glucose; amino acid.

1. Introduction

The purpose of this chapter is to present basic principles involved in measurement of uterine, umbilical, and uteroplacental uptake rates of different classes of nutrients (glucose and selected amino acids) by application of the Fick principle. This chapter will deal with studies in the sheep, although this methodology has been applied to pregnant females of many species as large as the horse and cow and as small as the guinea pig *(1–3)*.

The Fick principle is an example of the law of conservation of matter. Specifically, for a given substance, the amount that enters an organ equals the amount that leaves the organ minus the amount that was consumed by the organ plus the amount that was added by the organ. Application of the Fick principle involves computing the product of organ blood flow rate times the whole blood concentration difference of the substance in question across the organ. The placenta is unique in that it is perfused by two circulations, the (maternal) uterine circulation and the (fetal) umbilical circulation. The uterine circulation delivers nutrient substrates (e.g., oxygen, glucose, amino acids) through

From: *Methods in Molecular Medicine, Vol. 122: Placenta and Trophoblast: Methods and Protocols, Vol. 2*
Edited by: M. J. Soares and J. S. Hunt © Humana Press Inc., Totowa, NJ

its arterial circulation to the uterus for uterine and placental uptake, metabolism, and flux to the umbilical circulation. The uterine circulation also is responsible for the removal of waste products (CO_2 and urea) excreted from the fetus and placenta into the uterine venous circulation. The umbilical circulation takes up nutrient substrates from the placenta through the umbilical venous circulation (umbilical uptake) and distributes these substrates to fetal organs and tissues through the fetal systemic circulation. Waste products from fetal metabolism are then delivered to the placenta for transfer to the uterine venous circulation. These different fluxes of substances, specifically nutrient substrates, are net fluxes. They are regulated by the delivery rate of the substrate to the uteroplacenta and the transfer mechanisms into and across the uteroplacenta; simple diffusion as for oxygen and water, facilitated diffusion or transport via protein transporters as for glucose, and active diffusion or transport as for amino acids *(4–6)*.

It is important to note that for in vivo studies, because the uterine circulation supplies both the uterus and the placenta on the maternal side and these two flows cannot be separately measured, fluxes of substrates and waste products through the placenta cannot be resolved specifically. What is isolated is the uterus plus the placenta, or the uteroplacenta, which represents those tissues interposed between the uterine and umbilical circulations. Fortunately for most metabolic substances, based on isolated placental studies, microsphere blood flow measurements, and cell studies, between 70 and 80 % of uteroplacental uptake, transfer, and metabolism is accounted for by the placenta itself *(7,8)*. Thus, the terms uteroplacenta and placenta are often used interchangeably, although they have different absolute anatomical, physiological, and metabolic characteristics. For all nutrient substrates, application of the Fick principle to measure uterine, umbilical, and uteroplacental net uptake rates is accomplished by measuring uterine and umbilical net uptake rates and calculating uteroplacental net uptake rate as the difference between uterine and umbilical net uptake rates, where a negative result would represent a net production rate *(9–11)*.

2. Materials

2.1. Surgical Preparation of the Pregnant Sheep

1. Buprenorphine (0.01 mg/kg, subcutaneously [SC]).
2. Diazepam (0.11 mg/kg, intravenously [IV]).
3. Ketamine (4.4 mg/kg, IV).
4. Isoflurane (1–3%).
5. Buprenex (6 mg intramuscularly [IM] per dose).

6. Ampicillin (500 mg).
7. Heparin.
8. Saline.
9. Surgical equipment and various syringes (18–20 gauge).
10. Polyvinyl catheters.
11. Anesthetic gas inhalation machine.
12. Pulse oximeter.
13. Heparin and ethylenediamine tetraacetic acid (EDTA)-treated collection syringes.
14. Blood gas analyzer (e.g., Radiometer ABL 520, Brønshøj, Denmark).
15. Glucose/lactate analyzer (e.g., Yellow Springs Instruments 2700 Select, Yellow Springs, OH).

2.2. Measuring Uterine and Umbilical Blood Flow

2.2.1. Chemicals and Reagents

1. Tritiated water.
2. Saline.
3. Heparin.
4. Plasma solubilizer.
5. Liquid scintillation counting (LSC) cocktail.

2.2.2. Equipment Equipment

(This list will be common to the remaining techniques presented under in **Subheadings 2.3, 2.4.**, and **2.5.**)

1. Infusion pumps.
2. Timers.
3. Various syringes and catheter attachments.
4. Centrifuge capable of plasma separation.
5. Various collection tubes, centrifuge tubes and scintillation vials.
6. Vortex.
7. Liquid scintillation counter.

2.3. Measuring Uterine, Umbilical, and Uteroplacental Glucose Uptake in the Steady State Situation

2.3.1. Chemicals and Reagents

1. [6-^{3}H]glucose (250–500 μCi) and [U-^{14}C]glucose (250–500 μCi) dissolved in 30 mL of saline.
2. Saline.
3. Heparin.
4. Plasma solubilizer.
5. LSC cocktail.

2.4. Bolus Method to Determine Steady State and Unidirectional Flux Rates of a Non-metabolizable Amino Acid

2.4.1. Chemicals and Reagents

1. The labeled substrate of choice, generally dissolved in 10 mL of saline.
2. Saline.
3. Heparin.
4. Plasma solubilizer.
5. LSC cocktail.

2.5. Uteroplacental Uptake and Utilization of an Amino Acid (Threonine) Using Simultaneous Intravenous Infusions

2.5.1. Chemicals

1. Tritiated water.
2. A solution of L-[U-^{14}C]threonine (98% pure) and L-[U-^{13}C]threonine (131 mCi · mmol^{-1}) in saline for fetal infusion.
3. A preparation of L-[1-^{13}C]threonine (99% pure) in saline for maternal infusion.
4. Saline.
5. Heparin.
6. Plasma solubilizer.
7. LSC cocktail.

2.5.2. Equipment (In Addition to Those Described in Under **Subheading 2.2.2.**)

1. High-performance liquid chromatography (HPLC) for amino acid determinations.
2. Gas chromatograph-mass spectrometer.

3. Methods

3.1. Surgical Preparation of the Pregnant Sheep (see Note 1)

1. After 24 h fasting and 12 h without water, buprenorphine (0.01 mg/kg, SC) and diazepam (0.11 mg/kg, IV) are administered prior to the administration of anesthetic.
2. Approximately 1 h later, animals are sedated with ketamine (4.4 mg/kg, IV) and then placed on isoflurane (1–3%) inhalation following intubation.
3. Following securing the animal to the operating table, the uterus is exposed through a midline abdominal incision.
4. The uterine vein draining the pregnant horn is isolated by shunt dissection and a catheter is inserted (*see* **Note 5**).
5. The fetus is then exposed through an approximately 6-cm incision of the uterine wall, and polyvinyl catheters (1.4 mm outer diameter, *see* **Note 2**) are placed in the fetal pedal artery and vein and in the umbilical vein (*see* **Note 3**).
6. An additional catheter is placed in the amniotic cavity to allow amniotic antibiotic prophylaxis delivery to the fetus (*see* **Note 4**).

7. The uterine incision is closed with sutures, allowing the fetal catheters to move back and forth through the wound.
8. The maternal femoral artery, vein are then exposed through a grain incision and are also catheterized (*see* **Note 5**).
7. All catheters are then tunneled subcutaneously to a pouch secured to the animal's flank.
8. Following surgery, sheep are placed in individual carts with free access to water, feed and mineral blocks, depending upon experimental protocol.
9. Buprenex should be administered for pain relief every 12 h (6 mg IM per dose).
10. Ampicillin (500 mg) is injected daily into the amniotic cavity for the first 3 d after surgery.
11. Following surgery, daily samples are collected from mother and fetus and analyzed for glucose and lactate concentrations (heparin treated syringes) and also pH, PO_2, PCO_2 readings (EDTA-treated syringes) to monitor maternal and fetal well being.
12. Animals are allowed to recover from laparotomy for at least 5 d before study (*see* **Note 6**).
13. Catheters are then maintained patent with daily-heparinized saline flushes (35 U heparin $\cdot$ mL^{-1}).

3.2. Measuring Uterine and Umbilical Blood Flow (see Note 7)

1. On the day of study, a solution of tritiated water (^3H_2O, ~ 325 μCi, *see* **Note 8**) is administered at a rate of 5 mL $\cdot$ hr^{-1} following a three 3-mL priming dose in the fetal pedal vein. The infusion rate is determined with ^3H_2O syringe volume recordings at regular time intervals.
2. The ^3H_2O infusion begins 90 min before blood flow sampling commences to ensure a steady state concentration difference across the umbilical and uterine circulations during the course of the four-sample collection study period.
3. At steady state, four sets of 1-mL blood samples are drawn from maternal femoral artery (A), uterine vein (V), umbilical vein (v), and fetal artery (a) for analysis of maternal and fetal ^3H_2O concentrations. These four sets of samples are drawn over approximately 60–100 min with 15 –25 min spacings between the sampling draws.
4. Samples are also collected at each sampling from mother and fetus and analyzed for glucose and lactate concentrations and also pH, PO_2, PCO_2 and O_2 content determinations, to ensure physiological steady state during the experimental period.
5. For ^3H_2O whole blood analysis, 0.1-mL plasma samples are solubilized in 1.0 mL of a solubilizer and subsequently mixed with a suitable LSC cocktail. Blood ^3H_2O concentrations are calculated by using the relation of blood water content to hematocrit.
6. Determined tracer concentration is plotted against time (*see* **Note 9**).
7. The rate of tracer accumulation in the fetus is then determined from the slope of the fetal arterial plasma tracer concentration vs. time relationship. This rate of

fetal tracer accumulation can be subtracted from the infusion rate to obtain the actual transplacental flux rate of the tracer, which along with the concentration differences of the tracer across the umbilical circulations can be used to calculate umbilical blood flow rate (*see* **Note 10**).

8. A separate sample is collected at each steady state sampling period for measurement of the hematocrit, which is determined as packed cell volume.
9. Plasma flows are calculated using uterine or umbilical flow multiplied by one minus the fractional maternal or fetal hematocrit, respectively (*see* **Note 11**).
10. The placenta must be weighed at autopsy immediately after the physiological studies to express blood flow rates per unit mass.

3.3. Measuring Uterine, Umbilical, and Uteroplacental Glucose Uptake in the Steady State Situation

1. Prepare animal as described for surgery and conduct blood flow determinations.
2. Following measurement of umbilical and uterine blood flows, a 30 mL normal saline mixture of [6-^{3}H]glucose (250–500 µCi) and [U-^{14}C]glucose (250–500 µCi) is infused at a constant rate into a fetal femoral vein catheter, as a primed-constant infusion (*see* **Note 12**).
3. To calculate the maternal rate of glucose production (equal to maternal glucose utilization rate at steady state, unless there is exogenous glucose infused intravenously into the mother, in which case, utilization rate exceeds the infusion rate by the rate of maternal glucose production) 30 mL normal saline mixture of [6-^{3}H]glucose (250–500 µCi) is infused into the maternal femoral vein. Fetal glucose utilization rate is measured simultaneously by infusing [U-^{14}C]glucose (250–500 µCi) into the fetal femoral vein; fetal utilization rate is calculated as the ratio of infusion rate minus net loss to the placenta divided by the fetal arterial glucose specific radioactivity.
4. Whole blood samples from the maternal artery, uterine vein, umbilical vein, and fetal artery are then drawn simultaneously at approximately 60, 90, 120, 150, and 180 min after the beginning of the infusion (*see* **Note 13**).
5. The samples are then prepared and analyzed for ^{3}H$_2$O, glucose, and radioactive glucose concentrations, in a similar manner as described above previously for ^{3}H$_2$O determinations.
6. Radioactive glucose is measured as the gluconic acid derivative to avoid contamination by fructose (*see* **Note 14**).
7. At the end of the study, the ewe and fetus are euthanzied and tissue weights collected.
8. The fetuses are autopsied for tissue collection and weight measurements, and catheter location should also be confirmed.
9. Tracer and tracee uterine, umbilical and uteroplacental fluxes are then calculated (*see* **Notes 15** and **16**).

3.4. Bolus Method to Determine Steady State and Unidirectional Flux Rates of a Non-metabolizable Amino Acid. (see Note 17)

1. Prepare animal as described for surgery and conduct blood flow determinations.
2. Following blood flow determination sample collection, the radioactive non-metabolizable amino acid is dissolved in 10 mL of saline and injected as a bolus over a 1-min period into the maternal femoral vein.
3. During and after the bolus, blood samples (1 mL) are drawn simultaneously from the four vessels, A, V, v, and a. The sequence for the 16 sampling times should be: 0, 0.5, 1, 1.5, 2, 3, 4, 5, 10, 20, 30, 60, 90, 120, 150, and 180 min after the bolus injection (*see* **Note 18**). This sampling regimen ensures that the peak radioactivity in maternal plasma for the non-metabolizable amino acid can be determined.
4. Collected blood samples are then centrifuged, and for radioactivity measurements, plasma samples are solubilized and then mixed with a suitable LSC cocktail. Disintegrations per minute (dpm) are then measured for 10 min in a liquid scintillation analyzer.
5. For placental radioactivity content determinations, approximately 50 mg of ground placental tissue, collected at autopsy, is thawed and prepared for radioactivity determination in a liquid scintillation analyzer (*see* **Note 19**).
6. Calculate flux (clearance) of amino acid from mother to the fetus (*see* **Note 20**).

3.5. Uteroplacental Uptake and Utilization of an Amino Acid (Threonine) Using Simultaneous Intravenous Infusions (see Note 21)

1. Prepare animal as described for surgery.
2. On the day of study, the fetuses are infused at a constant rate ($0.085 \text{ mL} \cdot \text{min}^{-1}$) via the pedal vein catheter with a solution of L-[U-^{14}C]threonine (98% pure, ~ $0.4 \text{ μCi} \cdot \text{min}^{-1}$); L-[U-^{13}C]threonine (131 mCi $\cdot$ mmol^{-1}, ~ 2.0 μmol $\cdot$ min^{-1}) and tritiated water (2.1 μCi $\cdot$ min^{-1}), all mixed in normal saline.
3. At the same time, maternal sheep are infused at a constant rate via the femoral vein catheter with L-[1-^{13}C$_1$]threonine (99% pure, ~ 9.0 μmol·min^{-1}) dissolved in normal saline.
4. At 30-min intervals beginning 2 h after the start of the infusions, blood samples for ^{3}H$_2$O concentrations, blood gas determinations, glucose and lactate concentrations, and natural, stable and radioactive amino acid concentrations and enrichments are drawn simultaneously from the A, V, a, and v catheters, for a total of four samples. An initial sample set obtained before the start of the infusions is used for blank enrichment measurements.
5. For ^{3}H$_2$O whole blood analysis, 0.1-mL plasma samples are solubilized in 1.0 mL of a solubilizer and subsequently mixed with a suitable LSC cocktail as discussed in the blood flow determination section previously. Blood flow is converted to plasma flow as mentioned previously (*see* **Note 11**).

6. Samples are also collected at each sampling from mother and fetus and analyzed for glucose and lactate concentrations as well as pH, PO_2, PCO_2, and O_2 content determinations, to ensure physiological steady state during the experimental period.
7. Samples are also collected for the natural plasma concentration of the amino acid of interest and concentrations and uptakes determined (*see* **Note 22**), stable isotope enrichments of the amino acid of interest to calculate fluxes (*see* **Note 23**) and whole blood $^{14}CO_2$ as a measure of amino acid oxidation (*see* **Note 24**).
8. Following completion of sample collections, an autopsy is performed and the fetus, placental cotyledons, and uterine tissues are collected and weighed separately.

4. Notes

1. The techniques described here are for a near term single pregnancy in sheep. Surgery on younger animals is possible, but requires smaller catheters and different mode and location of placement. Fetuses younger than 80 days of gestation usually require catheterization of the fetal peripheral circulation (i.e., through umbilical branch vessels entering and leaving individual cotyledous of placentomes, rather than directly into the fetus) as previously described *(12)*.
2. Most investigators use polyvinyl catheters (1.4 mm outer diameter for 135 days gestational age 2–4 kg fetuses).
3. The tip of the umbilical venous catheter is placed in the common umbilical vein, generally about approx 2.5 to 3 cm from the junction of the umbilical cord and the skin surface in a 2–4 kg fetus, or directly into the common umbilical vein after exposure through a skin incision just caudal to the umbilicus.
4. Fetal pedal or brachial veins also can be catheterized at the same time for infusion of test substances, tracers, and replacement blood if required.
5. Catheters for the uterine circulation include a maternal hind limb (femoral) artery (representative of the uterine artery) and one of the uterine veins. Usually, a third- or fourth-order uterine vein is exposed high in the broad ligament of the pregnant horn and the catheter is advanced so that its tip extends approximately 3–5 cm beyond the ovary. Placement of the catheter in this position ensures sampling of blood that is representative of the uterine drainage, while minimizing any possible dilution of this sample with back flow from the inferior vena cava. A femoral vein catheter also is placed directly when the femoral artery catheter is inserted. Both can be done through one femoral skin incision. The femoral vein catheter serves as an infusion catheter for test substances and tracers.
6. Animals are recovered from surgery for at least 5 d before study as earlier observations indicated that both fetus and mother often were in negative nitrogen balance for this long *(13)*. However, it should be noted that these earlier studies were conducted using spinal anesthesia, as opposed to current studies, and it is likely that animals are in fact in normal nitrogen balance within 3 d post surgery.
7. The Fick principle requires accurate measurement of uterine and umbilical blood flow at the same time that substrate concentrations are sampled from the uterine artery and vein and the umbilical artery and vein *(9)*. Current approaches to these

measurements with Doppler ultrasound determinations are not sufficiently accurate for this purpose. Both Doppler and electromagnetic flow probe determinations as used in the sheep preparation do not satisfy the requirement that they measure total uterine or umbilical blood flow, since their measurements can only be taken across one single vessel at one time. Indicator or tracer methods do measure total flow rates simultaneously with sampling during a steady state period and have been the mainstay of in vivo blood flow measurements. Furthermore, they can be continued for long periods and repeated as often as needed. Microspheres also can be injected at the time of sampling to accurately estimate blood flow, but repeated measures are less reliable, thereby confining their use to one or two experimental periods.

8. Several inert or relatively inert solutes can be used to determine blood flow in the pregnant animal. Most studies have used antipyrine, ethanol (EtOH), or tritiated water (^3H_2O) *(11,14)*. Each of these has a flow-limited clearance, in that the placental permeability to these compounds is very high and the major determinant of how much of these compounds are transferred or cleared across the placenta is a direct function of blood flow. Tritiated water is radioactive and is readily measured, though for accurate measurements, generally one mL of whole blood is required. EtOH, on the other hand, requires only 0.3 mL of blood, is not radioactive, and allows the experimental design to incorporate tritiated tracer substances for study at the same time. One problem with the use of EtOH is the determination of EtOH concentrations through enzymatic determination and spectrophotometer analysis is time consuming and calls for careful measurements as small experimental errors can greatly alter arteriovenous concentration differences. Antipyrine, although an excellent inert solute for these types of studies is the least used of the three, because systems for its concentration determination are not readily available.

9. A substance that is inert (non-metabolizable) and diffuses across membranes as fast as it arrives at the membrane can be used to determine umbilical and uterine blood flow rates when infused into the fetus at a constant rate. During such an infusion, the accumulation rate of the substance can be measured as the slope of its increasing concentration over the early phase of infusion; or, one can wait until the substance has equilibrated in the fetal fluids and tissues, at which time its infusion rate into the fetal circulation equals its disappearance rate out of the fetus, termed a steady state. Because the fetus swallows large amounts of amniotic fluid, any tracer that enters the amniotic fluid, either by diffusion across skin and umbilical cord tissue or from fetal urine, re-enters the fetus. Thus, transplacental diffusion represents the only escape of the tracer from the fetal circulation and infusion rate equals disappearance rate. Using the Fick principle calculation, the disappearance rate of the tracer from the fetal circulation, measured as the infusion rate of the tracer into the fetal circulation, divided by arteriovenous concentration difference across the placenta (umbilical arterial – umbilical venous tracer concentration) represents the rate of umbilical blood flow ($mL \cdot min^{-1} \cdot kg \ fetus^{-1}$).

10. The rapid rise in concentration that occurs within the fetal circulation establishes the transplacental concentration gradient that facilitates the movement of the solute across the placental tissues into the uterine circulation, thus preventing rapid accumulation within the fetus. This gradient also serves to establish a steady-state condition in which the arteriovenous differences between the umbilical artery and vein and the maternal artery and uterine vein are constant.

11. For substances that are carried in red blood cells (RBC) as well as plasma and have a very rapid exchange rate across the RBC membranes (e.g., glucose), whole blood concentrations should be measured along with uterine and umbilical whole blood flow rates. For substances that are carried only in the plasma, or if the substrate is carried in the RBCs but has a negligible rate of exchange across the RBC membrane (e.g., amino acids), plasma concentrations should be measured along with uterine and umbilical plasma flow rates (*15*). Plasma flows are calculated using uterine or umbilical flow multiplied by one less the fractional maternal or fetal hematocrit, respectively (*16*).

12. The ratio of prime dose to constant infusion rate has been determined from earlier experiments that provided estimates of maternal and fetal glucose turnover rates and pool sizes (*17*). Briefly, one-fifth to one-fourth of the tracer infusate is injected as a priming dose, followed by a constant infusion of $0.1 \text{ mL} \cdot \text{min}^{-1}$. Data collected using this format show that constant specific activities, indicative of a steady state situation, are observed in all sampling vessels within 90 min of the priming injection.

13. Previous studies have determined that steady-state conditions for glucose and tracer glucose are achieved and maintained at these times.

14. To measure glucose radioactivity, whole blood is hemolyzed and deproteinized with $ZnSO_4$ and $Ba(OH)_2$. Samples are then incubated for one 1 h at 37°C and then passed through a 2.0-mL bed volume anion exchange column. Equal aliquots of the supernatant are then incubated for one 1 h at 37°C with an excess of glucose oxidase to convert the glucose to gluconic acid and then passed through identical columns. The glucose oxidase step avoids contamination of the glucose determination with radioactive fructose.

    The columns are then washed with 3.0 mL of water and the collected eluates evaporated to dryness to remove ^3H_2O. Dried samples are then resuspended in water, scintillation fluid is added, and samples are placed in a liquid scintillation analyzer. The determined cpms are corrected to dpms with appropriate blanks and external standard quench and efficiency corrections. The radioactivity of glucose is then calculated as the difference in dpm between the two column eluates, glucose having been retained on the second column as gluconate as described (*17*).

15. Glucose tracer and tracee fluxes; the determination of the relative uptakes is given by these formulae:

    • Uterine net substrate uptake rate (mmole/min) = uterine blood flow rate (mL/min) × [uterine arterial-venous substrate concentration difference, mmole/mL blood].

- Umbilical net substrate uptake rate (mmole/min) = umbilical blood flow rate (mL/min) × [umbilical venous-arterial substrate concentration difference, mmole/mL blood].
- Uteroplacental net substrate uptake rate (mmole/min) = uterine – umbilical net substrate uptake rate (mmole/min).
- Maternal glucose production (for tracer glucose infused into the maternal femoral vein) = tracer infusion rate (dpm/min)/maternal arterial glucose specific activity (dpm/mg).
- Maternal glucose production (for tracer glucose infused into the fetal femoral vein) = glucose utilization of the non-uterine maternal tissues + net uterine glucose uptake, where glucose utilization of the non-uterine maternal tissues = net maternal tracer uptake rate (dpm/min)/maternal arterial glucose specific activity (dpm/mg) and where net maternal tracer uptake = uterine blood flow × uterine venous-arterial blood tracer glucose concentration difference.

16. The difference between uterine and umbilical net uptake rates represents the net rate of glucose consumption by the uteroplacental tissues. The uteroplacenta comprises the maternal and fetal vasculature, uterine tissues (e.g., epithelium, myometrium, and endometrium), and the trophoblast or placenta *(18)*. The fraction of uteroplacental net substrate uptake (consumption) rate that is strictly placental (trophoblast) has not been determined; however, as previously mentioned, blood flow *(19)*, Fick principle *(20)*, and tracer *(17)*, estimates indicate that most (at least 70–80%) of net uteroplacental substrate uptake is placental.

17. The purpose of this experimental approach is to determine unidirectional and steady-state flux rates for a substrate across the placenta. Following a bolus injection of a tracer (radiolabeled or stable isotope) of the substrate of interest into the maternal or fetal circulation, repeated sampling over 20–30 min in the opposite circulation (uterine vein for a fetal injection or umbilical vein for a maternal injection) allows calculation of the area under the curve (AUC) for concentration vs time. This rapid distribution period provides a quantitative estimate of the immediate rate of substrate transport across the placenta, which then can be used, for example, to determine the relationship between transporter concentration and unidirectional transport rate. Both metabolizable and non-metabolizable tracers can be used, although if metabolizable tracers are used, measurement of metabolic products (e.g., carbon-labeled CO_2, lactate, and fructose for a metabolizable glucose tracer in sheep) and subtraction from the calculated total rate of transport are required to determine the net rate of tracer substrate transport independent of metabolism. The metabolizable tracer does, however, provide the opportunity for insight into the rates of transport vs. metabolism, and might be useful for determining how these different pathways are altered when placental function changes. In the details provided the example of a non-metabolizable amino acid is presented. Non-metabolizable amino acids represent a class of analogues that allow examina-

tion of placental amino acid transport in isolation, without confounding variables introduced by placental and fetal metabolism.

18. Relatively large volumes of blood often are required for analytical measurements during Fick principle and tracer studies of uteroplacental substrate uptake, metabolism, and transfer. This can produce considerable blood loss in the sampling process, particularly in the fetal circulation, leading to hypovolemia and pathophysiological consequences. Fetal blood transfusions can be used in such studies to maintain fetal blood volume and normal circulation during the steady state sampling periods. Donor fetuses are especially useful for long-term transfusion studies, providing fetal hemoglobin to prevent changes in the oxygen-hemoglobin dissociation curve and thus fetal oxygenation. For shorter studies of two 2 to six 6 h, however, maternal blood transfusion does not appear to produce measurable adverse effects on fetal physiological or metabolic conditions. Fetal transfusions during the steady state period could introduce sufficient blood that could dilute the inert solute tracer concentrations, upsetting the arteriovenous concentration differences. This usually is not a problem if transfusion volumes are limited to 8–10 mL, as because the transfusion of 8–10 mL represents no more than an approx 2% alteration in blood volume of a 3.5-kg fetus. A period of 10–15 min after the transfusion before the next sample is taken has not been associated with measurable changes in the arteriovenous differences of metabolic substrates or their tracers before and after the transfusion.

19. Whole placentomes are dissected into maternal (caruncle) and fetal (cotyledon) components, snap frozen in liquid nitrogen, and stored at –70°C. At the time of radioactivity determination, approx 6–10 grams of sample is ground under liquid nitrogen and approximately 50 mg of ground placental tissue thawed and dissolved in 2 mL of a commercial tissue solubilizer, and incubated at 60°C overnight. Samples are then allowed to cool, after which 200 mL of 30% peroxide is added and samples reheated at 60°C for 5 h. After cooling, 20 mL of a compatible liquid scintillation fluid is added and samples are left overnight. The radioactive content (dpm) is then counted for 10 min in a liquid scintillation analyzer.

20. Calculation of steady state and unidirectional flux rates, using a non-metabolizable amino acid as an example. For these calculations, we prefer to use the term *clearance*, which takes into account arterial concentrations of a test substrate during the measurment period. As in many experimental settings this may have been manipulated by the investigator, especially in the situation of a bolus injection. The transplacental clearance of our non-metabolizable amino acid example, Aminocyclopentane-1-carboxylic acid (ACP), or the clearance to the fetus from the mother $(C_{f,m}, \text{ mL/min})$ is calculated according to the equation:

$$C_{f,m} = f \cdot \frac{\int_0^{180} (\gamma - \alpha)_t \, dt}{\int_0^{180} A_t \, dt}$$

where f is umbilical plasma flow, $(\gamma - \alpha)_t$ is the ACP concentration difference between umbilical venous and arterial plasma at time t (min) and A_t is the maternal arterial plasma ACP concentration at time t. The integral in the numerator of the function is the area under the curve of a plot of $(\gamma - \alpha)$ vs t for the 0- to 180-min period, with 0 being the time of the bolus ACP injection. The integral in the denominator is the area under the curve of a plot of A vs. t for the same time period. Areas are estimated using Area Under Curve (AUC) determinations software.

For the purpose of graphic representation, in each animal the 16 sets of maternal and fetal ACP clearance measurements (C_t) are used to calculate 16 data points. The C_t values are then plotted against time. Each C_t value represents umbilical uptake of ACP at sampling time t, normalized for placental weight and the integral of maternal arterial ACP concentration:

$$C_t = f \cdot \frac{(\gamma - \alpha)_t}{\left(100 g_{placenta}\right) \cdot \overline{A}}$$

where $\overline{A} = \int_0^{180} A_t dt / 180$

This calculation represents only that movement to the fetus and a total placental ACP clearance calculation should also be determined. At 180 min after ACP injection into the maternal circulation, an appreciable amount of ACP is present in the placenta, and at higher concentrations than in the 180 min maternal plasma samples *(21,22)*. Therefore, the net uptake of ACP by the placenta from the maternal circulation has two components, i.e., the quantity crossing the basal membrane into the umbilical circulation (umbilical uptake) and the quantity retained by the placenta. The latter quantity was used to calculate a placental retention clearance (C_r):

$$C_r = \frac{P_{180}}{\int_0^{180} A_t dt}$$

where P_{180} is the quantity of ACP present in the whole placenta at 180 min. The total placental clearance of ACP from the maternal circulation (C_{tot}) was then calculated as the sum of C_r and $C_{f,m}$:

$$C_{tot} = C_r + C_{f,m}$$

For purpose of comparison between animals, the C_{tot}, C_r, and $C_{f,m}$ clearances should be expressed per 100 g placenta.

21. Simultaneous infusion studies are used to determine substrate fluxes, including maternal and fetal disposal and clearance rates, as well as substrate metabolism parameters (CO_2 production) and the flux from mother to fetus, and the back flux of the substrate of study from the fetus back to the placenta. These are complex studies requiring maternal and fetal infusions, similar to the glucose studies described in under **Subheading 3.3.**

22. In the following three sets of notes and accompanying equations, the amino acid of choice is threonine, and the symbols A, V, a, v, will be used to indicate maternal artery, uterine vein, fetal artery, umbilical vein, as previously outlined, and

now we will add the symbols I, f, p, and m to represent infusate, fetus, placenta, and mother, respectively. For the purpose of calculating umbilical and uterine threonine uptakes, the concentrations of plasma threonine measured by the amino acid analyzer were corrected by subtracting the concentrations of tracer threonine. Currently, our amino amino-acid concentrations are determined in the following manner. Plasma is quickly thawed, deproteinized with a solution of 10% sulfosalicylic acid, with L-norleucine added as internal standard, and buffered with LiOH to pH 2.2. Samples are then centrifuged at 14,000g for 10 min, and the supernatant fraction is filtered through a Millipore filter and loaded onto a high-performance liquid chromatography (HPLC) column with refrigerated autosampler. The samples are then analyzed by cation exchange column with gradient change from three different buffers isothermally. Ninhydrin is used as color reagent, and a dual wavelength spectrophotometer with wavelengths of 440 and 570 nm is used for concentration determinations.

Fetal and maternal coefficients of threonine extraction across the umbilical (COE_f) and uterine (COE_m) circulations are estimated according to the formulas:

$$COE_f = (Thr_v - Thr_a) / Thr_a$$

$$COE_m = (Thr_A - Thr_V) / Thr_A$$

where Thr represents the corrected plasma threonine concentration. The uterine uptake of threonine (μmol/min) is calculated using uterine plasma flow (*see* **Note 11**) and the arteriovenous concentration difference of plasma threonine across the uterine circulation $(\Delta Thr)_{A-V}$.

$$\text{uterine threonine uptake} = \text{uterine plasma flow } (\Delta Thr)_{A-V}$$

The equation assumes that maternal plasma is the only blood compartment exchanging threonine with the pregnant uterus, which is supported by other findings in sheep plasma (*15*). Similarly, umbilical threonine uptake is calculated using umbilical plasma flow,

$$\text{umbilical threonine uptake} = \text{umbilical plasma flow } (\Delta Thr)_{v-a}$$

where $(\Delta Thr)_{v-a}$ is the venous-arterial concentration difference of plasma threonine across the umbilical circulation.

23. The fetal plasma threonine disposal rate (DR) is calculated using the infusion rate of L-[U-^{13}C]threonine into the fetus

$$DR = (100\ I^* / MPE_a^f) - I$$

where I^* is the fetal infusion rate of L-[U-^{13}C]threonine, I is the infusion rate of threonine (both tracer and tracee), and MPE_a^f is the steady-state molar percent enrichment of the fetally infused threonine in fetal arterial plasma. Stable isotopic enrichments are analyzed with a gas chromatograph-mass spectrometer in the electron impact mode, in 250 μL of acidified plasma using 50 n*M* of L-norleucine as internal standard. The amino acid fraction is separated from other fractions on a 1.5-cm cation-exchange resin column (50W × 8, 100–200 mesh, hydrogen form) eluted with 1 mL of 15% NH_4OH. Percentage recoveries of basic, neutral, and acidic amino acids are tested with corresponding radiolabeled amino acids and varied from 80 to 92%. Samples are dried, derivatized with 15% tert-butyldimethylsilyl, or (TBDMS), and injected in triplicate on a gas chromatograph equipped with a 30-m DB-1 0.25-mm-ID inner diameter, 0.25-mm film thickness, with helium as the carrier gas, and a Mass Selective Device.

Enrichments of plasma amino acids are calculated by comparing the difference in peak area ratios between enriched and unenriched samples according to the formula molar percent enrichment (MPE) (%) =

$$\frac{100 \times (\text{ratio of enriched sample - ration of unenriched sample})}{[(\text{ratio of enriched sample - ratio of unenriched sample}) + 1]}$$

where MPE expresses the relative abundance of the enriched tracer in excess of that occurring naturally. Peaks are then read at mass-to-charge ratios (m/z).

The maternal plasma threonine DR is calculated using the infusion rate of tracer threonine in the mother and an equation analogous to the DR equation above for fetal DR. In both mother and fetus, plasma threonine clearance was calculated as the DR-to-plasma arterial concentration ratio and expressed as $mL \cdot min^{-1} \cdot kg$ body wt^{-1}. The direct flux of maternal threonine into the fetal systemic circulation (flux$_{f,m}$) is calculated according to the equation:

$$(\text{flux}_{f,m}) = (DR) \cdot MPE_a^m \div MPE_A^m \cdot \left(100 - MPE_A^m\right) / \left(100 - MPE_a^m\right)$$

where MPE_a^m and MPE_A^m are molar percent enrichments of maternally infused L-[1–$^{13}C_1$]threonine in fetal arterial and maternal arterial plasma, respectively.

The loss of tracer threonine molecules $\left(r_{p,f}^{13Thr}\right)$ to the placenta from the fetal circulation is calculated as the product of umbilical plasma flow (f) times the concentration difference of fetally infused tracer threonine (^{13}Thr) between umbilical arterial (a) and venous (v) blood.

$$r_{p,f}^{13Thr} = f\left(\Delta^{13}Thr\right)_{a-v}$$

The $r_{p,f}^{13Thr}$ rate is then used to estimate the fraction of fetally infused tracer taken in by the placenta. Back flux of fetal threonine into the placenta can then be calculated as the product of the fraction times fetal DR.

24. Nutrients taken up by the placenta either can be transported to the fetus or metabolized, or both. The Fick principle can also be used to quantify the metabolism of carbon consumed by the placenta to CO_2 as the difference between the rates of uterine and umbilical CO_2 excretion, each of those calculated as the product of umbilical or uterine blood flow rate and the umbilical arterial-venous or the uterine venous-arterial CO_2 concentration difference *(23)*. Measurement of blood CO_2 concentrations is technically difficult, so these values are commonly calculated using ^{14}C- or ^{13}C-labeled tracers of the nutrient substrate and measuring labeled $^{14}CO_2$ or $^{13}CO_2$ concentrations.

To measure $^{14}CO_2$ activity, whole blood samples of approximately 0.3–0.4 mL are injected anaerobically into a small glass vial which is glued with epoxy to the inside wall of a plastic scintillation vial containing 1.0 mL of tissue solubilizer, as described *(24)*. Briefly, following this, about 0.5 mL of 1.0 N HCl is added anaerobically to the blood to liberate all of the CO_2, which is trapped in the solubilizer as a stable carbamate. The vial is then incubated overnight at room temperature on an orbital shaker. After this incubation period, 15 mL of LSC 99:1 with methanol is added and the radioactivity counted.

The rate of $^{14}CO_2$ $\left(r_{p,f}^{14CO_2}\right)$ produced from tracer threonine and excreted by the fetus via the umbilical circulation (dpm/min) was measured as the product of umbilical blood flow (f) and the concentration difference between umbilical arterial and venous $^{14}CO_2$ blood concentrations

$$r_{p,f}^{14CO_2} = f \cdot \left(\Delta^{14}CO_2\right)_{a-v}$$

The fetal threonine oxidation fraction (ϕ_f) is calculated as

$$\phi_f = r_{p,f}^{14CO_2} \div I**$$

where I** is the infusion rate of L-[U-^{14}C]threonine. This fraction represents the fraction of the infused tracer threonine carbon excreted as $^{14}CO_2$ via the umbilical circulation. Umbilical excretion of CO_2 (μmol/min) derived from fetal plasma threonine carbon $\left(R_{p,f}^{CO_2}\right)$ was estimated as

$$R_{p,f}^{CO_2} = DR \cdot 4 \cdot \phi_f$$

DR is multiplied by 4 to convert the micromoles of threonine to micromoles of threonine carbon.

The rate of $^{14}CO_2$ produced from fetal tracer threonine and excreted into the mother via the placenta $R_{p,m}^{14CO_2}$ is measured as the product of uterine blood flow (F) and the concentration difference between uterine venous and maternal arterial $^{14}CO_2$ blood concentrations

$$r_{p,m}^{14CO_2} = F \cdot \left(\Delta^{14}CO_2\right)_{V-A}$$

The uterine threonine oxidation fraction (ϕ_U) can then be defined as

$$\phi_U = r_{p,m}^{14CO_2} \div I**$$

This fraction represents the fraction of fetally infused tracer threonine carbon excreted as $^{14}CO_2$ via the uterine circulation. The fetal plus placental production of CO_2 (μmol/min) derived from fetal plasma threonine carbon $\left(R_{p,m}^{CO_2}\right)$ is estimated as

$$R_{p,m}^{CO_2} = DR \cdot 4 \cdot \phi_U$$

Acknowledgments

This work was supported by National Institutes of Health grant HD28794 (WWH, PI) and National Institutes of Health grant HD41505 (TRHR, Co-I).

The authors also wish to acknowledge all of the staff and trainees at University of Colorado Health Sciences Center Perinatal Research Center, past and present, who have made so many of the techniques discussed in this chapter common practice. Particularly, we wish to thank Drs. Giacomo Meschia and Frederick Battaglia who pioneered the techniques discussed in this chapter and under whose mentorship many of us learned to understand and use them. The ease with which we use these techniques today is a reflection of their mentorship and should in no way diminish the complex biology which we study by using techniques that we often take for granted.

References

1. Bissonnette, J. M., Hohimer, A. R., Cronan, J. Z., and Black, J. A. (1979). Glucose transfer across the intact guinea-pig placenta. *J. Dev. Physiol.* **1,** 415–426.
2. Ferrell, C. L. and Reynolds, L. P. (1992). Uterine and umbilical blood flows and net nutrient uptake by fetuses and uteroplacental tissues of cows gravid with either single or twin fetuses. *J. Anim. Sci.* **70,** 426–433.
3. Fowden, A. L., Taylor, P. M., White, K. L., and Forhead, A. J. (2000). Ontogenic and nutritionally induced changes in fetal metabolism in the horse. *J. Physiol.* **528(Pt 1),** 209–219.
4. Battaglia, F. C. and Meschia, G. (1986). Fetal and placental metabolism: Part II Amino acids and lipids, in *An Introduction to Fetal Physiology*, Academic Press, Orlando, FL, pp. 100–135.
5. Battaglia, F. C. and Meschia, G. (1986). Transplacental diffusion:Basic concepts, in *An Introduction to Fetal Physiology*, Academic Press, Orlando, FL, pp. 28–49.
6. Regnault, T. R. H., de Vrijer, B., and Battaglia, F. C. (2003). Transport and metabolism of amino acids in placenta. *Endocrine* **19,** 23–41.
7. Battaglia, F. C. and Meschia, G. (1988). Fetal nutrition. *Annu. Rev. Nutrition* **8,** 43–61.
8. Hay, W. W. J. (1996). Placental function. I, in *Scientific Basis of Pediatric and Perinatal Medicine,* (Gluckman, P. D. and Heymann, M. A., eds.), Edward Arnold Ltd, London, pp. 213–227.
9. Meschia, G., Cotter, J. R., Makowski, E. L., and Barron, D. H. (1967). Simultaneous measurement of uterine and umbilibal blood flows and oxygen uptakes. *Quart. J. Exp. Physiol.* **LII,** 465–482.
10. Meschia, G., Battaglia, F. C., and Bruns, P. D. (1967). Theoretical and experimental study of transplacental diffusion. *J. Applied Physiol.* **22,** 1171–1178.
11. Wilkening, R. B., Anderson, S., and Meschia, G. (1984). Non-steady state placental transfer of highly diffusible molecules. *J. Dev. Physiol.* **6,** 121–129.
12. Bell, A. W., Battaglia, F. C., and Meschia, G. (1987). Methods for chronic studies of circulation and metabolism in the sheep conceptus at 70-80 days gestation. In , in *Animal Models in Fetal Medicine, Vol. 6,* (Nathanielsz, P. W., ed.), Perinatology Press, Ithaca, NY, pp. 38–54.

13. Gresham, E. L., James, E. J., Raye, J. R., Battaglia, F. C., Makowski, EL, and Meschia, G. (1972). Production and excretion of urea by the fetal lamb. *Pediatrics* **50,** 372–379.

14. Bonds, D. R., Anderson, S., and Meschia, G. (1980). Transplacental diffusion of ethanol under steady state conditions. *J. Dev. Physiol.* **2,** 409–416.

15. Chung, M., Teng, C., Timmerman, M., Meschia, G., and Battaglia, F. C. (1998). Production and utilization of amino acids by ovine placenta in vivo. *Am. J. Physiol.* **274,** E13–E22.

16. Regnault, T. R. H., de Vrijer, B., Galan, H. L., Davidsen, M. L., Trembler, K. A., Battaglia, F. C., et al. (2003). The relationship between transplacental O2 diffusion and placental expression of PlGF, VEGF and their receptors in a placental insufficency model of fetal growth restriction. *J. Physiol.* **550,** 641–656.

17. Hay, W. W. J., Sparks, J. W., Quissel, B. J., Battaglia, F. C., Meschia, G., and Quissell, B. J. (1981). Simultaneous measurments of umbilical uptake, fetal utilisation rate and fetal turnover rate of glucose. *Am. J. Physiol.* **240,** E662–E668.

18. Battaglia, F. C. and Meschia, G. (1986). Uteroplacental blood flow, in *An Introduction to Fetal Physiology*, Academic, Orlando, FL, pp. 212–229.

19. Makowski, E. L., Meschia, G., Droegemueller, W., and Battaglia, F. C. (1968). Measurement of umbilical arterial blood flow to the sheep placenta and fetus in utero. Distribution to cotyledons and the intercotyledonary chorion. *Circulation Res.* **23,** 623–3631.

20. Simmons, M. A., Battaglia, F. C., and Meschia, G. (1979). Placental transfer of glucose. *J. Dev. Physiol.* **1,** 227–243.

21. de Vrijer, B., Regnault, T. R., Wilkening, R. B., Meschia, G., and Battaglia, F. C. (2004). Placental uptake and transport of ACP, a neutral nonmetabolizable amino acid, in an ovine model of fetal growth restriction. *Am. J. Physiol. Endocrinol. Metab.* **287,** E1114–1124.

22. Jozwik, M., Teng, C., Timmerman, M., Chung, M., Meschia, G., and Battaglia, F. C. (1998). Uptake and transport by the ovine placenta of neutral nonmetabolizable amino acids with different transport system affinities. *Placenta* **19,** 531–538.

23. Hay, W. W. J. and Sparks, J. W. (1988). Tracer methods for studying fetal metabolism in vivo. I, in *Animal Models in Fetal Medicine, Vol. 6,* (Nathanielsz, P. W., ed.). Perinatology Press, Ithaca, NY, pp. 133–177.

24. Van Veen L. C., Hay, W. W. J., Battaglia, F. C., and Meschia, G. (1984). Fetal CO_2 kinetics. *J. Dev. Physiol.* **6,** 359–365.

13

In Vitro Models for Studying Trophoblast Transcellular Transport

Claudia J. Bode, Hong Jin, Erik Rytting, Peter S. Silverstein, Amber M. Young, and Kenneth L. Audus

Summary

In vitro models have proven to be effective in studying the placental transporters that play a role in the exchange of nutrients, waste products, and drugs between the maternal and fetal circulations. Although primary cultures of trophoblast cells can be used to perform uptake, efflux, and metabolism studies, only the rodent HRP-1 and the human BeWo cell lines have been shown to form confluent monolayers when grown on semi-permeable membranes. Protocols for the revival, maintenance, passage, and growth of BeWo cells for transporter expression and transcellular transport studies are provided.

Key Words: Trophoblast cells; BeWo cell; transcellular transport; efflux mechanisms.

1. Introduction

As the fetus develops within the uterus, its sole link to the mother's blood circulation is through the placenta. Serving as a barrier between the mother and the fetus, the placenta mediates the transfer of nutrients and metabolic waste products while also secreting hormones that maintain pregnancy. The vectorial exchange of these compounds occurs because of the polarized nature of the placenta, and specifically the rate-limiting, single cell layer called the syncytiotrophoblast (1–3). In the process of forming the syncytiotrophoblast, blastocyst-derived cytotrophoblast stem cells invade the uterus to reach the maternal blood supply. Ultimately, the terminal differentiation of these cytotrophoblasts results in the complete fusion of lateral cell membranes, such that a polarized multinucleated syncytium forms (4). The maternal-facing plasma membrane of the syncytium consists of a microvillous brush border membrane that is in direct contact with maternal blood. On the opposite side, the basal membrane faces the fetal circulation and lacks microvillar projections. The two sides of the syncytium are not only structurally distinct, but also differ in the localization of transporters, enzymes, and hormone receptors.

From: *Methods in Molecular Medicine, Vol. 122: Placenta and Trophoblast: Methods and Protocols, Vol. 2*
Edited by: M. J. Soares and J. S. Hunt © Humana Press Inc., Totowa, NJ

In order to investigate the transport of nutrients, drugs, and pathogens across the placental syncytium, it is essential to utilize an effective in vitro model system in which cultured cells form a confluent monolayer on semi-permeable supports. Primary cultures of undifferentiated human cytotrophoblast cells can be isolated from term placentas *(5)*. These cells syncytialize spontaneously when cultured and provide a good in vitro model system to successfully study uptake, efflux, metabolism, and hormone secretion. Unfortunately, instead of forming a tight-junctioned monolayer appropriate for transport studies, these nonproliferative, multinucleated cells form aggregates with large intercellular spaces when grown on semi-permeable membranes. In order to address this obstacle, Hemmings et al. have prepared confluent cell layers of syncytiotrophoblasts on semi-permeable supports *(6)*. This technique involves plating highly purified primary cultures of cytotrophoblasts in three successive cycles of seeding and differentiation. Although this method produces multiple overlapping layers of syncytialized cells, these cultures possess areas of microvillar projections on the apical surface and function as a barrier to low and high-molecular-weight molecules.

There are a variety of other experimental trophoblast systems available, including immortalized cell lines derived from normal and malignant tissues (reviewed in King et al. *[7]*). More recently, trophoblast cell lines have been developed from human embryonic stem cells *(8)* and the mouse trophectoderm and later extraembryonic ectoderm *(9)*. Although trophoblast cells derived from human embryonic stem cells propagate poorly, likely because of as-yet unidentified growth factors, it is a potentially attractive biological resource because these cells form syncytia, express a range of trophoblast markers, and secrete placental hormones *(8)*. In addition, stem-cell-derived cytotrophoblasts may provide a model for the early placenta, in contrast with primary cultures of cytotrophoblasts and choriocarcinoma-derived cell lines, which display characteristics of third-trimester placentas. As for in vitro model systems for studying trophoblast transcellular transport, currently there are only two trophoblast cell lines that have been shown to form confluent monolayers when grown on semi-permeable membranes, including the human BeWo cell line *(10)* and the rodent HRP-1 cell line *(11)*.

The HRP-1 cell line is derived from normal midgestation rat chorioallantoic placenta. The HRP-1 cell line expresses cellular markers of and is morphologically similar to labyrinthine trophoblast cells *(11)*. This cell line has been used to study the expression and/or function of fatty acid, glucose, glutamate, and organic anion transport systems *(12–16)*. Because HRP-1 cells express the cytochrome P450 CYP1A1 isozyme, these cells also serve as a useful in vitro model for placental metabolic studies *(11)*.

The human, choriocarcinoma-derived, BeWo cell line *(17)* forms a confluent, polarized monolayer that provides a good in vitro model system to study the transcellular distribution of nutrients and drugs across the placental trophoblast *(10)*. The BeWo cell line is easy to maintain by passage and grows in a relatively short period of time. BeWo cells also demonstrate hormonal secretion properties common to typical trophoblasts and display many of the characteristics of third-trimester trophoblasts *(18)*. In contrast with primary cultures of cytotrophoblasts, BeWo cells are unable to spontaneously differentiate and consist predominantly of undifferentiated cytotrophoblasts with a few syncytialized cells *(19)*. Although treatment with forskolin or cyclic-adenosine monophosphate will stimulate BeWo cells to syncytialize *(19)*, these treatments cause cellular aggregation and destroy monolayer confluency. Fortunately, undifferentiated BeWo cells are morphologically similar to primary cultures of trophoblasts, exhibiting close cell apposition and microvillar projections on the apical side of the monolayer *(10)*. Furthermore, the monolayer is polarized in the expression of apical and basolateral marker enzymes and transporters in a manner consistent with primary trophoblasts *(20)*. Overall, the BeWo cell line has been successfully utilized to investigate the asymmetric transcellular transport of multiple nutrients and compounds, including amino acids *(21–23)*, glucose *(24,25)*, cholesterol *(26)*, folic acid *(27)*, fatty acids *(10)*, transferrin *(28,29)*, serotonin *(30)*, choline *(31)*, and immunoglobin G *(32)*.

Transport studies can be performed in Transwell® inserts, Side-bi-Side™ diffusion chambers, or a similar setup (**Fig. 1**). Detailed instructions for carrying out transplacental transport experiments with BeWo cells in Transwell inserts appear in the protocols that follow. Outlined procedures include cell revival, maintenance of the BeWo cells in culture, freezing cells, plate preparation, seeding the cells, and transport protocols.

2. Materials

1. The BeWo cell line was originally derived from a human choriocarcinoma. The BeWo clone (b30) in use in our laboratory was obtained from Dr. Alan Schwartz (Washington University, St. Louis, MO). The original BeWo cell line is also available through American Type Culture Collection (ATCC; Manassas, VA, cat. no. CCL-98); however, it does not have the same monolayer-forming behavior in culture as the Schwartz clone.
2. Cell culture medium. This is prepared using Dulbecco's modified Eagle's medium (DMEM) (with L-glutamine and 4500 mg glucose/L, without sodium bicarbonate; Sigma Chemical Co., St. Louis, MO, cat. no. D-5648), heat-inactivated fetal bovine serum (FBS) (Atlanta Biologicals, Norcross, GA), penicillin/streptomycin (10,000 U/mL; Invitrogen, Carlsbad, CA), and MEM nonessential amino acids (Invitrogen).

A

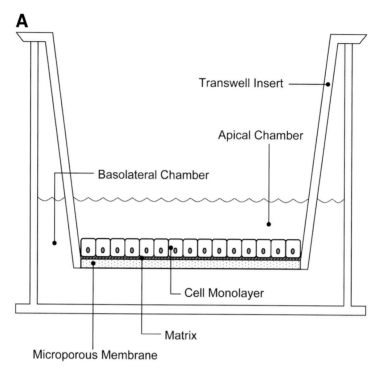

B

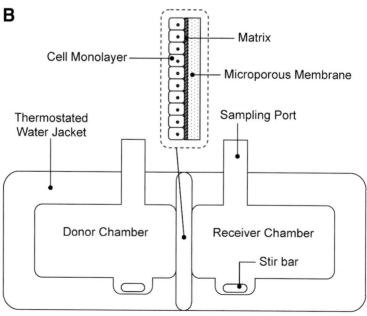

3. HBSS-Glc. Hanks' balanced salt solution (HBSS) with sodium bicarbonate and without phenol red (Sigma, cat. no. H-8264) containing 25 mM D-glucose.
4. Tissue culture flasks (25, 75, 150 cm^2). Available from Corning Costar (Corning, NY).
5. Trypsinization solution. Trypsin–ethylenediamine tetraacetic acid (EDTA) (10X) (Sigma, cat. no. T-4174) diluted as stated in Methods in 1X PBS. PBS is prepared from 10X phosphate buffered saline (PBS), pH 7.4, without calcium chloride, without magnesium chloride (Invitrogen, cat. no. 70011-044).
6. Freezing canister. Nalgene Cryo 1° Freezing Container (Nalgene Nunc International, Rochester, NY, cat. no. 5100-0001).
7. Freezing medium. Cell culture medium containing 10% dimethylsulfoxide (DMSO).
8. Lysis buffer. The formulation is listed in Methods. Use Triton X-100 (Sigma, cat. no. T-9284). Ensure that lysis conditions are compatible with detection methods for the substrate used.
9. Human placental collagen (Fluka Chemical, Milwaukee, WI, cat. no. WA13270).
10. Protease inhibitor cocktail. Complete Mini Protease Inhibitor Cocktail Tablets (Roche Diagnostics, Indianapolis, IN, cat. no. 1 836 153).
11. 12-well Transwell polycarbonate plates (Corning Costar, cat. no. 3460).
12. Trypan Blue (0.4% solution, Sigma, cat. no. T-8154).
13. BCA Protein assay (Pierce, Rockford, IL, cat. no. 23227).
14. Hot box/incubator. Several options are available; we use the Boekel Jitterbug (Boekel Scientific, Feasterville, PA).
15. Fibronectin. Dissolve 5 mg of lyophilized fibronectin (Sigma) in 20 mL of sterile 1X PBS. The solution may be warmed to 37°C for brief periods to ensure dissolution. The stock (250 µg/mL) should be stored at 4°C and is stable for up to 2 mo. Immediately before use, a working solution of fibronectin (50 µg/mL) is prepared by diluting the stock solution 1:4 in sterile PBS.
16. Poly-D-lysine (PDL) hydrobromide (MW 70,000-150,000; Sigma, cat. no. P-6407).

Fig. 1. (*opposite page*) Diagrams of Transwell® inserts (**A**) and Side-bi-Side™ diffusion chambers (**B**) used in transcellular transport experiments. In the 12-well Transwell plates described in the text, the apical chamber holds 0.5 mL of transport buffer and the basolateral chamber holds 1.5 mL. For both the Transwell inserts and Side-bi-Side apparatus, the membrane separating the two chambers is coated with a matrix, such as human placental collagen, and cells are seeded at the appropriate cell density. Both chambers can be sampled for analysis. To achieve uniform mixing, Transwell plates should be placed on a rotating platform; stir bars are placed within the Side-bi-Side diffusion chambers.

3. Methods

3.1. BeWo Cell Culture Medium

1. Dissolve the contents of one bottle (enough for 1 L which is 13.4 g) DMEM powdered media in 870 mL of double-distilled water (ddH$_2$O).
2. Supplement with 3.5 g NaHCO$_3$ and stir for 20 min.
3. Adjust the pH to 7.4 using 1 N HCl.
4. Filter media through a 0.22-μm disposable filter in a laminar flow hood (*see* **Note 1**).
5. Add 10 mL of 200 mM L-glutamine, 10 mL of 10,000 U/mL penicillin with 10 mg/mL streptomycin and 10 mL of 10 M nonessential amino acids to media.
6. Add FBS for 10% (v/v) (*see* **Note 2**).

3.2. BeWo Cell Revival From Liquid Nitrogen

1. Warm all the solutions needed for cell culture, e.g., DMEM and PBS, to 37°C.
2. Remove a vial of frozen BeWo cells from a liquid nitrogen storage tank and thaw the cells in a 37°C water bath.
3. Immediately after the cells are thawed, transfer the cell suspension to a 15-mL falcon tube containing 10 mL DMEM, and mix the cell suspension gently.
4. Centrifuge to pellet the cells at 335g for 8 min at room temperature.
5. Aspirate the supernatant and resuspend the cell pellet in 10 mL of media.
6. Centrifuge again, remove the supernatant and gently resuspend the cell pellet in 8 mL of media using a sterile Pasteur pipet.
7. Place the entire cell suspension into a 25-cm^2 tissue culture flask and label the flask with the cell line, passage number, and date.
8. Grow cells in a 37°C incubator supplied with 5% CO$_2$ and 95% relative humidity (*see* **Note 1**).
9. When the cells reach 70–80% confluence, the monolayer can be treated with trypsin to detach and disperse the cells.
10. Aspirate media from 25-cm^2 tissue culture flask using a sterile Pasteur pipet.
11. Wash flask with 5 mL of PBS twice in order to remove serum.
12. Detach the cells from a 25-cm^2 flask by incubating the cells with 5 mL of 1X trypsin-EDTA solution in PBS for 30 s and then aspirate off all but few drops of the liquid (*see* **Note 3**).
13. Place the flask in the 37°C incubator for approx 2 min.
14. Take the 25-cm^2 flask out of the incubator and examine the cell layer under the microscope to ensure that cells have detached from the substratum and "ball up."
15. Suspend the cells uniformly in 12 mL of media and transfer the entire cell suspension to seed cells in a 75-cm^2 tissue culture flask. Label the flask with the cell line, passage number, and date.
16. When the cells become 70–80% confluent, passage cells to a 150-cm^2 tissue culture flask.
17. Detach and disperse cells as described in **Subheading 3.2.**, **steps 10–14**, except use about 10 mL of the trypsin–EDTA solution.

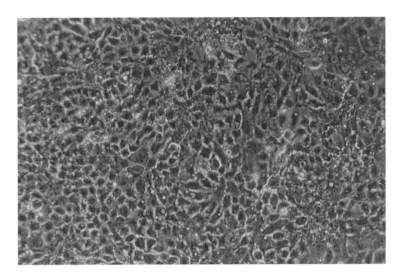

Fig. 2. Morphology of BeWo cells in culture. The BeWo cells form a monolayer when they are approx 100% confluent. Magnification 200×.

18. Suspend the cells uniformly in 10 mL of media and seed 5 mL of such cell suspension into one 150-cm^2 tissue culture flask, which has 20 mL of media in it. Label the flask with the cell line, passage number and date.
19. Subsequent passages can be performed and are described as follows.

3.3. BeWo Cell Passage

1. Aspirate media from flask of cells to be passaged and wash flask with 10 mL of PBS twice.
2. Detach and disperse cells with trypsin-EDTA solution (2 mL of 10X trypsin-EDTA stock solution in 9 mL of PBS). Place in a 37°C incubator for approx 3–5 min and visually confirm cell detachment (*see* **Note 4**).
3. Add 10 mL of DMEM in the flask to stop trypsinization. Suspend cells and transfer entire cell suspension into a 50-mL Falcon tube.
4. Centrifuge to pellet the cells at 300g for 8 min at room temperature.
5. Aspirate the supernatant media and resuspend the cell pellet in 10 mL of DMEM.
6. Seed 1 mL of this cell suspension to each 150-cm^2 tissue culture flask, which has 25 mL of media in it (*see* **Note 5**).
7. Add one to the passage number shown on the initial frozen vial from liquid nitrogen. Label the flask with the cell line, passage number, and date.
8. Feed the cells the next day and every other day subsequently.
9. Visualize cells under a microscope. The morphology of cells is shown in **Fig. 2**.

3.4. BeWo Cell Storage

1. Obtain the cell pellet from trypsinization of a 150-cm^2 flask as described in **Subheading 3.3., steps 1–4**.
2. Suspend cells in 10 mL of DMEM media, determine the cell density, and create a cell suspension with 1×10^6 cells/mL in DMEM containing 10% DMSO.
3. Locate and label 2 mL tissue culture vials appropriate for deep-freezing.
4. Transfer 1.5 mL of cell suspension to each vial.
5. Freeze cells by placing in a freezing canister and placing in a –80°C freezer for 12 h. Cell vials should then be transferred to a liquid nitrogen storage container for long-term storage (*see* **Note 6**).

3.5. Efflux and Uptake Transporter Expression in BeWo Cells

Efflux transporters can be characterized by examining their expression at the level of protein in cultured cells, identifying substrates of the transporter by measuring transmonolayer permeability in a Transwell system (**Fig. 1**) and determining inhibitors of the transporter using uptake assays. All these techniques can also be applied to study uptake transporters.

1. Plate cells in either 75-cm^2 or 150-cm^2 tissue culture flasks as described under **Subheading 3.3.**
2. Harvest cells when they are approx 80% confluent.
3. Rinse cells with 5 mL of prewarmed (37°C) PBS three times.
4. Scrape cells from flask in 5 mL of PBS using a cell scraper and transfer the cells to a 15-mL Falcon tube.
5. Rinse the flask with another 5 mL of PBS and combine with the scraped cells.
6. Resuspend by pipetting up and down with a 5-mL pipet to break up cell clumps.
7. Count the cells using the trypan blue exclusion method.
8. Pellet cells by centrifugation at 335g for 15 min in a refrigerated centrifuge.
9. Resuspend cell pellet in fresh lysis buffer (1% Triton X-100, 20 mM Tris-HCl, pH 8.0, 150 mM NaCl, protease inhibitor cocktail, 1 mM phenylmethylsulfonyl fluoride [PMSF]) to give a cell density at 1×10^8 cells/mL lysis buffer.
10. Incubate the cell lysate on ice for 30 min. Vortex briefly midway through incubation.
11. Centrifuge at 18,300g for 10 min at 4°C.
12. Collect supernatant, which contains solubilized protein and store aliquots at –80°C.
13. Determine protein concentrations using standard assays (e.g., BCA assay).
14. Transporter protein expression can be detected using standard procedures for Western blot analysis.

3.6. Growth of BeWo Cells in Transwell Plates

1. Prepare a stock solution of the coating material by dissolving human placental collagen in 0.1% acetic acid solution (1 mg in 0.345 mL) and store at 4°C. Prepare a working solution of the coating material immediately before use by diluting the stock solution 1:3 in 70% ethanol (one part human placental collagen in 0.1 % acetic acid and three parts 70% ethanol).

2. Pipet 70 μL of the coating material on the membrane of each well for a 12-well Transwell plate (adjust the volume for plates with different size wells), making sure that the membrane is coated evenly.
3. Dry for 2–3 h in a laminar flow hood with lid open (no ultraviolet [UV] light).
4. Sterilize the plates for 1 h under UV light with the lid open. Longer exposure times can cause the membranes to split.
5. If the plate is to be used immediately, skip to **step 7** below. Otherwise, wrap the plates in aluminum foil and store at 4°C. The plates may be used up to one week after coating with collagen.
6. If coated plates were stored in the refrigerator, allow the plates to warm to room temperature for approx 30 min before use.
7. Prewet the membranes with the addition 1 mL of prewarmed PBS (37°C) to the apical chamber and 2 mL to the basal chambers for 30–45 min.
8. Meanwhile, prepare cells for plating as described under **Subheading 3.3.** and determine the density of viable cells using trypan blue exclusion.
9. Calculate the dilution of the cell suspension needed to get a seeding density of 50,000 to 100,000 cells per mL.
10. Dilute the cells with DMEM to get the proper seeding density and mix well to ensure uniformity.
11. Aspirate PBS from both apical and basolateral chambers.
12. Seed the apical chamber with 0.5 mL per well of cell suspension using a repeat pipettor. Shake to evenly distribute the cells.
13. Add 1.5 mL of media in the basolateral chamber.
14. Feed cells the next day and every other day subsequently. Media on both the apical and basolateral sides should be replaced at each feeding.
15. Transport assays can be performed when the cells become confluent, which usually takes 5–6 d.

3.7. Transporter Assays

1. Warm up a bench-top incubator and all cell culture solutions to be used in the transport assay to 37°C for 30–45 min before preparing cells.
2. Solutions for pre-incubation and incubation steps should be prepared and warmed to 37°C. Generally, HBSS containing 25 mM L-glucose (HBSS-Glc) is the medium used for transport when using fluorescent substrates. The pre-incubation solution usually consists of HBSS-Glc along with any inhibitors that may be used in the experiment; the incubation solution should be identical to the pre-incubation solution except for the inclusion of the transporter substrate (*see* **Note 7**).
3. Remove media and wash the cells twice with prewarmed (37°C) HBSS-Glc (0.5 mL for apical chambers and 1.5 for basolateral chambers for a 12-well Transwell plate).
4. Aspirate HBSS-Glc from all the chambers.
5. Incubate cells in the appropriate pre-incubation solution for 30–60 min at 37°C on a rotating platform (*see* **Note 8**).
6. Aspirate the pre-incubation solution.

7. Add dosing solution to either the apical or basolateral chamber. For apical (A) to basolateral (B) transport, load 0.5 mL of drug/substrate to the top and 1.5 mL buffer to the bottom. Load the drug/substrate to the bottom for B to A transport.

8. At designated time points, sample 100 μL from the receiver chamber (to measure A to B transport, sample from the basolateral side; to measure B to A transport, sample from the apical side). Place the samples in a 96-well plate for fluorescent assay or scintillation vials, as appropriate.

9. Replace the sample withdrawn with 100 μL of fresh buffer identical to that originally added to that compartment.

10. Continue taking time points until designated time has elapsed.

11. To determine the rate of paracellular transport, [^{14}C]-sucrose flux can be measured. This is usually done after a fluorescence experiment, but can be performed concurrently with the primary experiment when using a [^{3}H]-labeled compound.

12. Fluorescence analysis or scintillation counting can then be performed for each time point.

3.8. Calculation of Apparent Permeability Coefficients

Apparent permeability coefficient for the monolayers of cells, P_{app} (in cm/s), can be calculated according to the following equation: $P_{app} = \Delta Q / \Delta t / (A * C_0)$, where $\Delta Q / \Delta t$ is the linear appearance rate of mass in the receiver solution, A is the membrane/cell surface area, and C_0 is the initial concentration of the test compound. The net efflux of a test compound can be assessed by calculating the ratio of P_{app} in the basolateral to apical direction vs P_{app} in the apical to basolateral direction *(33)*.

3.9. Growth of BeWo Cells on Standard Cell Culture Plates

1. Prepare a PDL coating solution in 28% ethanol (5 μg/mL).

2. Pipet coating solution to each well of culture plates, for example 100 μL per well for a 12-well plate.

3. Shake the plate to coat the bottom of the well evenly and dry for 3 h in a laminar flow hood with the lid open (no UV light).

4. Sterilize the plates for 1 h under UV light. The plates could be used right away by skipping to **step 6** or kept in the refrigerator up to 2 wk if wrapped in aluminum foil.

5. If PDL coated plates were stored in the refrigerator, warm up the plate to room temperature for about 30 min before use.

6. Add 1 mL of PBS to each well of 12 well plates and leave in a laminar flow hood for 30 min.

7. Aspirate PBS and add three drops fibronectin (50 μg/mL in PBS).

8. Shake the plates to spread the fibronectin and coat the wells evenly.

9. Dry the plates in hood for about 45 min.

10. Meanwhile, prepare cell suspension as described under **Subheading 3.3.** and determine viable cell density by using the trypan blue exclusion method.

11. Calculate the dilution of the cell suspension needed to get a density of 50,000 to 100,000 cells per mL and prepare a cell suspension of the proper seeding density by dilution with DMEM.

12. Remove excess fibronectin from the well by washing with 1 mL of DMEM.

13. Seed with 0.5 mL of cell suspension per well for 12 well plates using a repeat pipettor.

14. Add another 1 mL of DMEM to each well of a 12-well plate and shake to evenly distribute the cells.

15. Feed with 1.5 mL of DMEM every 2 d.

16. Use cells for uptake assay when they are at least 70–80% confluent; this usually occurs 5–6 d after plating.

3.10. Uptake Assays on Standard Cell Culture Plates

Uptake assays can be performed as described *(34)* with some modifications.

1. Warm up the bench top incubator and HBSS-Glc to 37°C for 30–45 min before preparing cells.

2. Place some HBSS-Glc on ice (approx 36–40 mL for a 12-well plate or 72–80 mL if using a 12-well Transwell plate).

3. Prepare solutions for pre-incubation and uptake as described previously for transport assays (*see* **Subheading 3.7.**).

4. Remove media and wash the cells twice with prewarmed (37°C) HBSS-Glc (1 mL per well for a 12-well plate or if using a 12-well Transwell plate, 0.5 mL for apical chamber and 1.5 mL for basolateral chamber).

5. Aspirate HBSS-Glc from all the wells.

6. Incubate cells in pre-incubation solutions for 30–45 min at 37°C in the bench top incubator on a rotating platform (add pre-incubation solution into both apical and basolateral chambers for a 12-well Transwell plate).

7. Aspirate the pre-incubation solution and initiate the uptake with the addition of 1 mL of the uptake incubation solution ± inhibitor to each well for a 12-well plate. For a 12 Transwell plate, either add 0.5 mL of uptake incubation solution ± inhibitor into apical chamber and 1.5 mL of HBSS-Glc ± inhibitor into the basolateral chamber or vice versa.

8. Incubate the cells in the incubation solution for the desired time period; this will depend on the substrate transmembrane permeability.

9. Remove the culture plate from the incubator and aspirate the uptake incubation solution.

10. Wash cells in each well three times with ice cold HBSS-Glc to stop uptake and remove excess substrate.

11. Add 1 mL of lysis buffer (0.5% Triton X-100 in 0.2 N NaOH; *see* **Note 9**) to each well for a 12-well plate. For a 12 Transwell plate, add 0.5 mL of lysis buffer into the apical chamber.

12. Cover and incubate the plate in the bench top incubator at 37°C for 2 h, or at 4°C overnight.

13. Mix the contents of each well by pipetting.
14. Assay the lysate from each well to determine the amount of substrate present and the protein concentration.
15. Uptake can be normalized to the number of cells in each well by expressing the data as: concentration of substrate/protein concentration. It is important that each data point be determined by substrate and protein determinations from the same well.

4. Notes

1. Unless otherwise noted, procedures should be performed under a laminar flow hood for sterile conditions. Cell lysis (**Subheading 3.5.**) and transporter (**Subheading 3.7.**) and uptake (**Subheading 3.10.**) assays may be performed in nonsterile surroundings. Culture conditions are 37°C, 5% CO_2, and 95% relative humidity.
2. The medium can be divided into two aliquots and filtered into 500-mL bottles. FBS (50 mL for 10% v/v) should be added to one bottle and the other stored without FBS until ready for use. Once serum is added, the medium may be used for up to 2 wk.
3. During the revival period and for several subsequent passages, the BeWo cells are treated with greater care. The cells are detached from the flasks by rapid exposure to 1X trypsin-EDTA and immediately resuspended. Centrifugation is avoided during this time to improve cell survival and attachment rates.
4. Once normal culture conditions are reached, the cells are passaged at a higher trypsin concentration. The final concentration used to passage BeWo is roughly 1.8X trypsin-EDTA (2 mL 10X trypsin-EDTA and 9 mL PBS).
5. Cell density is not precisely determined for seeding BeWo flasks. Adding 1 mL of suspension is a good place to start, but the amount may need to be adjusted accordingly. If cells reach confluency before 4–5 d, decrease the amount. Likewise, increase the amount of suspension added if it is more than 6 d before the cells are ready for passage.
6. Using a freezing canister filled with isopropyl alcohol (*see* Materials) will help to freeze the cell suspension more gradually and improve cell viability upon revival.
7. Radiolabeled compounds are common substrates for transport and uptake assays. These experiments may be performed under nonsterile conditions, but personal protective equipment and shielding appropriate for the selected isotope must be used.
8. Pre-incubation with an inhibitor may be necessary depending on its particular effect on the chosen transporter. Initial assays with a positive control should be performed to determine whether or not pre-incubation is needed.
9. Lysis buffer including NaOH may quench some fluorescent compounds, such as calcein. An alternative lysing solution is 2% Triton X-100.

Acknowledgments

This work was supported in part by National Institute of Child Health and Human Development (NICHD) (HD39878-03), by National Institutes of Health (NIH) Institutional Research and Academic Career Development Awards (IRACDA) (GM-63651, C. J. B.), and by a Madison and Lila Self Predoctoral Fellowship award (E. R.).

References

1. Stulc, J. (1989) Extracellular transport pathways in the haemochorial placenta. *Placenta* **10,** 113–119.
2. Sibley, C. P. (1994) Mechanisms of ion transfer by the rat placenta—a model for the human placenta. *Placenta* **15,** 675–691.
3. Enders, A. C. and Blankenship, T. N. (1999) Comparative placental structure. *Adv. Drug Delivery Rev.* **38,** 3–15.
4. Ringler, G. E. and Strauss, J. F. III (1990) In vitro systems for the study of human placental endocrine function. *Endocrine Rev.* **11,** 105–123.
5. Kliman, H. J., Nestler, J. E., Sermasi, E., Sanger, J. M., and Strauss, J. F. III (1986) Purification, characterization, and in vitro differentiation of cytotrophoblasts from human term placentae. *Endocrinology* **118,** 1567–1582.
6. Hemmings, D. G., Lowen, B., Sherburne, R., Sawicki, G., and Guilbert, L. J. (2001) Villous trophoblasts cultured on semi-permeable membranes form an effective barrier to the passage of high and low molecular weight particles. *Placenta* **22,** 70–79.
7. King, A., Thomas, L., and Bischof, P. (2000) Cell culture models of trophoblast II: trophoblast cell lines—a workshop report. *Placenta* **21,** S113–S119.
8. Xu, R. H., Chen, X., Li, D. S., Li, R., Addicks, G. C., Glennon, C., Zwaka, T. P., and Thomson, J. A. (2002) BMP4 initiates human embryonic stem cell differentiation to trophoblast. *Nat. Biotechnol.* **20,** 1261–1264.
9. Tanaka, S., Kunath, T., Hadjantonakis, A. K., Nagy, A., and Rossant, J. (1998) Promotion of trophoblast stem cell proliferation by FGF4. *Science* **282,** 2072–2075.
10. Liu, F., Soares, M. J., and Audus, K. L. (1997) Permeability properties of monolayers of the human trophoblast cell line BeWo. Am. J. Physiol. 42, C1596–C1604.
11. Shi, F. L., Soares, M. J., Avery, M., Liu, F., Zhang, X. M., and Audus, K. L. (1997) Permeability and metabolic properties of a trophoblast cell line (HRP-1) derived from normal rat placenta. *Exp. Cell Res.* **234,** 147–155.
12. Knipp, G. T., Liu, B., Audus, K. L., Fujii, H., Ono, T., and Soares, M. J. (2000) Fatty acid transport regulatory proteins in the developing rat placenta and in trophoblast cell culture models. *Placenta* **21,** 367–375.
13. Das, U. G., Sadiq, H. F., Soares, M. J., Hay, W. W., and Devaskar, S. U. (1998) Time-dependent physiological regulation of rodent and ovine placental glucose transporter (GLUT-1) protein. *Am. J. Physiol.* **43,** R339–R347.

14. Rajakumar, R. A., Thamotharan, S., Menon, R. K., and Devaskar, S. U. (1998) Sp1 and Sp3 regulate transcriptional activity of the facilitative glucose transporter isoform-3 gene in mammalian neuroblasts and trophoblasts. *J. Biol. Chem.* **273,** 27,474–27,483.

15. Novak, D., Quiggle, F., Artime, C., and Beveridge, M. (2001) Regulation of glutamate transport and transport proteins in a placental cell line. *Am. J. Physiol.* **281,** C1014–C1022.

16. Zhou, F., Tanaka, K., Soares, M. J., and You, G. F. (2003) Characterization of an organic anion transport system in a placental cell line. *Am. J. Physiol.* **285,** E1103–E1109.

17. Pattillo, R. A. and Gey, G. O. (1968) The establishment of a cell line of human hormone-synthesizing trophoblastic cells in vitro. *Cancer Res.* **28,** 1231–1236.

18. Friedman, S. J. and Skehan, P. (1979) Morphological differentiation of human choriocarcinoma cells induced by methotrexate. *Cancer Res.* **39,** 1960–1967.

19. Wice, B., Menton, D., Geuze, H., and Schwartz, A. L. (1990) Modulators of cyclic AMP metabolism induce syncytiotrophoblast formation in vitro. *Exp. Cell Res.* **186,** 306–316.

20. Zhao, H. Y. and Hundal, H. S. (2000) Identification and biochemical localization of a Na-K-Cl cotransporter in the human placental cell line BeWo. *Biochem. Biophys. Res. Commun.* **274,** 43–48.

21. Furesz, T. C., Smith, C. H., and Moe, A. J. (1993) ASC system activity is altered by development of cell polarity in trophoblast from human placenta. *Am. J. Physiol.* **265,** C212–C217.

22. Moe, A. J., Furesz, T. C., and Smith, C. H. (1994) Functional characterization of L-alanine transport in a placental choriocarcinoma cell line (BeWo). *Placenta* **15,** 797–802.

23. Way, B. A., Furesz, T. C., Schwarz, J. K., Moe, A. J., and Smith, C. H. (1998) Sodium-independent lysine uptake by the BeWo choriocarcinoma cell line. *Placenta* **19,** 323–328.

24. Shah, S. W., Zhao, H., Low, S. Y., McArdle, H. J., and Hundal, H. S. (1999) Characterization of glucose transport and glucose transporters in the human choriocarcinoma cell line, BeWo. *Placenta* **20,** 651–659.

25. Vardhana, P. A. and Illsley, N. P. (2002) Transepithelial glucose transport and metabolism in BeWo choriocarcinoma cells. *Placenta* **23,** 653–660.

26. Schmid, K. E., Davidson, W. S., Myatt, L., and Woollett, L. A. (2003) Transport of cholesterol across a BeWo cell monolayer: implications for net transport of sterol from maternal to fetal circulation. *J. Lipid Res.* **44,** 1909–1918.

27. Takahashi, T., Utoguchi, N., Takara, A., Yet al. (2001) Carrier-mediated transport of folic acid in BeWo cell monolayers as a model of the human trophoblast. *Placenta* **22,** 863–869.

28. van der Ende, A., du Maine, A., Schwartz, A. L., and Strous, G. J. (1989) Effect of ATP depletion and temperature on the transferrin-mediated uptake and release of iron by BeWo choriocarcinoma cells. *Biochem. J.* **259,** 685–692.

29. van der Ende, A., du Maine, A., Schwartz, A. L., and Strous, G. J. (1990) Modulation of transferrin-receptor activity and recycling after induced differentiation of BeWo choriocarcinoma cells. *Biochem. J.* **270,** 451–457.
30. Prasad, P. D., Hoffmans, B. J., Moe, A. J., Smith, C. H., Leibach, F. H., and Ganapathy, V. (1996) Functional expression of the plasma membrane serotonin transporter but not the vesicular monoamine transporter in human placental trophoblasts and choriocarcinoma cells. *Placenta* **17,** 201–207.
31. Eaton, B. M. and Sooranna, S. R. (1998) Regulation of the choline transport system in superfused microcarrier cultures of BeWo cells. *Placenta* **19,** 663–669.
32. Ellinger, I., Schwab, M., Stefanescu, A., Hunziker, W., and Fuchs, R. (1999) IgG transport across trophoblast-derived BeWo cells: a model system to study IgG transport in the placenta. *Eur. J. Immunol.* **29,** 733–744.
33. Gao, J.N., Hugger, E.H., Beck-Westermeyer, M.S., and Borchardt, R.T. (2000) Estimating intestinal mucosal permeation of compounds using Caco-2 cell monolayers. *Current Protocols in Pharmacology* **Supplement 8,** 7.2.1.–7.2.23.
34. Silverstein, P. S. Karunaratne, D. N., and Audus, K. L. (2003) Uptake studies for evaluating activity of efflux transporters in a cell line representative of the blood-brain barrier. *Current Protocols in Pharmacology* **Supplement 23,** 7.7.1–7.7.14.

14

In Vitro Methods for Studying Human Placental Amino Acid Transport

Placental Plasma Membrane Vesicles

Jocelyn D. Glazier and Colin P. Sibley

Summary

Isolated plasma membrane vesicles from human placenta allow transporter-mediated mechanisms across individual plasma membranes to be identified and characterized in vitro. This approach is reliant on isolating each of the trophoblast plasma membranes, either the maternal-facing microvillous plasma membrane (MVM) or the fetal-facing basal membrane (BM) in a relatively pure form. Purity of the isolated trophoblast plasma membranes can be confirmed by the use of protein membrane markers, which have a polarized distribution to either membrane. The isolated trophoblast plasma membranes are then encouraged to vesiculate by applying a shear force, to yield enclosed plasma membrane vesicles across which the uptake or efflux of radiolabeled solute (e.g., amino acid) can be measured. The advantage of this technique is that it allows characterization of transporter activity and expression in a defined plasma membrane, independent of any metabolic processes, and can be utilized for a variety of different solutes. The disadvantage is that membrane transporter activities are usually measured in the absence of regulatory factors and may not be reflective of in vivo fluxes.

Key Words: Placenta; syncytiotrophoblast; microvillous plasma membrane; basal plasma membrane; vesicle; transport; amino acid.

1. Introduction

"Vesicles" are pieces of vesiculated plasma membrane across which the uptake or efflux of radiolabeled solute (e.g., amino acid) can be measured. For influx or uptake, radiolabeled substrate would be added to the incubation medium, and for efflux the vesicles would be preloaded with radiolabeled substrate and incubated in a label-free buffer. The radiolabel content within the vesicles is then determined following separation from the extravesicular buffer by rapid filtration.

From: *Methods in Molecular Medicine, Vol. 122: Placenta and Trophoblast: Methods and Protocols, Vol. 2*
Edited by: M. J. Soares and J. S. Hunt © Humana Press Inc., Totowa, NJ

This approach has the advantages of defining individual transport mechanisms without the complication of placental metabolism, and allows the experimental conditions on either side of the membrane to be precisely set. The disadvantages are plasma membrane vesicles lack intracellular constituents, limiting their usefulness when examining regulatory processes using signalling cascades, and although a transport mechanism might be identified in a particular plasma membrane, estimation of the contribution that transporter activity makes to in vivo transplacental flux is not possible.

The first step is to isolate each of the trophoblast plasma membranes, the maternal-facing microvillous plasma membrane (MVM) or the fetal-facing basal membrane (BM) in a relatively pure form. To do this, reliance is put on the functional and biochemical polarity of these two plasma membranes, as well as their biophysical properties. The most common approaches to isolate MVM from human placenta involve stirring the tissue to shear off MVM *(1)* or homogenization followed by Mg^{2+} treatment and differential centrifugation *(2)*. The latter approach offers the opportunity for BM to be harvested alongside *(3)*, or, alternatively, this can be achieved separately using a sonication procedure *(4–6)*. The isolated membranes are then vesiculated by passage through a fine-gage needle, forcing membrane ends to reseal generating vesicles of heterogeneous size *(2,4)*. MVM vesicles tend to reseal in the same membrane orientation as in vivo with respect to cytoplasm *(2)*, whereas BM vesicles adopt mixed membrane orientation *(3,4)*. This is not a limitation, because amino acid transporters inserted in plasma membranes can function symmetrically, dependent on prevailing gradients *(7)*.

Influx of radiolabeled solute is more commonly measured in MVM and BM vesicles, with rate of influx normalized to membrane protein content as a proxy of membrane surface area *(8)*. The underlying assumption in using this technique is that the membrane vesicle isolation procedure preserves transporter integrity and capacity within these membranes, a notion supported by the widespread use of MVM and BM vesicles from human placenta and the identification of multiple amino acid transporters within these membranes *(8–10)*.

2. Materials

2.1. MVM Isolation (see Note 1)

2.1.1. Buffers and Reagents

1. Mannitol buffer: 300 mM mannitol, 1 mM MgCl$_2$, 10 mM HEPES/Tris, pH 7.4 at 4°C.
2. MgCl$_2$ (solid) and 1 M MgCl$_2$ (*see* **Note 2**).
3. Intravesicular buffer (IVB; *see* **Note 3**).

4. Protein assay reagents (*see* **Note 4**).
5. Alkaline phosphatase (AP) assay reagents (*see* **Note 5**).

2.1.2. Equipment

1. Electric homogenizer.
2. Centrifuge (*see* **Note 6**).
3. Hand homogenizer.
4. Stirrer.

2.2. BM Isolation (see Note 7)

2.2.1. Buffers and Reagents

1. Phosphate-buffered saline (PBS).
2. 50 mM Tris-HCl, pH 6.9 (*see* **Note 8**).
3. 5 mM Tris-HCl, pH 6.9 (*see* **Note 9**).
4. 10 mM Na$_4$EDTA/sucrose/Tris (pH 7.4; *see* **Note 10**).
5. Ethanol (for ice-ethanol bath).
6. IVB (*see* **Note 3**).
7. Protein assay reagents (*see* **Note 4**).
8. ^{3}H-dihydroalprenolol (DHA) binding assay reagents (*see* **Note 11**).

2.2.2. Equipment

1. Stirrer.
2. Electric mincer.
3. Sonicator (Vibra-Cell VCX400; 20kHz frequency, maximum amplitude 127 µm) with three-quarter-inch high-gain probe.
4. Centrifuge (*see* **Note 12**).
5. Vacuum pump.

2.3. Amino Acid Uptake Assay (see Note 13)

2.3.1. Buffers and Reagents (see Note 14)

1. Intravesicular buffer (*see* **Notes 3** and **15**):
   a. For neutral amino acids: 290 mM sucrose, 5 mM Tris-base, 5 mM HEPES, pH 7.4.
   b. For cationic amino acids: 100 mM mannitol, 50 mM KCl, 50 mM choline chloride, 20 mM HEPES-Tris, pH 7.4.
2. Extravesicular buffer (*see* **Notes 13** and **15**):
   a. For neutral amino acids: 145 mM NaCl or KCl, 5 mM Tris-base, 5 mM HEPES, pH 7.4.
   b. For cationic amino acids: 50 mM NaCl with 50 mM KCl or 100 mM KCl, 100 mM mannitol, 20 mM HEPES-Tris, pH 7.4.

3. Substrate (*see* **Note 13**):

Radiolabeled amino acids at suitable concentrations in extravesicular buffer (EVB) (*see* **Note 16**).

Amino acid transporter	Initial	Final	Reference
Neutral amino acids	330 μM ^{14}C-MeAIB	165 μM ^{14}C-MeAIB	13
	40 μM ^{14}C-leucine	20 μM ^{14}C-leucine	14
Cationic amino acids	0.24 μM ^{3}H-arginine	0.2 μM ^{3}H-arginine	12

4. Stop buffer (*see* **Note 17**):
    a. For neutral amino acids: 130 mM NaCl, 10 mM Na$_2$HPO$_4$, 4.2 mM KCl, 1.2 mM MgSO$_4$, 0.75 mM CaCl$_2$, pH 7.4 at 4°C.
    b. For cationic amino acids: 200 mM NaCl, 20 mM Na$_2$HPO$_4$, 3.6 mM KH$_2$PO$_4$, pH 7.4.

5. 2-Ethoxyethanol (Cellosolve).

2.3.2. Equipment

Vacuum pump.

3. Methods

3.1. MVM Isolation (see Note 18)

1. Take a radial segment of human placenta (~100 g wet weight) and remove chorionic plate.
2. Homogenize in 2.5 vol of ice-cold mannitol buffer until a smooth homogenate is obtained.
3. Retain sample of homogenate (~5 mL) for protein and AP activity (*see* **Note 19**).
4. Add solid MgCl$_2$ to a final concentration of 10 mM and stir on ice for 10 min.
5. Spin at 2300g for 15 min at 4°C, retain supernatant and spin at 23,500g for 40 min at 4°C.
6. Weigh pellet and resuspend in 2.5 vol of ice-cold mannitol buffer using hand homogenizer on ice.
7. Repeat **steps 4** and **5**; (*see* **Note 2**).
8. Take final MVM pellet, weigh, and resuspend in 4 vol of IVB using hand homogenizer on ice (*see* **Note 3**).
9. Vesiculate MVM by passing suspension through fine-gage needle (25-gage) 15–20 times. Store at 4°C until assay (*see* **Notes 19** and **20**).

3.2 BM Isolation (see Note 21)

1. Take placenta and remove chorionic and basal plates, cut into chunks, and place in ice-cold PBS.
2. Retain a piece of placenta (~1.5 g) for later analysis for DHA binding (*see* **Note 11**). Prepare a homogenate from this for subsequent assay (*see* **Note 19**).

3. Wash placental tissue four times in 500 mL ice-cold PBS (use chilled buffers throughout procedure, unless otherwise stated).

4. All remaining procedures are conducted in the cold room unless otherwise stated. Mince tissue with an electric domestic mincer.

5. Wash tissue four times in 500 mL ice-cold PBS, draining each time through nylon mesh, 100-μm pore size (*see* **Note 22**).

6. Stir vigorously in 500 mL PBS for 60 min (to shear away MVM).

7. Drain tissue onto nylon mesh and repeat washes as in **step 5** (*see* **Note 22**).

8. Wash tissue four times with 500 mL 50 m*M* Tris-HCl (pH 6.9; *see* **Note 22**). Filtrate should appear red.

9. Divide tissue into approx 15-g portions and place each in 100 mL 50 m*M* Tris-HCl (pH 6.9).

10. Sonicate each portion in turn (to disrupt syncytial integrity) at 90% maximum amplitude for 10 s with the probe immersed to a depth of 1 cm in an ice-ethanol bath (done in laboratory at room temperature). Drain tissue onto nylon mesh.

11. Return tissue to the cold room, wash tissue once with 500 mL 50 mM Tris-HCl, pH 6.9 (*see* **Note 22**).

12. Wash tissue four times with 500 mL 5 m*M* Tris-HCl, pH 6.9 (*see* **Note 22**). Tissue should now appear very pale.

13. Stir tissue in 1 L 5 m*M* Tris-HCl (pH 6.9) for 30 min (to remove syncytial contents).

14. Drain tissue onto nylon mesh and wash twice with 500 mL 5 m*M* Tris-HCl, pH 6.9 (*see* **Note 22**).

15. Return tissue to laboratory at room temperature, incubate tissue in 500 mL EDTA/sucrose/Tris (pH 7.4) for 10 min. Stir occasionally.

16. Still at room temperature, drain well and divide tissue into approx 15-g portions and place each in 100 mL EDTA/sucrose/Tris (pH 7.4) for 20 min, stirring every 5 min.

17. Sonicate each portion in turn (to release BM) at 100% maximum amplitude for 20 s with the probe immersed to a depth of 1 cm in an ice-ethanol bath (done in laboratory at room temperature). Drain tissue onto six layers of cotton gauze. Filtrate should appear turbid.

18. Centrifuge filtrate at 4000*g* for 10 min at 4°C, retain supernatant, and spin at 10,000*g* for 30 min at 4°C to pellet intracellular organelles.

19. Spin supernatant at 100,000*g* for 45 min to pellet BM.

20. Take BM pellet, weigh and resuspend in 4 vol of IVB using hand homogenizer on ice (*see* **Note 3**).

21. Vesiculate BM by passing suspension through fine-gage needle (25-gage) 15–20 times. Store at 4°C until assay (*see* **Notes 19** and **20**).

3.3. Amino Acid Uptake Assay (see Note 23)

1. Adjust the protein concentration of MVM and BM vesicles to 10 mg/mL with IVB.

2. Set up some plastic tubes in duplicate with an aliquot of EVB containing radiolabeled substrate. There are several conditions that one may wish to investigate:

time course, effect of inhibitor or ion substitution, competitive inhibition by other (unlabeled) amino acids (*see* **Notes 24** and **25**).

3. Set up some tubes for "blanks," in which an equal volume of IVB will replace vesicle suspension (*see* **Note 26**).

4. To each tube, containing EVB with radiolabeled substrate add 20 μL MVM or BM vesicle suspension (~200 μg protein; *see* **Note 27**). Angle the tube almost horizontally; and carefully apply the vesicle suspension droplet to the side of the tube, above, but clearly separated from, the EVB. The viscosity of the vesicle droplet should allow it to stick to the tube side without mixing with the EVB.

5. At time zero, mix the tube contents quickly by vortex. Have the timer scrolling near the vortex.

6. At a suitable time point (*see* **Note 28**), stop the uptake by the addition of 2 mL ice-cold stop solution, and vortex immediately.

7. Quickly remove 2×1 mL from the assay tube and apply to a presoaked Millipore (in stop buffer) filter (HAWP, pore size 0.45 μm; *see* **Note 29**) under vacuum. The vesicle protein is retained by the filter and separated from the radiolabeled substrate in the EVB, which is sucked through the filter.

8. Wash filter with 10 mL ice-cold stop buffer, applied with a syringe over the filter surface.

9. Remove filter and place in prelabeled scintillation vial with 2 mL 2-ethoxyethanol to dissolve filter.

10. Add scintillation fluid and count.

11. Count 3×5 μL EVB radiolabeled stock as standards (*see* **Note 30**).

12. Convert counts to moles of substrate (*see* **Note 30**), correct for nonspecific (protein-free) binding (*see* **Note 26**), and normalize to the amount of membrane protein applied to the filter to give uptake values expressed as moles/mg protein.

4. Notes

1. The method used routinely in our laboratory to isolate MVM is the Mg^{2+}-precipitation method *(2)*. This relies on the characteristic of MVM having a highly negative surface charge density, such that in the presence of Mg^{2+} the charge of the cation is accommodated, whereas plasma membranes of intracellular organelles and BM (with lower negative surface charge density) cross-link under these conditions and can be separated by centrifugation.

2. 1 *M* $MgCl_2$ can be used for second cycle Mg^{2+} treatment rather than solid $MgCl_2$.

3. Choice of IVB will depend on amino acid transporter system being studied. Details are given under "Amino Acid Uptake Assay."

4. We routinely use the Lowry method to assay protein, but other assays could be used. Expect to recover approx 0.5 mg and 0.22 mg protein/g placenta for MVM and BM respectively.

5. AP is used as a marker of MVM and an indicator of MVM purity. AP activity is measured in MVM and normalized to that in the initial placental homogenate. This AP "enrichment factor" (MVM/homogenate) should be >12 and usually falls within the range of 18–23. The assay is performed by measuring the increase in

absorbance at 410 nm over 2 min following addition of 50 μL protein (1/300 or 1/40 dilution of MVM or homogenate respectively) to 2.5 mL diethanolamine (DEA) buffer (1 M DEA, 0.5 mM MgCl$_2$, pH 9.8) in a cuvet, with the reaction initiated by addition of 0.25 mL substrate (3 tablets × 5 mg p-nitrophenylphosphate tablets [Sigma] in 4 mL DEA buffer). Generation of the yellow product, p-nitrophenol, is measured by an increase in absorbance at 410 nm.

6. The centrifuge must be able to perform top speed spin of 23,500g for 40 min at 4°C.

7. This isolation procedure has to be performed in the cold room at 4°C.

8. 50 mM Tris-HCl buffer made by adding 7.5 g Tris-HCl and 0.5 g Tris-base in 1 L and adjusting to pH 6.9 at 4°C with 1 M HCl.

9. 5 mM Tris-HCl buffer made by dilution of 50 mM Tris-HCl buffer with pH adjusted to 6.9 at room temperature with either 1 M HCl or 1 M NaOH.

10. EDTA/sucrose/Tris buffer is made freshly on day of use by first preparing sucrose/Tris buffer (85.6 g sucrose/7.5 g Tris-HCl/0.5 g Tris-base in 1 L adjusted to pH 6.9 at room temperature with concentrated HCl). Then dissolve 3.802 g Na$_4$EDTA (10 mM) in 835 mL sucrose/Tris buffer, adjust to pH 7.4 at room temperature with concentrated HCl, and make up to 1 L with H$_2$O.

11. Enrichment of ^{3}H-DHA binding (binding to BM/initial placental homogenate prepared from a ~1.5-g chunk) is used as a marker of BM purity. Enrichment factors should be >20 and routinely fall between 25- and 35-fold. ^{3}H-DHA binding to placental homogenates (1 mg protein) and BM (100 μg protein) is performed in Tris/Mg buffer (22 mM Tris-base, 28 mM Tris-HCl, 25 mM MgCl$_2$, pH 8.0) with 10 nM ^{3}H-DHA at 30°C for 30 min in the presence and absence of 30 μM propranolol. The reaction is stopped with 2 mL ice-cold Tris/Mg buffer (as previously described but pH 6.9), passed through two Whatman GF/C filters under vacuum and washed with 2 × 9 mL ice-cold Tris/Mg buffer (pH 6.9). Alternatively, adenylate cyclase can be used as a BM marker *(3)*.

12. The centrifuge must be capable of performing top speed spin of 100,000g for 45 min at 4°C.

13. In order to decide on buffer composition for amino acid uptakes, the first consideration is whether the transport system under investigation is Na$^+$-dependent or not as this will necessitate measuring uptake under conditions in which Na$^+$ is present or absent (usually replaced by K$^+$ or choline). Second, if the amino acid is positively charged (cationic), in order to preclude any transmembrane electrical gradient generating a driving force *(11)*, equalization of any potential difference across the vesicular membrane is achieved by pre-incubation of the vesicles with 4 μM valinomycin in K$^+$-containing buffer for 1 h at room temperature *(12)*. Third, the affinity of the transport system dictates the substrate concentration used, and in order to measure uptake rates at initial rate, this should be below the K$_m$ value reported in the literature although it should be bourn in mind this might vary between different cell types (*see* **Note 16**).

14. Presented here are conditions for neutral amino acid uptake *(13,14)* and cationic amino acid uptakes *(12)*, previously performed in our laboratory. Essentially, the

same approach could be applied to examine the uptake of any amino acid into MVM and BM (*see* **Note 16**).

15. Most IVBs for vesicle studies have an osmolality of approx 300 mOsm/kg H_2O which has to matched to the EVB, otherwise vesicles will shrink or swell if the EVB is not iso-osmotic. Vesicle size determines the intravesicular space available for substrate uptake and so needs to be kept constant. In fact, manipulation of vesicular size by exposure to EVBs of various osmotic strengths is a useful means of determining that uptake is into an osmotically active intravesicular space rather than just simply binding to the membrane *(15–17)*.

16. If a Na^+-dependent transport system is being investigated two EVB radiolabeled substrate stocks ± Na^+ are required. The nonmetabolizable analogue MeAIB is often used as substrate for the neutral amino acid system A transporter. Other amino acid substrates have been used at the following final concentrations to investigate uptake mechanisms in MVM and BM (alanine, 20, 87 or 100 µM *(18–21)*; methionine, 20 µM *(17,20)*; glycine, 0.6 or 20 µM *(16,17,20)*; tryptophan, 2 µM *(22)*; histidine, 100 µM *(23)*; glutamine, 100 µM *(23)*; cysteine, 5 µM *(19)*; lysine, 0.1, 0.2, 1, 2, 10, or 20 µM *(17,20,24–28)*; proline, 20 or 188 µM *(15,17,20)*; glutamate, 1, 2, 10, or 20 µM *(17,20,29,30)*; aspartate, 20 µM *(29)*; taurine, 0.5 or 1 µM *(31,32)*.

17. This should be kept on ice, thereby rapidly quenching transporter activity by a sharp fall in temperature. The stop buffer also serves as wash buffer.

18. The procedure is given as Method 3 in **ref. 2**.

19. Store homogenate and vesicles at 4°C until assay, but perform all assays (protein, markers, amino acid uptakes) within 24–48 h.

20. Some laboratories freeze MVM and BM vesicles and then perform uptake assays subsequently, but for some amino acid transporters this has a deleterious effect and uptakes are compromised with loss of activity *(33)*. Hence, we prefer to use nonfrozen vesicles for transport assays that have been stored at 4°C (*see* **Note 19**).

21. Essentially this method involves three steps: mincing of tissue followed by removal of MVM by agitation, an ultrasonication cycle to disrupt syncytial integrity and release of cellular contents and another ultrasonication cycle in the presence of EDTA to disassociate BM from underlying basal lamina, as outlined in **ref. 6**.

22. Thorough washing and draining of the tissue and removal of blood clots are critical to the success of this method.

23. Uptakes are measured under *zero-trans* conditions and the temperature at which uptakes are performed might vary depending on the system being studied and its maximal velocity and kinetic properties. Routinely we perform uptakes at room temperature, but sometimes (e.g., in the case of 20 µM leucine), we perform amino acid uptakes at 4°C (cold room) in order to be able measure uptake at initial rate *(14)*. Others have found that by decreasing the concentration of leucine to 0.25 µM, uptakes can be performed at 37°C *(28)*.

24. The volume of EVB can be varied and may well be different for different uptake protocols. It is worth bearing in mind that a bigger EVB volume means using

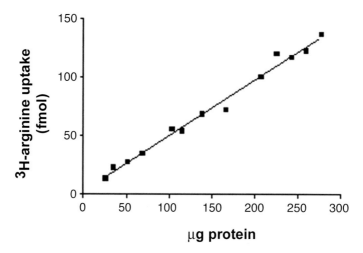

Fig. 1. Linearity of arginine uptake into microvillous plasma membrane (MVM) vesicles with variable MVM protein. Uptake of 0.2 μM ^{3}H-arginine into MVM where the amount of protein in the assay was varied. There was a significant positive correlation between uptake and MVM protein in assay ($r^2 = 0.99$, $p < 0.001$).

    more isotope. The volume selected will depend on whether it is desirable to alter the buffer composition to apply different treatments, for which solubility considerations could dictate. We routinely use 20 µL EVB for neutral amino acids and 100 µL EVB for cationic amino acids.

25. The number of tubes will depend on the protocol and whether a time course is being performed or simply some different buffer conditions at an initial rate. Be sure to pipet the radiolabeled substrate neatly to the bottom of the tube to prevent premature mixing with the vesicle suspension.

26. By replacing membrane protein in vesicle suspensions with IVB, an estimate of how much radiolabel is nonspecifically bound in the absence of protein can be determined and corrected for in the calculation of uptakes.

27. We routinely use approx 200 µg protein, but this might need to be modified depending on the level of transporter expression in the plasma membrane and its kinetic properties. It is worth performing uptakes with membrane protein titrated, so as to ascertain over what range uptake is linear with respect to membrane protein. This is useful reference data in the situation of MVM or BM protein being limited (**Fig. 1**).

28. In order to decide on this time point, it is necessary to perform preliminary experiments establishing a time course over which uptake is linear, defining uptake under initial rate conditions. A time point that falls within this period is then selected. Practically, it is difficult to add stop buffer before 15 s has elapsed and so we commonly use 30 s as our time point, usually performing a time course over 1 min.

29. Have precut, 1-inch filter squares presoaked in stop buffer on ice.
30. The standard count is used to convert counts to moles substrate.

References

1. Smith, N. C., Brush, M. G., and Luckett, S. (1974) Preparation of human placental villous surface membrane. *Nature* **252,** 302–303.
2. Glazier, J. D., Jones, C. J. P., and Sibley, C. P. (1988) Purification and Na$^+$ uptake by human placental microvillus membrane vesicles prepared by three different methods. *Biochim. Biophys. Acta* **945,** 127–134.
3. Illsley, N. P., Wang, Z.-Q., Gray, A., Sellers, M. C., and Jacobs M. M. (1990) Simultaneous preparation of paired, syncytial, microvillous and basal membranes from human placenta. *Biochim. Biophys. Acta* **1029,** 218–226.
4. Kelley, L. K., Smith, C. H., and King, B. F. (1983) Isolation and partial characterization of the basal cell membrane of human placental trophoblast. *Biochim. Biophys. Acta* **734,** 91–98.
5. Smith, C. H. and Kamath, S. G. (1994) Trophoblast basal and microvillous membrane isolation. *Placenta* **15,** 779–781.
6. Glazier, J., Ayuk, P., Grey, A.-M., and Sides, K. (1998) Syncytiotrophoblast basal plasma membrane isolation. *Placenta* **19,** 443–444.
7. Weigensberg, A. M. and Blostein, R. (1985) Na$^+$-coupled glycine transport in reticulocyte vesicles of distinct sideness: stoichiometry and symmetry. *J. Membr. Biol.* **86,** 37–44.
8. Jansson T. (2001) Amino acid transporters in the human placenta. *Pediatr. Res.* **49,** 141–147.
9. Kudo, Y. and Boyd, C. A. R. (2002) Human placental amino acid transporter genes: expression and function. *Reproduction* **124,** 593–600.
10. Cariappa, R., Heath-Monnig, E., and Smith, C. H. (2003) Isoforms of amino acid transporters in placental syncytiotrophoblast: plasma membrane localization and potential role in maternal/fetal transport. *Placenta* **24,** 713–726.
11. Shennan, D. B. and Reid, D. (1991) Endogenous transmembrane electrical gradients associated with human placental microvillous membrane vesicles. *Exp. Physiol.* **76,** 277–280.
12. Ayuk, P. T.-Y., Sibley, C. P., Donnai, P., D'Souza, S., and Glazier, J. D. (2000) Development and polarization of cationic amino acid transporters and regulators in the human placenta. *Am. J. Physiol. Cell Physiol.* **278,** C1162–C1171.
13. Mahendran, D., Donnai, P., Glazier, J. D., D'Souza, S.W., Boyd, R. D. H., and Sibley, C. P. (1993) Amino acid (system A) transporter activity in microvillous membrane vesicles from the placentas of appropriate and small for gestational age babies. *Pediatr. Res.* **34,** 661–665.
14. Kuruvilla, A. G., D'Souza, S. W., Glazier, J. D., Mahendran, D., Maresh, M. J., and Sibley, C. P. (1994) Altered activity of system A amino acid transporter in

microvillous membrane vesicles from placentas of macrosomic babies born to diabetic women. *J. Clin. Invest.* **94,** 689–695.

15. Boyd, C. A. R. and Lund, E. K. (1981) L-proline transport by brush border membrane vesicles prepared from human placenta. *J. Physiol.* **315,** 9–19.

16. Dicke, J. M., Verges, D., Kelley, L. K., and Smith, C. H. (1993) Glycine uptake by microvillous and basal plasma membrane vesicles from term human placentae. *Placenta* **14,** 85–92.

17. Kudo, Y., Yamada K., Fujiwara, A., and Kawasaki, T. (1987) Characterization of amino acid transport systems in human placental brush-border membrane vesicles. *Biochim. Biophys. Acta* **904,** 309–318.

18. Johnson, L. W. and Smith, C. H. (1988) Neutral amino acid transport systems of microvillous membrane of human placenta. *Am. J. Physiol. Cell Physiol.* **254,** C773–C780.

19. Hoeltzli, S. D. and Smith, C. H. (1989) Alanine transport systems in isolated basal plasma membrane of human placenta. *Am. J. Physiol. Cell Physiol.* **256,** C630–C637.

20. Kudo, Y. and Boyd, C. A. R. (1990) Characterization of amino acid transport systems in human placental basal membrane vesicles. *Biochim. Biophys. Acta* **1021,** 169–174.

21. Iioka, H., Hisanaga, H., Moriyama, I. S., et al. (1992) Characterization of human placental activity for transport of L-alanine, using brush border (microvillous) membrane vesicles. *Placenta* **13,** 179–190.

22. Kudo, Y. and Boyd, C. A. R. (2001) Characterisation of L-tryptophan transporters in human placenta: a comparison of brush border and basal membrane vesicles. *J. Physiol.* **531.2,** 405–416.

23. Karl, P. I., Tkaczevski, H., and Fisher, S. E. (1989) Characteristics of histidine uptake by human placental microvillous membrane vesicles. *Pediatr. Res.* **25,** 19–26.

24. Eleno, N., Devés, R., and Boyd, C. A. R. (1994) Membrane potential dependence of the kinetics of cationic amino acid transport systems in human placenta. *J. Physiol.* **479.2,** 291–300.

25. Furesz , T. C., Moe, A. J., and Smith C. H. (1991) Two cationic amino acid transport systems in human placental basal plasma membranes. *Am. J. Physiol. Cell Physiol.* **261,** C246–C252.

26. Furesz , T. C., Moe, A. J., and Smith, C. H. (1995) Lysine uptake by human placental microvillous membrane: comparison of system y⁺ with basal membrane. *Am. J. Physiol. Cell Physiol.* **268,** C755–C761.

27. Furesz, T. C. and Smith, C. H. (1997) Identification of two leucine-sensitive lysine transport activities in human placental basal membrane. *Placenta* **18,** 649–655.

28. Jansson, T., Scholtbach, V., and Powell, T. L. (1998) Placental transport of leucine and lysine is reduced in intrauterine growth restriction. *Pediatr. Res.* **44,** 532–537.

29. Moe, A. J. and Smith, C. H. (1989) Anionic amino acid uptake by microvillous

membrane vesicles from human placenta. *Am. J. Physiol. Cell Physiol.* **257,** C1005–C1011.

30. Hoeltzli, S. D., Kelley, L. K., Moe, A. J., and Smith, C. H. (1990) Anionic amino acid transport systems in isolated basal plasma membrane of human placenta. *Am.J. Physiol. Cell Physiol.* **259,** C47–C55.

31. Norberg, S., Powell, T. L., and Jansson, T. (1998) Intrauterine growth restriction is associated with a reduced activity of placental taurine transporters. *Pediatr. Res.* **44,** 233-238.

32. Miyamoto, Y., Balkovetz, D. F., Leibach, F. H., Mahesh, V. B., and Ganapathy, V. (1988) $Na^+ + Cl^-$ -gradient-driven, high affinity, uphill transport of taurine in human placental brush-border membrane vesicles. *FEBS Lett.* **231,** 263–267.

33. Karl, P. I., Teichberg, S. and Fisher, S. E. (1991) Na^+-dependent amino acid uptake by human placental microvillous membrane vesicles: importance of storage conditions and preservation of cytoskeletal elements. *Placenta* **12,** 239–250.

15

In Vitro Methods for Studying Human Placental Amino Acid Transport

Placental Villous Fragments

Susan L. Greenwood and Colin P. Sibley

Summary

A method is described for measuring amino acid uptake by the syncytiotrophoblast of the human placenta in vitro using taurine as an example. Small fragments of placental villous tissue (2–3 mm^3) are tied to a comb that enables them to be moved in concert between a series of incubation and wash buffers. The fragments are incubated in control or Na$^+$-free Tyrode's buffer containing ^{3}H taurine for timed intervals. Following incubation, the tissue is washed, lysed in water to release the accumulated isotope, and finally denatured in NaOH to determine protein. The water lysate is counted for radioactivity and the Na$^+$-dependent component of ^{3}H taurine uptake calculated as the difference between uptake in control and Na$^+$-free conditions. Because the taurine transport protein (system β) is Na$^+$-dependent, the Na$^+$-dependent component of ^{3}H taurine uptake gives a measure of system β activity in the microvillous membrane of the syncytiotrophoblast. The method described here in relation to taurine can be applied to other Na$^+$-dependent amino acid transport systems. An advantage of the fragment model is that syncytiotrophoblast metabolism and signaling are retained. A disadvantage is that fragments contain many cell types and carrier-mediated amino acid uptake may be into several compartments including syncytiotrophoblast.

Key Words: Placenta; syncytiotrophoblast; microvillous plasma membrane; villus; transport; amino acid; taurine.

1. Introduction

Studies of amino acid transport by the human placenta using in vitro preparations of intact villous tissue were first described more than 30 yr ago. These early studies used either placental villous slices (approx 0.3–0.5 mm thick) prepared using a Stadie-Riggs microtome *(1–3)* or small fragments of villi (4–5 mm) which were pooled to a weight of approx 250 mg *(4–7)*. Villous fragments were considered to be the better preparation and yielded more consistent results than slices, which were difficult to prepare with uniform composition

From: *Methods in Molecular Medicine, Vol. 122: Placenta and Trophoblast: Methods and Protocols, Vol. 2*
Edited by: M. J. Soares and J. S. Hunt © Humana Press Inc., Totowa, NJ

and weight *(3,4)*. Amino acid uptake was determined by incubating slices or fragments in radiolabeled amino acids for varying lengths of time and then measuring the radioactivity in a tissue extract. In both models, separate estimates of extracellular water were made in parallel using radiolabeled inulin *(5)* and the amino acid uptake into cellular (specific uptake) and extracellular (nonspecific accumulation) tissue compartments were calculated by correcting for the inulin space.

The method described in this chapter is based on these early studies but differs in two respects. First, amino acid uptake is measured into individual villous fragments (wet weight approx 10 mg) using a modification of the procedure described by Shennan and McNeillie *(8)* to study volume regulation of amino acid efflux. The unique feature of their technique was to tie a small fragment of placental villous tissue into a bundle with fine thread, which was then used to transfer the tissue through a series of solutions. In the method described here, the tissue bundles are tied to metal hooks that are attached to a Perspex comb to further facilitate transfer of the fragments *(9–11)*. The arrangement allows three fragments to be manipulated simultaneously and transferred quickly and precisely through uptake and wash solutions.

The second difference between the procedure described here and earlier studies is in the estimation of the nonspecific component of tissue amino acid accumulation. We describe the method for amino acid uptake into fragments using taurine as an example and exploit the knowledge that the transport protein for taurine, system β, is Na^+-dependent. Radiolabeled taurine uptake into villous fragments is measured in control and Na^+-free conditions and the latter is used to estimate the nonspecific accumulation of the amino acid into cellular and extracellular compartments. This approach avoids the problems associated with the use of inulin to measure extracellular space in the placenta *(5)*.

The method described below is a procedure to determine the time course of Na^+-dependent ^{3}H taurine uptake into human placental villous fragments. Essentially, uptake is measured in triplicate over 2–30 min with tissue bathed at 37°C in control and Na^+-free Tyrode's buffer (choline chloride replaces NaCl: *see* **Note 1**) containing tracer concentrations of ^{3}H taurine. After exposing the fragments to ^{3}H taurine, they are washed rapidly in ice-cold buffer, to inhibit transport and remove extracellular isotope, and then lysed in water to release the exchangeable radiolabeled amino acid that has been accumulated by the tissue. Finally the fragments are denatured in NaOH for determination of protein. Na^+-dependent taurine uptake is calculated (uptake in Na^+-free conditions subtracted from that in control) and expressed per mg fragment protein. The assumptions are made (1) that ^{3}H taurine accumulation in Na^+-free conditions reflects nonspecific diffusion into cells and extracellular fluid and (2) that Na^+-dependent ^{3}H taurine uptake is a measure of taurine transport into the syncytiotrophoblast by system β in the microvillous membrane. As the fragments contain a mixture of cell types (e.g., macrophages, endothelium, smooth muscle cells) it is possible that each of the cell types within the fragments make some contribution to measured uptake. However, the microvillous membrane is likely to be the major contributor because it is the first plasma membrane encountered by tracer and has the greatest overall surface area (*see* **Note 2**).

Villous fragments are relatively quick to prepare and study and, once the amino acid uptake properties have been established, amino acid transport activity can be compared in large numbers of placentas *(12)*. An advantage of this preparation is that cellular machinery remains intact and fragments have been used to assess the electrochemical driving forces, which are a determinant of amino acid uptake *in situ* and to study regulation of placental amino acid transport by hormones and reactive oxygen species *(9–11,13)*. Villous fragments may be used for transport studies on placentas from first trimester and tissue from early or late gestation can be maintained in long-term explant culture for studies of chronic regulation *(14; see* **Note 3**). The fragment method can be applied to studying amino acid transport by placentas of other species *(15,16)*. The method described here in relation to taurine has been applied to other Na^+-dependent transporters *(9,12,17)* and could be used, with modification, to examine other amino acid transport systems (*see* **Note 4**).

2. Materials

2.1. Buffers and Reagents

1. Tyrode's buffers (prepare 5 L and make fresh weekly: store at 4°C when not in use):
   a. Control Tyrode's buffer: 135 mM NaCl, 5 mM KCl, 1.8 mM CaCl$_2$, 1.0 mM MgCl$_2$ (6H$_2$O), 1.0 mM MgSO$_4$, 10 mM HEPES, 5.6 mM glucose. Adjust to pH 7.4 with 10 M NaOH. Osmolality approx 295 mOsm/Kg H$_2$O.
   b. Na^+-free Tyrode's buffer as above but replace NaCl with 135 mM choline chloride. Adjust to pH 7.4 with 10 M KOH. Check osmolality and adjust to 295 mOsm/Kg H$_2$O by the addition of choline chloride.

2. DMEM:Tyrode's mix (Prepare 1 L and make fresh weekly: store at 4°C when not in use). Mix one part Dulbecco's modified Eagle's medium (DMEM) and three parts control Tyrode's solution to maintain tissue. DMEM (Invitrogen, Carlsbad, CA, cat. no. 12320) contains 5.5 mM D-glucose, 25 mM HEPES buffer, 110 mg/L sodium pyruvate, vitamins and the following amino acids: 100 µM arginine, 50 µM cysteine, 1000 µM glutamine, 100 µM glycine, 50 µM histidine, 200 µM isoleucine, 200 µM leucine, 200 µM lysine, 50 µM methionine, 100 µM phenylalanine, 100 µM serine, 20 µM threonine, 20 µM tryptophan, 100 µM tyrosine, and 200 µM valine. Add 150 µM taurine.

3. Incubation solution with ^{3}H taurine: 250 µCi ^{3}H taurine stock (in 250 µL aqueous solution: Amersham Biosciences, Chalfont St.Giles, UK) is supplied at a specific

activity of 19 Ci/mmol (taurine 52.63 μM). For incubation solutions, prepare a 1 in 1000 dilution with control and Na$^+$-free Tyrode's as required (*see* **Subheading 3.2.8.**) to give an isotope concentration of 1 μCi/mL (52.63 pmol/mL taurine) (*see* **Note 5**).

4. Ice-cold wash solutions: prepare control or Na$^+$-free Tyrode's on ice as required (*see* **Subheading 3.1.2.**).
5. Tissue lysis buffer: 500 mL 0.3 M NaOH and 500 mL 0.3 M HCl for lysing tissue and protein assay.
6. Bio-Rad protein assay reagent concentrate (Bio-Rad Laboratories Ltd., Hemel Hempstead, UK).

2.2. Equipment

1. Glass Pasteur pipet attached to vacuum pump to aspirate radioactive solutions to waste.
2. Scintillation fluid (Optiphase Hisafe 2).
3. Glass scintillation vials (volume 23 mL).
4. Water bath, β-scintillation counter, spectrophotometer
5. Pipet aid.
6. Perspex combs with hooks (**Fig. 1**) (University of Manchester Central Workshop). The dimensions are appropriate for use with scintillation vials (*see* **Subheading 2.2.3.**) when housed in aluminum scintillation vial racks (*see* **Subheading 2.2.7.**).
7. 10x aluminum scintillation vial racks (6 × 6) (VWR International, Poole, UK, cat. no. 402/0690/00).
8. Two pairs watchmakers forceps; one pair fine and one pair medium scissors.
9. Petri dishes, cotton thread.

3. Methods
3.1. Prepare the Following in Advance of the Arrival of a Placenta

1. 36 ties of cotton thread to secure the tissue fragments to the hooks on the Perspex combs (**Fig. 1**). Cut 2-inch lengths of cotton and loosely form a double loop that can be pulled tight later.
2. Wash solutions: beakers containing 800 mL of control and 800 mL Na$^+$-free Tyrode's on ice; store at 4°C until the start of the experiment.
3. 36 scintillation vials with 4 mL DMEM:Tyrode's in which to maintain the tissue at room temperature prior to experimentation.
4. 36 scintillation vials with 4 mL DMEM:Tyrode's in which to pre-incubate the tissue at 37°C; place in scintillation vial racks in the water bath.
5. 18 scintillation vials with 4 mL control and 18 vials with 4 mL Na$^+$-free Tyrode's to prewash the tissue for 2 min prior to measuring uptake (*see* **Note 6**). Place in scintillation vial racks in the water bath.
6. Incubation solutions: prepare incubation solutions by adding 37 μL of ^{3}H taurine stock in 37 mL (1 in 1000 dilution) of control or Na$^+$-free Tyrode's buffer. Pre-

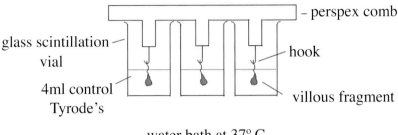

Fig. 1. Experimental arrangement to manipulate small fragments of villous tissue for measurement of radiolabelled amino acid uptake. The tissue is tied to stainless steel hooks attached to a comb that is supported on glass vials housed in racks in a water bath. The tissue can easily be exposed to solutions of different composition by moving the comb between vials.

pare nine scintillation vials with 4 mL control incubation solutions (label 1–3, 7–9, 13–15) and nine vials with 4 mL Na⁺-free incubation solutions (label 4–6, 10–12, 16–18) and place in the scintillation vial racks in the water bath.

7. Prepare two racks, each containing 36 scintillation vials, and keep on ice to pre-cool in preparation for the ice-cold washes.
8. Prepare 36 scintillation vials containing 4 mL distilled water to lyse the tissue fragments at the end of the experiment.
9. Prepare 36 scintillation vials containing 4 mL 0.3 M NaOH to dissolve the tissue fragments 18 h after completion of the experiment (cap until required).

3.2. On Arrival of the Placenta

1. Remove six 1-cm square samples of the full thickness of the placenta, sampling at random from different cotyledons, and place into DMEM:Tyrode's buffer at room temperature (*see* **Note 7**) . Taking each cube, remove the chorionic and basal plates and discard. Wash the remaining villous tissue three times in 50 mL DMEM:Tyrode's to remove maternal blood.
2. Using small scissors remove six to eight chunks of villous tissue from each cube approx 5 mm in diameter and place them into fresh DMEM:Tyrode's in a Petri dish. Refine the size of the fragments to approx 4 mm³ by snipping off loose villi on the edge of the clumps. Prepare 36 evenly sized fragments (*see* **Note 8**) (12 time points in triplicate) to allow uptake to be measured at six time points (2, 5, 10, 15, 20, and 30 min) in the presence and absence of Na⁺ (*see* **Note 9**).
3. Taking one Perspex comb at a time, support it in a petri dish and secure a fragment onto a hook using watchmakers forceps to knot the cotton thread (**Fig.1**). Place the tissue in the preprepared double loop in the thread then tighten. Once the tissue is tied, trim it to a final size of approx 2 mm³. Cut one of the loose ends of thread close to the knot and discard. Form a loop in the remaining thread, slip

it over a hook, tie it securely using a double knot, and then cut off the excess thread. Keep the tissue moist at all times and manipulate it using the thread thereby handling the tissue as little as possible. Before tightening, adjust the length of the cotton such that the fragment hangs approx 1 cm directly below the hook once the thread is knotted; this will ensure that the tissue is completely immersed in DMEM:Tyrode's solution when the comb is supported on the vials (**Fig. 1**).

4. When tissue has been secured onto three hooks of one comb, support the comb on the pre-prepared vials containing 4 mL DMEM:Tyrode's solution and leave at room temperature until all the fragments are tied in place.

5. The three fragments on each comb allow measurements to be made in triplicate at each time point. Label each comb with the incubation time (2, 5, 10, 15, 20, 30 min control or Na$^+$-free) and transfer all the combs to scintillation vials containing DMEM:Tyrode's prewarmed to 37°C in the water bath .

6. Allow the tissue to stabilize in DMEM:Tyrodes at 37°C for 30 min before commencing uptake measurements.

7. Before initiating uptake, wash each set of triplicates in either control or Na$^+$-free Tyrode's as appropriate for 2 min. Transfer the fragments to the prewarmed scintillation vials in the water bath and time the wash with a stopwatch.

8. Immediately after completion of the wash, transfer each set of triplicates to the vials containing prewarmed incubation solutions to initiate uptake and start the stopwatch. Each set of incubation vials can be used twice (to reduce the isotope cost) in the following way to minimize the difference in exposure to tissue between the vials: for control incubations use vials 1–3 for 30 min and 2 min uptakes; vials 7–9 for 15 min and 10 min uptakes; vials 13–15 for 20 min and 5 min uptakes. For Na$^+$-free incubations use vials 4–6 for 30 min and 2 min; vials 10–12 for 15 min and 10 min; vials 16–18 for 20 min and 5 min.

9. Fill six precooled scintillation vials with 12 mL ice-cold control or Na$^+$-free Tyrode's as appropriate. At the end of the timed uptake, keep the stopwatch running and immediately transfer the fragments to three vials of ice-cold wash for exactly 15 s and gently agitate the tissue (*see* **Note 10**). Repeat the wash by transferring to the second three wash vials for exactly 15 s and finally place the tissue, still attached to the comb, in the preprepared vials containing 4 mL distilled water to lyse for 18 h (*see* **Note 11**).

10. Discard the used wash vials and replace with new precooled vials ready to fill with ice-cold wash for the next set of triplicate fragments and repeat the process until the uptakes are completed.

11. At the end of the experiment, remove 2 × 100 µL aliquots from each incubation to measure the radioactivity (*see* **Note 12**). Add the 100-µL aliquot, 3.9 mL of distilled water, and 16 mL of Optiphase HiSafe 2 scintillation fluid to each vial. Shake to ensure good mixing.

12. After lysing in water for 18 h, remove the tissue and count the water lysate by adding 16 mL of scintillation fluid to each vial. Shake to ensure good mixing.

13. Detach the villous fragments from the hooks by cutting the thread and allowing the fragments to fall into the scintillation vials containing 4 mL 0.3 *M* NaOH. Cap the vials and place in an oven at 37°C for a minimum of 10 h to dissolve the tissue.

14. After lysing in 0.3 M NaOH, remove 2×80 µL aliquots for protein assay with the Bradford method using Bio-Rad protein reagent (*see* **Subheading 3.3.**). Count the remaining lysate by adding 16 mL scintillation fluid to the vial and mixing well.

15. Count the samples and standards on a β scintillation counter for a minimum of 5 min using window settings appropriate for tritium. Prepare background samples of 4 mL H_2O or 0.3 M NaOH and 16 mL scintillation fluid.

16. Express the results as xmol ^3H taurine uptake/mg fragment protein/incubation time. Use the counts in the corresponding tissue incubation solution, and the concentration of taurine, to calculate counts per nmol taurine (counts in 1 mL incubation solution/nmol taurine in 1 mL incubation solution). Take the counts in the 4 mL water lysate sample and divide by the counts per nmol taurine. The Na^+-dependent component of uptake is the difference between uptake in control and Na^+-free Tyrode's. Perform the same calculation on the NaOH lysate to estimate the counts still associated with the tissue (nonexchangeable or bound taurine; *see* **Note 13**) remembering to correct for the volume removed for the protein assay.

3.3. Protein Assay

1. Warm Bio-Rad reagent to room temperature.
2. Prepare 10 mg/10 mL bovine serum albumin (BSA) in 0.3 M NaOH. Make a 1 in 4 dilution of this stock BSA with 0.3 M NaOH to give a standard solution of 0.25 mg/mL.
3. Label small glass test tubes for tissue lysate samples (in duplicate) plus 12 for standards (see below; six in duplicate).
4. Prepare standards in duplicate of 0–20 µg BSA content by diluting the standard solution with 0.3 M NaOH.
5. Prepare 2×80 µL fragment lysate samples.
6. Add 320 µL 0.3 M NaOH and 400 µL 0.3 M HCl to each standard and sample tube and vortex.
7. Add 200 µL Bio-Rad reagent and vortex.
8. 5 min after adding Bio-Rad reagent, read the samples using a spectrophotometer at a wavelength of 595 nm.
9. Note that the fragment protein lysates are radioactive and take the necessary precautions during the assay and for disposal of waste. It is recommended that disposable cuvets be used to read the samples.
10. Calculate the sample protein content by interpolation from the standard curve and multiply by 50 (fragments lysed in 4 mL 0.3 M NaOH) to give fragment protein content in µg.

4. Notes

1. To examine nonspecific amino acid uptake in the absence of extracellular Na^+, we substituted Na^+ in Tyrode's with choline. Choline is transported across the syncytiotrophoblast microvillous membrane and it is possible that there are consequences of choline uptake, which might impact on amino acid transport although this has not been evaluated. It might be of use to compare choline substitution with an alternative cation, e.g., *n*-methyl-D-glucamine (NMDG). Alternatively,

the nonspecific component of uptake can be examined using a high concentration of a nonlabeled competing substrate. In this regard, it is reassuring that ^{3}H taurine uptake in the presence of 10 mM β-alanine, a substrate for system β, is identical to the uptake in the absence of Na$^+$ (choline substitution) *(10,13)*. The latter approach avoids the pitfalls of exposing tissue to Na$^+$- free solutions over long periods of time that could induce cellular swelling and change the passive permeability properties of the tissue leading to inaccurate estimates of the nonspecific component of uptake.

2. Amino acid uptake has been measured into cytotrophoblast cells isolated from term placenta to examine system A activity using the principles of the methods described for villous fragments *(18)*. A method for preparation of cytotrophoblast cells for amino acid uptake studies and their morphological and biochemical differentiation in culture, has been described *(19–21)*.

3. Short term regulation (over 2 h) of system β and system A (Na$^+$-dependent uptake of ^{14}C methylaminoisobutyric acid, MeAIB) by hormones and reactive oxygen species has been demonstrated using the fragment method *(9–11)*. The method can also be applied to placental villous tissue following explant culture and this allows investigation of chronic (long-term) regulation of amino acid transport. The procedure for explant culture and the morphological and biochemical characteristics of the tissue maintained over 11 d is described in *(14)*. Following this method, with the exception that three explants each of 0.3 mg protein were cultured per Netwell, we showed that taurine uptake on day 7 of culture exhibited transport characteristics typical of system β that were qualitatively identical to those in fresh tissue (Na$^+$- and Cl$^-$-dependent; inhibition by β-alanine *[22]*). Experiments examining regulation of amino acid transport should be performed at the initial rate of uptake. Initially a time course of uptake should be performed so that modulators can be examined over the linear phase. Having chosen a time point at which uptake is linear, kinetic studies to examine K_m and V_{max} could be performed using a range of substrate concentrations, although this may be limited in practice because of the time required to dissect and tie sufficient fragments (*see* **Note 9**).

4. The method can be used to measure the uptake of any radiolabelled amino acid, but the distinction should be made (1) between accumulation into cellular and extracellular compartments and (2) uptake by specific transport proteins in the cell membrane and nonspecific diffusion, including that through tissue damaged by dissection. The strategy we employed for system A and system β, both Na$^+$-dependent transporters, was to determine the Na$^+$-dependent component of uptake and we attributed this to specific carrier mediated transport. For system β, we also confirmed the Cl$^-$-dependency of transport using Cl—free Tyrode's (gluconate replacement *[13]*). The method has been used to examine the activity of system A using radiolabeled substrates such as MeAIB (^{14}C MeAIB; nonmetabolized *[9]*) or ^{3}H glycine *(17)* (*see* **Note 3**).

Competitive inhibition using high concentrations of unlabeled substrate has been used to determine the contribution of an amino acid transport system, which has more than one substrate. For example, the contribution of system A to glycine uptake has been assessed by examining the degree by which its accumulation is inhibited in the presence of MeAIB, a specific substrate for system A, at concentrations which will saturate the transporter (10 mM) **(17)**.

5. ^{3}H taurine was used at 1 µCi/mL because this level of activity gave counts significantly above background in the tissue lysate samples over the shortest uptake periods in the absence of Na$^+$. We have also measured Na$^+$-dependent ^{14}C MeAIB, ^{14}C aminoisobutyric acid (AIB) and ^{3}H glycine uptake into villous fragments, to investigate system A activity, using 0.5 µCi/mL **(9,17)**. In all these cases the tracer concentration of the substrate is well below the K$_m$ for system β and system A in syncytiotrophoblast microvillous membrane vesicles. The specific activity of radiolabeled amino acids can differ slightly between batches, and the dilution of the stock should be adjusted to achieve the same concentration of amino acid in the final incubation rather than the same activity.

6. The 2-min prewash in Na$^+$-free solution is performed to deplete tissue Na$^+$ prior to measuring uptake in Na$^+$-free conditions. In preliminary experiments, we found no further reduction in ^{3}H taurine uptake under Na$^+$-free conditions if the prewash period was extended for more than 2–10 min. On several occasions, we have performed experiments where we have been unable to detect a Na$^+$-dependent component of uptake. Two routine procedural errors were identified which accounted for this: (1) failure to agitate the tissue during the 2-min wash in Na$^+$ free solution (2) mistakenly adjusting the pH to 7.4 in Na$^+$-free Tyrode's with NaOH instead of KOH.

7. We have maintained the tissue in a DMEM:Tyrode's mix to keep a physiological concentration of amino acids in the extracellular environment and minimize depletion of cellular amino acids which might occur if tissue were maintained in Tyrode's alone during collection and dissection. It is important to avoid substrate deprivation as amino acid transporters in placental trophoblast exhibit adaptive regulation over a relatively short term **(23)**. In preliminary experiments, we demonstrated downregulation of Na$^+$-dependent taurine uptake after culturing explants for 7 d in high-taurine medium **(22)**.

8. Standardization of fragment size is important. **Figure 2** shows a significant negative correlation between Na$^+$-dependent and independent uptake of ^{3}H glycine per milligram fragment protein when plotted against protein over the range 0.1–0.5 mg. As fragment size increases (represented by an increase in protein), the surface area:volume ratio will fall. This could account for the negative correlation if amino acid uptake is a function of the surface area of the syncytiotrophoblast microvillous membrane. If several investigators are contributing to a data set, it is important to minimize differences in villous fragment size between individuals. Similarly, when comparing treatments, ensure that the fragment sizes in the treatment groups are comparable.

9. The time over which the overall experiment is performed is important. According to Soorana et al. **(24)**, syncytiotrophoblast deterioration is evident in villous

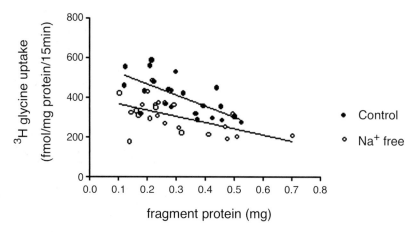

Fig. 2. There is a significant negative correlation between ^{3}H glycine uptake into placental villous fragments/mg protein with fragment protein when the tissue is bathed in control and Na^+-free Tyrodes ($n = 24$ fragments from four placentas). Least squares linear regression: control r^2 0.448 $p < 0.001$; Na^+-free r^2 0.306 $p < 0.005$.

     fragments of term placenta 6 h after delivery. Jansson et al. (*9*) performed scanning and transmission electron microscopy on tissue fragments following 3 h attachment to the hooks and reported normal syncytiotrophoblast ultrastructure. Based on these observations, it is recommended that experiments on fresh tissue be completed within 5 h of placental delivery

10. The particular advantage of this technique, and the reward for the tedium of tying each piece of tissue, is that each fragment is easily and accurately manipulated between the prewash, incubation, and stop solutions. Uptake is inhibited promptly and the extracellular isotope removed efficiently during the washes to avoid contamination. The wash process will remove most but not all the extracellular isotope and standardizing the volume and timing of the washes ensures that any residual extracellular isotope is similar for each tissue fragment.

11. In preliminary experiments, we determined the time course of isotope leaching from the tissue into the water lysate (at room temperature) and found no further loss of isotope after 18 h.

12. Standards are prepared from the incubation solution that have been in contact with the tissue and housed in the water bath at 37°C because a slight evaporation of the incubation solution can occur over time, and this must be taken into account when calculating the counts/$x$mol available for uptake.

13. We have found that the binding of ^{3}H taurine, ^{3}H glycine, ^{14}C AIB, and [14]C MeAIB is greater in the presence than absence of Na^+, higher at the shorter incubation times, and stabilizes over 10–30 min. In the presence of Na^+, the bound radiolabel represents 1–5% of the accumulated isotope over 10–30 min. Because it represents a small and constant proportion of the uptake, we have not routinely

corrected for binding. However, binding might be altered by experimental circumstances and should be evaluated when applying a new protocol.

Acknowledgments

We are very grateful to Mrs. Jean French for her expert assistance in preparing this manuscript.

References

1. Longo, L. D., Yuen, P., and Gusseck, D. J. (1973) Anaerobic, glycogen-dependent transport of amino acids by the placenta. *Nature* **243,** 531–533.
2. Miller, R. K. and Berndt, W. O. (1974) Characterization of neutral amino acid accumulation by human term placental slices. *Am. J. Physiol.* **227,** 1236–1242.
3. Schneider, H. and Dancis, J. (1974). Amino acid transport in human placental slices. *Am. J. Obstet. Gynecol.* **120,** 1092–1098.
4. Smith, C. H., Adcock, E. W 3rd, Teasdale, F., Meschia, G., and Battaglia, F. C. (1973) Placental amino acid uptake: tissue preparation, kinetics and preincubation effect. *Am. J. Physiol.* **224,** 558–564.
5. Smith, C. H. and Depper, R. (1974) Placental amino acid uptake. II. Tissue preincubation, fluid distribution, and mechanisms of regulation. *Pediat. Res.* **8,** 697–703.
6. Enders, R. H., Judd, M. R., Donohue, T. M., and Smith, C. H. (1976) Placental amino acid uptake. III. Transport systems for neutral amino acids. *Am. J. Physiol.* **203,** 706–710.
7. Steel, R. B., Smith, C. H., and Kelley, L. K. (1982) Placental amino acid uptake. V1. Regulation by intracellular substrate. *Am. J. Physiol.* **243,** C41–C51.
8. Shennan, D. B. and McNeillie, S. A. (1995) Volume activated amino acid flux from term human placental tissue: stimulation of efflux via a pathway sensitive to anion transport inhibitors. *Placenta* **16,** 297–308.
9. Jansson, N., Greenwood, S. L., Johansson, B. R., Powell, T. L., and Jansson, T. (2003) Leptin stimulates the activity of the system A amino acid transporter in human placental villous fragments. *J. Clin. End. Metab.* **88,** 1205–1211.
10. Roos, S., Powell, T. L., and Jansson, T. (2004) The human placental taurine transporter in uncomplicated and IUGR pregnancies: cellular localization, protein expression and regulation. *Am. J. Physiol. Regul. Integr. Comp.* **287,** R886–893; erratum **287,** R1517.
11. Khullar, S., Greenwood, S. L., McCord, N., Glazier, J. D., and Ayuk, P. T-Y. (2003) Nitric oxide and superoxide impair human placental amino acid uptake and increase Na^+ permeability: implications for fetal growth. *Free. Rad. Biol. Med.* **36,** 271–277.
12. Lewis, R., Barker, A. C., Godfrey, K. M., et al. (2002) Size at birth and system A activity in placental villous fragments. *Placenta* **23(7),** A.44.
13. Greenwood, S. L., Lambert, K. D., and Sibley, C. P. (2000) Na^+-dependent taurine uptake in human placental villous fragments. *J. Physiol. (Lond.)* **528.P,** 27.

14. Siman, C. M., Sibley, C. P., Jones, C. J. P., Turner, M. A., and Greenwood, S. L. (2001) The functional regeneration of syncytiotrophoblast in cultured explants of term placenta. *Am. J. Physiol.* **280,** R1116–R1122.

15. Champion, E. E., Bailey, S. J., Glazier, J. D., et al. (2003) Characterisation of long-term cat placental explant cultures for transport studies: uptake of taurine by system β. *J. Physiol. (Lond)* **547.P,** C53.

16. Champion, E. E., Bailey, S. J., Glazier, J. D., et al. (2001) Taurine uptake into cat placental tissue fragments. *Placenta* **22,** A42.

17. Champion, E. E., Glazier, J. D., Jones, C. J. P., Rawlings, J. D., Sibley, C. P., and Greenwood, S. L. (2001) Glycine uptake into human placental villous fragments. *J. Physiol. (Lond)* **535.P,** S032.

18. Nelson, D. M., Smith, S. D., Furesz, T. C., et al. (2003) Hypoxia reduces expression and function of system A amino acid transporters in cultured term human trophoblasts. *Am. J. Physiol.* **284,** C310–C315.

19. Greenwood, S. L., Brown, P. D., Edwards, D., and Sibley, C. P. (1993) Patch clamp studies of human placental cytotrophoblast cells in culture. *Troph. Res.* **7,** 53–68.

20. Clarson, L. H., Glazier, J. D., Greenwood, S. L., Jones, C. P., Sides, M. K., and Sibley, C. P. (1996) Activity and expression of Na+K+ATPase in human placental cytotrophoblast cells in culture. *J. Physiol. (Lond.)* **497.3,** 735–743

21. Greenwood, S. L., Clarson, L. H., Sides, M. K., and Sibley, C. P. (1996) Membrane potential difference and intracellular cation concentration in human placental trophoblast cells in culture. *J. Physiol. (Lond.)* **492.3,** 629–640.

22. Siman, C. M., Sibley, C. P., and Greenwood, S. L. (2001) Nutrient regulation of taurine uptake in term human placental villous explants. *Placenta* **22,** A46.

23. Jayanthi, L. D., Ramamoorthy, S., Maresh, V. B., Leibach, F. H., and Ganapathy,V. (1995) Substrate specific regulation of the taurine transporter in human placental choriocarcinoma cells (JAr). *Biochim. Biophys. Acta* **1235,** 351–360.

24. Soorana, S. R., Oteng-Ntim, E. O., Meah, R., Ryder, T. A., and Bajoria, R. (1999) Characterisation of human placental explants: morphological, biochemical and physiological studies using first and third trimester placenta. *Hum. Reprod.* **14,** 536–541.

16

Methods for Investigating Placental Fatty Acid Transport

Yan Xu, Thomas J. Cook, and Gregory T. Knipp

Summary

Fatty acids (FAs), especially essential fatty acids (EFAs) and their long chain polyunsaturated fatty acid (LCPUFAs) derivatives, are critical for proper fetal development. The fetus relies on the placental transfer of EFAs from the maternal circulation for development. In fact, fatty acid transfer is highly directional from the mother to the fetus. Significant changes in placental fatty acid transport and metabolism, the two primary processes that govern placental FA supply from mother to fetus, can subsequently result in aberrant fetal fatty acid/lipid homeostasis and dramatically increase the risk of abnormal fetal development. Besides passive diffusion, specific fatty acid transfer conferring proteins can actively mediate directional placental fatty acid uptake and transport. Enzymes for fatty acid β-oxidation and synthesis and the ones participating PUFA metabolism, including cytochrome P450 (mainly CYP4A), cyclooxygenases (COXs), and lipooxygenases (LOXs), have also been identified in the placenta. Methods for studying functional placental fatty acid uptake/transport/metabolism are discussed, focusing on an in vitro placental trophoblast model and long chain unsaturated fatty acids. The relevant theory of FA transport pathways, kinetic data analysis (uptake rates, permeability, influx/efflux ratio, K_m, and so on) and high-performance liquid chromatography identification are also discussed.

Key Words: Essential fatty acids; transport; metabolism; placenta; HRP-1 cells.

1. Introduction

Fatty acids are involved in energy storage *(1)* and are obligatory constituents of biological membranes *(2)*. In addition, fatty acids, particularly essential fatty acids (EFAs), are precursors of intracellular signaling molecules in the body and are involved in fetal organogenesis *(3–11)*. Thus, a proper balance of EFA supply to the fetus is important in guiding normal fetal development. Altered fetal EFA homeostasis dramatically increases the risk of abnormal fetal development, particularly with respect to the brains *(7)*, eyes *(8)*, lungs *(9,10)*, and cardiovascular systems *(11)*. The placenta regulates the exchange of nutrients, wastes and xenobiotics across the maternal–fetal interface, thus nourishing and protecting the fetus during development. For example, free fatty acid (FFA)

From: *Methods in Molecular Medicine, Vol. 122: Placenta and Trophoblast: Methods and Protocols, Vol. 2*
Edited by: M. J. Soares and J. S. Hunt © Humana Press Inc., Totowa, NJ

supply across the placenta is the main source of fetal EFAs, and is highly directional from mother to fetus *(5)*.

Placental transport and metabolism are two of the major processes contributing to the placental and fetal fatty acid homeostasis. Placental fatty acid transport has been documented by several research groups, emphasizing an active, directional mechanism mediated by several distinct fatty acid transporters that contribute to the directionality of EFA transfer that predicted by simple passive diffusion *(12,13)*. These fatty acid transfer-conferring proteins include fatty acid translocase/CD36 (FAT/CD36), fatty acid transport protein (FATP), plasma membrane fatty acid binding protein (FABPpm), and cytoplasmic fatty acid binding protein (FABP) *(12)*.

Although placental fatty acid metabolism has not been as extensively studied as transport, it has been demonstrated that the human placenta has high enzymatic activities for fatty acid β-oxidation and synthesis, leading to energy generation *(14,15)*. Additionally, three enzyme families participating in polyunsaturated fatty acid (PUFA) metabolism, including cytochrome P450 (mainly CYP4A) *(16,17)*, cyclooxygenases (COXs) *(18–20)*, and lipooxygenases (LOXs) *(20–22)* have also been identified in placental tissue and different cell models. Therefore, the placenta is important for the proper supply of EFAs and their derivatives as nutrients, for the generation of important bioactive molecules like eicosanoids and prostanoids, and potential detoxification of fetotoxic FA-based agents (**Fig. 1**).

It must be noted that most of the work detailing the role of placental EFA transport and metabolism has been performed with whole tissue studies, often utilizing perfusion techniques. There exists a need for the development of cell culture model systems that can form confluent monolayers and demonstrate trophoblast transport properties in vitro. This will enable researchers to utilize a relatively simple model that will reduce some issues that may obfuscate tissue models.

To address these issues, our discussion will be focused on a specific rat trophoblast cell model, HRP-1. HRP-1 cells were originally derived from explants of d 10.5 normal rat chorioallantoic placental tissue and exhibits selective features of the morphological and functional properties of trophoblast cells within the zone of the rat chorioallantoic placenta, where the majority of maternal–fetal nutrient/waste transfer occurs *(23,24)*. HRP-1 cells have

---

Fig. 1. (*opposite page*) Scheme of fatty acid transport and metabolism of fatty acids in placental cells. FAT/CD36, fatty acid translocase; FATP, fatty acid transport protein; FABPpm, plasma membrane fatty acid binding protein; FABPs, cytoplasmic fatty acid binding proteins; LPL, lipoprotein lipase; TAG, triacylglycerol *(12,39,47)*.

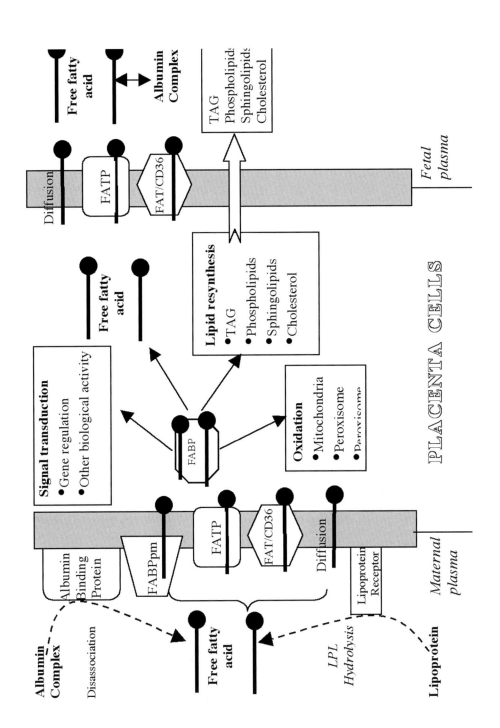

been previously demonstrated to form a monolayer of viable, polarized, fully differentiated cells and serves as a useful in vitro model of the placental barrier to study transport of nutrients, including fatty acids *(25)*, glutamate *(26)*, and glucose *(27)*. Here we describe the methods used in our laboratory to study the uptake, transport, and metabolism of fatty acids.

2. Materials

1. Chemicals: [1-^{14}C] arachidonic acid (AA; 55 mCi/mmol), [1-^{14}C] linoleic acid (LA; 55 mCi/mmol) and [1-^{14}C] α-linolenic acid (ALA; 55 mCi/mmol) were obtained from American Radiolabeled Chemicals Co. (St. Louis, MO); [1-^{14}C] docosahexaenoic acid (DHA; 56 mCi/mmol), [1-^{14}C] acid (SA; 56 mCi/mmol), and [1-^{14}C] oleic acid (OA; 54 mCi/mmol) were purchased from Moravek Biochemicals (Brea, CA); [^{14}C] mannitol (51 mCi/mmol), [^{3}H] mannitol (26.3 mCi/mmol), unlabeled fatty acids, fenofibrate, and dimethylsulfoxide (DMSO) were purchased from Sigma Chemical Company (St. Louis, MO). Type I rat tail collagen was obtained from BioRad (Hercules, CA). Other high-performance liquid chromatography (HPLC)-grade chemicals and solvents were obtained from Fisher Scientific (Atlanta, GA).
2. The HRP-1 trophoblast cell line was a generous gift from Dr. Michael J. Soares (University of Kansas Medical Center, Kansas City, KS).
3. Cell culture medium: RPMI-1640 culture medium (Mediatech Inc., Herndon, VA) supplemented with 10% heat-inactivated fetal bovine serum (FBS; Mediatech), 100 IU/ml of penicillin, and 100 µg/mL of streptomycin (Mediatech).
4. Uptake/transport buffer prepared with Hank's balanced salt solution (HBSS; Mediatech, containing 136.7 mM NaCl, 4.167 mM NaHCO$_3$, 0.385 mM Na$_2$HPO$_4$, 0.441 mM KH$_2$PO$_4$, 0.952 mM CaCl$_2$, 5.36 mM KCl, 0.812 mM MgSO$_4$, 5.5 mM D-glucose) supplemented with 10 mM HEPES (pH 7.4, Fisher Scientific) and stored at 4°C until use.
5. Stop buffer: prepared from uptake/transport buffer by addition of 0.1% bovine serum albumin (BSA; Sigma) and 200 µM phloretin (from a 1000X stock in ethanol), stored at 4°C and protected from light.
6. Wash buffer: phosphate-buffered saline (PBS; pH 7.4) from Mediatech and stored at 4°C until use.
7. Solubilizing reagents: 0.2 N NaOH and 0.2 N HCl.
8. Transwell® chambers (12-well cluster plates, polycarbonate, 0.4-µm pore size), 24-well tissue culture plates and T-75 cm^2 flasks were purchased from Corning Costar Corp. (Cambridge, MA).
9. Bicinchoninic acid (BCA) protein assay kit was obtained from Pierce Chemical Company (Rockford, IL).
10. Transepithelial electrical resistance (TEER) estimation was determined by the epithelial voltohmmeter (EVOM) (World Precision Instruments, Sarasota, FL).
11. HPLC mobile phase A: 0.1% acetic acid in filtered deionized water.
12. HPLC mobile phase B: 0.1% acetic acid in HPLC-grade acetonitrile.

13. HPLC column: Luna 5 µm C18, 250 × 4.6 mm (Phenomenex Inc, Torrance, CA).
14. β-RAM model 2 radio flow though detector (IN/US Systems Inc., Tampa, FL).
15. Chemstation software (Hewlett-Packard Company, Wilmington, DE).

3. Methods

3.1. Cell Culture

1. HRP-1 trophoblast cells are routinely maintained in 75-cm^2 flask in cell culture medium in an atmosphere of 5% CO_2 /95% air at 37°C in a humidified incubator. The cells are fed and passaged every 2 or 3 d (*see* **Note 1**).
2. The tissue culture plates and polycarbonate Transwell clusters (*see* **Note 2**) are coated with type I rat tail collagen at 5 µg/cm^2 for 1 h at room temperature under ultraviolet (UV) light before being washed twice with PBS on the same day of cell seeding (*see* **Note 3**). (Also, the Transwell clusters were incubated for another one hour in cell culture medium [37°C] for equilibrium.) For uptake/transport/metabolism study, HRP-1 trophoblast cells are seeded at 5 × 10^4 cells/well on 24-well tissue culture plates or 1.5 × 10^5 cells/well on Transwell 12-well-clusters (*see* **Note 1**). Cell culture medium is replaced daily with fresh medium and the cells are used on the second or the fourth days after seeding for uptake or transport studies, respectively. Prior to the start of an experiment, aspirate the cell culture medium and wash the cells twice with PBS 0.5 mL/well (incubating in the PBS for 1 min before removing).

3.2. Preparation of Albumin-Bound Fatty Acids

1. In order to mimic physiological conditions, the formation of complexes between long chain fatty acids and BSA in buffer is required (*see* **Note 4**). Dissolve the radiolabeled fatty acid in the uptake/transport buffer at 37°C, to which appropriate quantities of the corresponding unlabeled fatty acid are added in order to achieve the desired final concentration. Then add BSA from a 10X stock (dissolved in uptake/transport buffer) to obtain the desired fatty acid: BSA molar ratio (e.g., 1:1).
2. The FFA concentration at equilibrium with BSA can be calculated using the stepwise equilibrium method with the affinity constants, as published previously *(28,29)*.

3.3. Fatty Acid Uptake Studies

1. Both the cells and the uptake buffer are equilibrated at 37°C for 20 min.
2. Add the fatty acid/BSA stock solution (0.3 mL/well) to the cells to initiate the uptake experiment.
3. After incubation for a desired period of time, e.g., 15 min, uptake is stopped by rapidly washing the cells three times with ice-cold stop buffer (750 µL/well) followed by one rinse with ice-cold PBS (750 µL/well) (*see* **Note 5**).
4. Solubilize cells with 0.2 N NaOH (250 µL/well) for 20 min on a shaker at 37°C, and neutralize with 0.2 N HCl (250 µL/well) for 3 min.

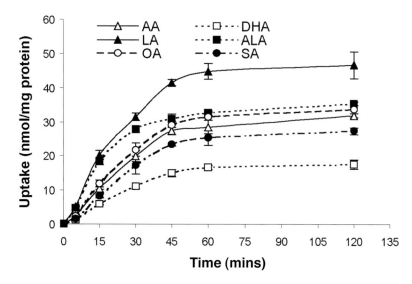

Fig. 2. Time-dependent study of fatty acid uptake in rat placental HRP-1 trophoblast cells. Uptake assays were performed with 200 µM of fatty acid (molar ratio of
fatty acid: bovine serum albumin = 1:1). AA, arachidonic acid; DHA, docohexaenoic
acid; LA, linoleic acid; ALA, α-linolenic acid; OA, oleic acid; SA, stearic acid. Data
shown are means ± SD ($n \geq 3$).

5. Remove an aliquot of 425 µL for scintillation counting and a 25 µL aliquot for
   the protein assay.
6. The protein concentration is determined by the BCA assay in order to normalize
   the radioactivity data.
7. For the time dependent uptake study, the total fatty acid concentrations as well as
   fatty acid/BSA molar ratios remain constant. The cells are incubated for different
   durations, for example, 5, 15, 30, 45, 60, and 90 min. Usually, there will be a
   linear time period followed by a plateau, where the linear region is required to get
   a nonsaturated value (**Fig. 2**).
8. For the concentration dependent uptake study, cells are incubated with a range of
   concentrations of the individual fatty acids and/or fatty acid/BSA ratios. The selected incubation time should be in the linear range of the time-dependent uptake
   curves for each substrate (**Fig. 2**). Demonstration of a plateau at high concentration in an uptake study is used as an indicator of a saturable kinetic process.
   Remember that several fatty acid transporters are expressed on the placental trophoblast cells as well as in other cell models (e.g., HRP-1 cells) (**13**). Therefore,
   the uptake of various fatty acid substrates in placental cells is affected by the total
   fatty acid transporter affinity, which is partially expressed by the Michaelis–
   Menten constant (K_m). It is important to note that this is an apparent K_m value
   potentially representative of several fatty acid transfer conferring proteins present

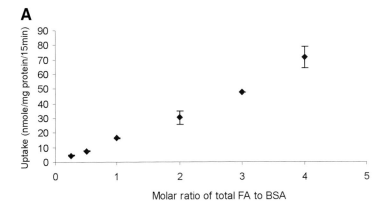

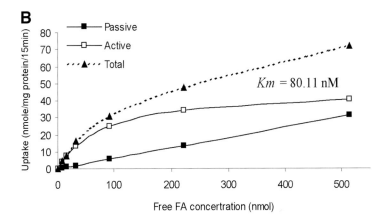

Fig. 3. Concentration-dependent, α-linolenic acid (ALA) uptake measured in rat placental HRP-1 trophoblast cells. Uptake assays were performed with a constant 200 μ*M* of bovine serum albumin (BSA) with different concentrations of total ALA to obtain the final molar ratios of fatty acid: BSA of 0.25, 0.5, 1.0, 2.0, 3.0, and 4.0) (**A**). **B** is plotted with the *x*-axis of concentration of free ALA, which was calculated using the stepwise equilibrium method and the affinity constants published previously *(28,29)*. The total uptake rate curve "—▲—" was separated to the active transport part "—□—" and the passive transport part "—■—". Fitting the data to equation "$V = V_{max} [S]/(Km + [S]) + P_{passive} [S]$" yields kinetic uptake parameters of a *Km* of 80.11 n*M*, a maximum uptake rate V_{max} of 46.72 nmol/mg protein/15 min and a passive membrane permeability coefficient $P_{passive}$ of 0.0609 l/mg protein/15 min. Data shown are means ± SD (*n* ≥3).

in the cells. K_m and other kinetic uptake parameters (e.g., V_{max}) could be determined by nonlinear least squares regression analysis using statistical software such as Sigma Plot (SPSS Inc, Chicago, IL) (**Fig. 3**).

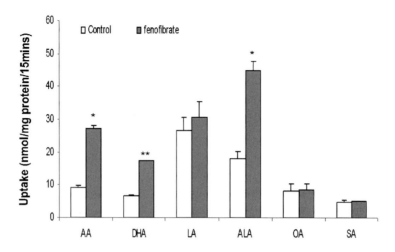

Fig. 4. Effect of fenofibrate on fatty acid uptake in rat placental HRP-1 trophoblast cells. Confluent HRP-1 cells were treated with 100 μ*M* of fenofibrate diluted in cell culture medium from a 1000 fold stock (in dimethylsulfoxide [DMSO]) and harvested at 24 h. Cells treated with DMSO alone were used as control. Immediately after treatment, 15 min uptake of 200 μ*M* of fatty acid (molar ratio of fatty acid: bovine serum albumin = 1:1) was assayed (AA, arachidonic acid; DHA, docosahexaenoic acid; LA, linoleic; ALA, α-linolenic; OA, oleic acid; SA, stearic acid). Data shown are means ± SD, (n =3 or 4, $*p < 0.01$, $**p < 0.001$).

9. The effects of different treatments that influence the expression and function of the related fatty acid transporters and thus the uptake rates of fatty acids could further be determined. For example, after incubation with fenofibrate (a known PPARα agonist and downstream fatty transporter inducer) at a concentration of 100 μ*M* in cell culture medium for 24 h, the uptake rates of long chain unsaturated fatty acids (AA and DHA) increase while there are no obvious changes in the uptake rates of saturated fatty acids (OA and SA) as shown in **Fig. 4**.

3.4. Check Monolayer Integrity (See Note 6)

3.4.1. TEER Estimation

1. The TEER value of the cell monolayers is determined by electrical resistance measurements at 37°C using EVOM.
2. EVOM probes should be equilibrated in PBS (37°C) for at least 15 min.
3. Cells grown on Transwell are washed twice for 10 min with PBS (37°C).
4. TEER is measured in PBS (37°C) during different stages of cell growth.
5. The TEER value is corrected for the resistances in the absence of cells (i.e., from the electrical system and the collagen-coated, polycarbonate membrane) by subtracting the TEER of a blank, collagen-coated Transwell.

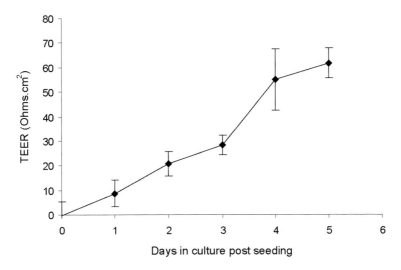

Fig. 5. Development of transepithelial electrical resistance (TEER) by HRP-1 monolayer cultures. TEER was measured at 37°C and in phosphate-buffered saline (PBS) buffer. Data shown are means ± SD (n = 3 or 4).

6. In our experience, TEER increases to a maximum of 50 to 60 $\Omega \cdot cm^2$ in 4–5 d (*see* **Fig. 5**). Thus, we have chosen 50 $\cdot \Omega \cdot cm^2$ as the critical point of cell integrity.

3.4.2. Mannitol Permeability Studies

1. Use [^{14}C] mannitol (3.92 *M*, 0.2 µCi/mL) in both apical to basolateral (AP–BL, AB) and basolateral to apical (BL–AP, BA) direction.
2. Compared with collagen-coated filter support only, mannitol permeability across the monolayer decreases more than 50% (about 3–5 × 10^{-5} cm/s) and there is no difference between the BA and AB directions, which is consistent with the previous report *(25)*.
3. In order to monitor the membrane integrity, [^3H] or [^{14}C] mannitol could be added to each dosing solution (see **Note 7**).

3.5. Fatty Acid Transport Studies

1. Transport studies are performed using [^{14}C] fatty acid at 0.1 µCi/mL diluted in transport buffer (pH 7.4). For all the studies, the apical and basolateral test solution volumes should be 0.5 and 1.5 mL, respectively.
2. System equilibration and transport studies are performed at 37°C while on a shaker (*see* **Note 8**).
3. Rinse and equilibrate cell monolayers for 30 min with the transport buffer prior to each study.
4. Following the addition of the test solution, withdraw samples at 15, 30, 45, 60, 75, 90, and 120 min with replacement of prewarmed transport buffer to maintain

constant volumes. The apical and basolateral sampling volumes are 50 μL and 150 μL, respectively, and all sample concentrations are corrected for dilution factors (*see* **Note 9**).

5. Collect 50 μL from donor chamber at 120 min for mass balance calculation.
6. Wash the cells twice with ice-cold transport buffer (750 μL/well) followed by one rinse with ice-cold PBS (750 μL/well).
7. Solubilize cells with 0.2 *N* NaOH (250 μL/well) for 20 min on shaker at 37°C, neutralize with 0.2 *N* HCL (250 μL/well) for 3 min, and aliquot for scintillation counting.
8. Calculation of permeability coefficients:
   The apparent permeability coefficients (P_{app}) are calculated using Equation 1:

$$P_{app} = \frac{dM_R}{dt} \frac{V_D}{[M_{D0}] \times A} \tag{1}$$

where $\dfrac{dM_R}{dt}$ = the slope of the linear region of amount of compound in receiver compartment versus time plot, V_D = donor volume, M_{D0} = starting donor amount, and A = the surface area of the membrane exposed to the compound (*see* **Note 10**). The permeability coefficient for the cell monolayer, P_{mono}, is calculated by

$$\frac{1}{P_{app}} = \frac{1}{P_{mono}} + \frac{1}{P_{blank}} \tag{2}$$

where P_{app} is the apparent permeability coefficient for the collagen-coated polycarbonate membranes in the presence of HRP-1 cell monolayer and P_{blank} is the apparent permeability coefficient for the collagen-coated polycarbonate membranes only. After obtaining the monolayer permeability of apical to basolateral transport $P_{mono(AB)}$ and the basolateral to apical (BA) transport $P_{mono(BA)}$, the permeability influx ratio R could be determined as

$$R = \frac{P_{mono(AB)}}{P_{mono(BA)}} \tag{3}$$

For a passively diffused compound, the AB and BA effective permeabilities should be similar and the influx ratio, R, would be approximately unity. For carrier-mediated transported compound, the $P_{mono(AB)}$ and $P_{mono(BA)}$ should be different based on the unidirectional transport mechanism and R is expected to be higher (absorptive transport) than or lower (secretory transport) than unity (*see* **Note 11**). Any treatments that influence the expression and function of the related transporter could change the ratio. In our fatty acid transport studies, the influx ratio of AA or DHA is less than one, whereas upon treatment with fenofibrate, both ratios increased, which suggests an increase in fatty acid transport to the fetus (**Fig. 6**).

3.6. Fatty Acid Metabolism Studies

There are two methods to analyze the samples collected during the fatty acid transport study. One is the scintillation counting, the other is using reverse-phase

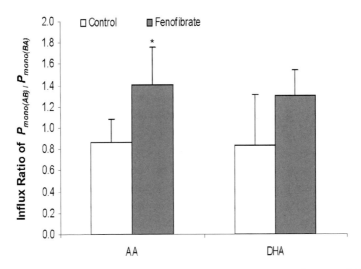

Fig. 6. Effects of fenofibrate on the fatty acid influx ratio of permeability in rat placental HRP-1 trophoblast cells. Confluent HRP-1 cells were treated with 100 µM of fenofibrate diluted in cell culture medium from a 1000-fold stock (in dimethylsulfoxide [DMSO]) and harvested at 24 h. Cells treated with DMSO alone were used as control. Immediately after treatment, transport study of 200 µM of fatty acid (molar ratio of fatty acid: bovine serum albumin = 1:1) was assayed (AA, arachidonic acid; DHA, docosahexaenoic acid). Data shown are means ± SD (n =3, *p < 0.05).

(RP)-HPLC analysis with radiochemical or tandem mass spectrometry (MS/MS) detection. The latter could also be used for separation and/or identification of possible fatty acid metabolites.

1. Prepare samples from the collections at different time points during the fatty acid transport experiments (**Subheading 3.5., steps 4–6**) (*see* **Note 12**).
2. HPLC condition for DHA analysis (*see* **Note 13**):

Time	Mobile phase A	Mobile phase B
0	30%	70%
20	10%	90%
25	10%	90%
27	30%	70%
30	30%	70%

   Flow rate (1 mL/min)
   Injection volume (100 µL)

3. Fatty acid signals detected by β-RAM radio flow through detector. (Data obtained by UV detector could be used as a further confirmation of the elution position of the fatty acid and its possible metabolites.)

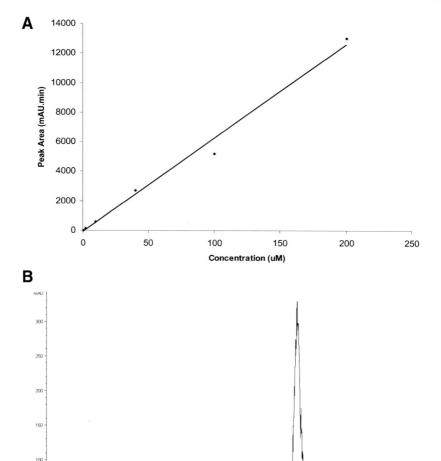

Fig. 7. High-performance liquid chromatography (HPLC) analysis of docosahexaenoic acid (DHA). **(A)** Standard curve for calculation of DHA concentration. Equation of linear regression is also shown. **(B)** Representative chromatography of DHA. Upper curve: sample from donor chamber at 2 h, peak area and corresponding DHA concentration is 8724.2 mAU min and 133.6 µ*M*, respectively. Lower curve: sample from receiver chamber at 2 h, peak area and corresponding DHA concentration is 859.6 mAU min and 10.9 µ*M*, respectively.

4. Analyze the chromatogram by integration and calculate the peak area or peak height. Compared with the standard curve (**Fig. 7A**), determine the corresponding fatty acid amount/concentration of the specific sample (**Fig. 7B**).

5. As under **Subheading 3.5.**, use Eqs. 1 and 2 to calculate the permeability coefficients, influx ratio etc. In our studies the permeabilities are similar to those determined by liquid scintillation counting. For example, the permeability of HRP-1 cells (after 24 h incubation with 100 μ*M* fenofibrate) to DHA in the apical to basolateral (AB) direction is 1.84×10^{-5} cm/s and 1.91×10^{-5} cm/s, by liquid scintillation counting and HPLC analysis, respectively.

6. If fatty acid metabolism is processed within the cells and the metabolites are released from the cell to the donor and/or receiver chamber, extra peaks besides the parent fatty acid would be shown on the chromatography. Usually, fatty acid metabolites are more polar and eluted earlier than the parent compounds. By comparing the chromatograms of the pure parent fatty acid and the experimental samples, metabolites could be characterized and further analyzed.

4. Notes

1. The properties of the cell monolayer have been suggested to vary depending on the cell culture conditions, such as the cell seeding density, the degree of confluence, the stage of cellular differentiation, the presence or absence of essential nutrients, and growth factors *(30,31)*. Therefore, both passive/active transport across the cell monolayer can be affected as a result of the change of monolayer integrity and altered expression levels of relevant transporters. The cell culture medium, seeding density, and growth days chosen here are for HRP-1 cells and are identical to the conditions used in our lab. A seeding density that is too high, and/or extended culture days might result in the formation of multiple layers or irregularly shaped tight junctions, in which case physical, chemical, or physiological characteristics of the cells could be changed and possibly lead to loss of polarization and/or inconsistent transport results. On the other hand, a seeding density that is too low would take more time to reach confluence, meaning lower efficiency and more labor. Therefore, it is highly recommended that the cell growth be monitored and the culture conditions optimized prior to the uptake/transport/metabolism study.

2. In transport studies with cell culture systems, a microporous substratum is necessary for cell attachment, growth, and differentiation. Although transparent polyester (PE) membranes allow for the routine examination of cells using a phase-contrast microscope, the reduced pore size density and other characteristics of the PE membrane may significantly alter the barrier properties of the cell monolayer including cell growth rate, morphology, density, TEER, functional expression of carriers, and other transport and metabolic properties of cells in culture *(32–34)*. For example, it has been reported that for highly lipophilic progesterone, the resistance attributed to PE filter (71%) was much higher than that of the PC (27%) in Caco2 cells *(35)*. Therefore, in conducting transport studies with cells cultured on microporous membranes, it is essential that the control experiment be conducted using the corresponding microporous membrane (as well as supporting matrix, if any) alone.

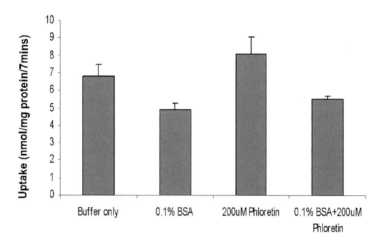

Fig. 8. Effects of the stop buffer on uptake rates of α-linolenic acid in rat placental HRP-1 trophoblast cells. Seven-minute uptake study of 200 μ*M* of α-linolenic acid (ALA) (molar ratio of fatty acid: bovine serum albumin = 1:1) was assayed on confluent HRP-1 cells. Data shown are means ± SD ($n \geq 3$).

3. We use collagen-coated wells in our uptake/transport/metabolism studies because we find that (1) HRP-1 cells grow too fast to strongly adhere to the membrane support of the transwells, thus they tend to detach even with only one PBS wash; (2) too rapid growth also brings the problem of uneven distribution of the HRP-1 cells when they come to confluence. Extracellular matrix components (e.g., collagen) have been suggested to accelerate cell proliferation, increase cellular contact areas, and induce cell differentiation and heterogeneity *(34,36,37)*. In our studies, we found that the formation of a more functionally consistent and tighter monolayer when seeding on collagen is consistent with previous reports.

4. In the fetal–maternal unit, FFAs originating in the maternal circulation are the major source of fatty acids for transport across the placenta *(38,39)* because triacylglycerols are not transported intact *(40,41)*. It is generally recognized that the protein–fatty acid complexes (albumin–fatty acid complex and lipoprotein complexes) decomposed into FFA at extracellular sites of placental trophoblast *(12,38)*. Subsequently, a number of fatty acid transporting systems located on the membrane of the cells can transport FFA into the cytoplasm. The physiological nonesterified fatty acid to albumin molar ratio in maternal plasma at term is about 1.3 *(42)*. Therefore, most of our experiments are studied with the ratio of fatty acid to BSA = 1.

5. The stop buffer contains 0.1% BSA and 200 *M* phloretin to remove fatty acid that adheres to the cell surface and to inhibit the influx of further fatty acid, and the efflux of internalized fatty acids, respectively *(28)* (**Fig. 8**). As shown in **Fig. 9**, washing more than three times does not further affect the cell-associated radioactivity. Therefore, we choose washing in triplicate with the stop buffer.

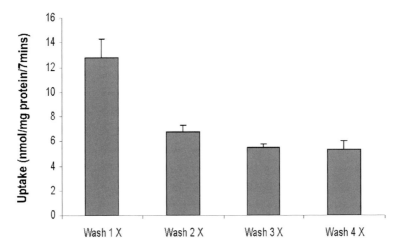

Fig. 9. Effects of wash times of stop buffer on α-linolenic acid uptake rates on rat placental HRP-1trophoblast cells. Seven-minute uptake study of 200 μ*M* of α-linolenic acid (ALA) (molar ratio of fatty acid: bovine serum albumin = 1:1) was assayed on confluent HRP-1 cells. Data shown are means ± SD (*n* = 3).

6. Prior to the transport study, the integrity of the monolayer should be confirmed. There are several methods to check the cell integrity, such as examination of the cell morphology by transmission electron microscope or cross-sectional analysis of fixed hematoxylin- and eosin Y-stained cells by light microscopy *(43)*. However, the most widely used techniques are TEER measurement and mannitol permeability determination, a marker of paracellular transport. As cells come to confluence and become well differentiated, tight junctions form between cells, thus TEER increases and the permeability coefficient of mannitol decreases *(43)*.

7. In the dual labeling of mannitol and fatty acid transport experiments, mannitol transports via paracellular pathway and can be used for checking cell monolayer integrity, whereas the fatty acid is highly lipophilic and transports via transcellular (passive and active) pathway. These two substances have no interaction in the transport study. However, the radiolabeled mannitol may interfere with the fatty acid metabolism study by exhibiting extra peaks on the chromatogram.

8. One disadvantage of the cell-inserted diffusion chamber is that this system is generally unstirred, thus creating a significant aqueous boundary layer (ABL) over the cell monolayer. For very lipophilic compounds (e.g., fatty acids), this ABL could be the diffusion barrier to flux of the solutes across the cell culture model system, thus yielding artificial data not representative of the in vivo situation *(35,43)*. Although mechanical stirring is suggested to obtain mixing, the unpredictable edge damage of the membrane leads to low reproducibility of the data. Our lab uses shakers to provide some kind of mixing while not being vigorous enough to cause membrane damage. On the other hand, we correct the data

(P_{app}) with the background (P_{blank}) provided by control wells (the filter resistance and also ABL resistance).

9. The correction factor for dilution of the receiver compartment is defined as and is calculated by

$$\frac{1}{X} = \sum_{n=1}^{a} (-1)^{n-1} \frac{B_{an}}{n} \left(\frac{S}{V}\right)^{n-1} \tag{4}$$

where X is the ratio of C2 to C1, C1 and C2 is the drug concentration in the receiver compartment at the time of sampling with or without sample taken, respectively), S = sample volume, V_D = total volume in the receiver compartment, a = sample number, B_{an} = the number corresponding to the Nth term in the ath row of Pascal's triangle.

10. Cellular measurements of the permeability usually focus on appearance or disappearance kinetics by carefully characterizing the concentration of the solute on only one side of the membrane barrier. As lipophilic compounds permeate across a cellular barrier, a fraction of the solute is retained by the barrier (as high as 54% has been detected for progesterone and propranolol [44]). Youdim et al. (45) recommend the use of Equation 5 to take into account compound retention in the cell monolayer:

$$P_{app} = \frac{dM_R}{dt} \frac{V_D}{\left(M_{DO} - M_{cells}\right) \times A} \tag{5}$$

where $\dfrac{dM_R}{dt}$ = the slope of the linear region of amount of compound in receiver compartment vs time plot, V_D = donor volume, M_{D0} = starting donor amount, A = the surface area of the membrane exposed to the compound, and M_{cells} = amount of compound retained by the membrane/cells, $[M_{cells} = M_{D0} - (M_{Dt} + \Sigma M_R)]$, where M_{Rt} is the amount in the receiver compartment and M_{Dt} is the amount in the donor compartment at the end of the experiment. However, this equation assumes that the compounds are stable and that the mass lost to the cells/membranes is calculated from the difference between the total starting amount and the amounts in donor and receiver compartment at the last sampling time (45). If any loss is due to compound breakdown or metabolism, it will affect the accuracy of the P_{app} calculation; analytical techniques that detect metabolites may be used to reduce these errors.

11. Different researchers use alternative terms to describe the direction of transport. In our lab, we use influx and efflux to refer to the directions relative to the polar cell monolayer, whereas secretory and absorptive transport in contrast to the systemic circulation (as to placenta, i.e., fetus circulation) (Fig. 10).

12. To avoid HPLC column flow problems, carefully prepare the buffer and the sample to prevent contamination. Fatty acid metabolite analysis requires further subcellular fatty acid/lipid separation.

13. RP-HPLC is widely used in biochemical analyses. Optimization of the separation conditions is important for good results. When chromatogram conditions are un-

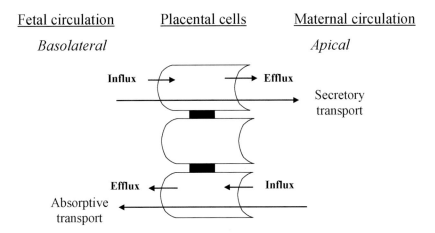

Fig. 10. Scheme of possible fatty acid transport pathways in the placental cells.

known, run the 60/60 gradient first, which means that the gradient starts at near 100% aqueous and ramps to 60% organic solvent in 60 min *(46)*. After separation, decrease the gradient to improve the separation and/or shorten the run time.

References

1. Uauy, R. and Hoffman, D. R. (2000) Essential fat requirement of preterm infants. *Am. J. Clin. Nutr.* **71(Suppl)**, S245–S250.
2. Uauy, R., Mena, P., and Valenzuela, A. (1999) Essential fatty acids as determinants of lipids requirements in infants, children and adults. *Euro. J. Clin. Nutr.* **53(Suppl)**, S66–S77.
3. Narumiya, S. and Fukushima, M. (1996) Site and mechanism of growth inhibition by PGs. *J. Pharmaco. Exp. Therap.* **239**, 500–511.
4. Ballabriga, A. (1994) Essential fatty acids and human tissue composition. An overview. *Acta Paediatrics* **402(Suppl)**, 63–68.
5. Hornstra, G., Al, M. D., van Houwelingen, A. C., and Foreman-van Drongelen M. M. (1995) Essential fatty acids in pregnancy and early human development. *Eur. J. Obstet. Gynecol. Reprod. Biol.* **61**, 57–62.
6. Schellenberg, J-C. and Kirkby, W. (1997) Production of prostaglandin F2a and E2 in explants of intrauterine tissue of guinea pigs during late pregnancy and labor. *Prostaglandin* **54**, 625–638.
7. Crawford, M. A., Costeloe, K., Ghebremeskel, K., Phylactos, A., Skirvin, L., and Stacey, F. (1997) Are deficits of arachidonic and docosahexaenoic acids responsible for the neural and vascular complications of preterm babies? *Am. J. Clin. Nutr.* **66 (Suppl)**, S1032–S1041.
8. Neuringer, M., Connor, W. E., Lin, D. S., Barsard, L., and Luck, S. (1986) Biochemical and functional effects of prenatal and postnatal w3 fatty acid deficiency on retina and brain in rhesus monkeys. *Proc. Natl. Acad. Sci. USA* **83**, 4021–4025.

9. Lane, D. M., McConathy, W. J., McCaffree, M. A., and Hall, M. (2002) Cord serum lipid and apolipoprotein levels in preterm infants with the neonatal respiratory distress syndrome. *J. Matern. Fetal Neonatal Med.* **11,** 118–125.

10. Barker, D. J. P., Godfrey, K. M., Fall, C., Osmond, C., Winter, P. D., and Shaheen, S. O. (1993) Relation of birth weight and childhood respiratory infection to adult lung function and death from chronic obstructive airways disease. *BMJ* **303,** 671–675.

11. Fall, C. H., Barker, D. J., Osmond, C., Winter, P. D., Clark, P. M. S., and Hales, C. N. (1992) Relation of infant feeding to adult serum cholesterol concentration and death from ischaemic heart disease. *BMJ* **304,** 801–805.

12. Dutta-Roy, A. K. (2000) Transport mechanisms for long-chain polyunsaturated fatty acids in the human placenta. *Am. J. Clin. Nutr.* **71(Suppl),** S315–S322.

13. Knipp, G. T., Ling, B., Audus, K. L., Fujii, H., Ono, T., and Soares, M. J. (2000) Fatty acid transport regulatory proteins in the developing rat placenta and in trophoblast cell culture models. *Placenta* **21,** 367–375.

14. Rakheja, D., Bennett, M. J., Foster, B. M., Domiati-Saad, R., and Rogers, B. B. (2002) Evidence for fatty acid oxidation in human placenta, and the relationship of fatty acid oxidation enzyme activities with gestational age. *Placenta* **23,** 447–450.

15. Shekhawat, P., Bennett, M. J., Sadovsky, Y., Nelson, D. M., Rakheja, D., and Strauss, A. (2003) Human placenta metabolizes fatty acids: implications for fetal fatty acids oxidation disorders and maternal liver diseases. *Am. J. Physiol. Endocrinol. Metab.* **284,** E1098–E1105.

16. Simpson, A. E., Brammar, W. J., Pratten, M. K., Cockcroft, N., and Elcombe, C. R. (1996) Placental transfer of the hypolipidemic drug, clofibrate, induces CYP4A expression in 18.5-day fetal rats. *Drug Metab. Dispos.* **24,** 547–554.

17. Xu, Y., Knipp, G. T., and Cook, T. J. (2005) Expression of CYP4A isoforms in developing rat placenta and trophoblast cell models. *Placenta* **26(2–3),** 218–225.

18. Johansen, B., Rakkestad, K., Balboa, M. A., and Dennis, E. A. (2000) Expression of cytosolic and secreted forms of phospholipase A (2) and cyclooxygenases in human placenta, fetal membranes, and chorionic cell lines. *Prostaglandins Other Lipid Mediat.* **60,** 119–125.

19. Wetzka, B., Nusing, R., Charnock-Jones, D. S., Schafer, W., Zahradnik, H. P., and Smith, S. K. (1997) Cyclooxygenase-1 and -2 in human placenta and placental bed after normal and pre-eclamptic pregnancies. *Hum. Reprod.* **12,** 2313–2320.

20. Xu, Y., Knipp, G. T., and Cook, T. J. (2004) Developmental expression in the rat placenta of enzymes involved in fatty acid metabolism. *Toxicological Sci.* **78(Suppl),** Abstract 349.

21. Joseph, P., Srinivasan, S. N., and Kulkarni, A. P. (1993) Purification and partial characterization of lipoxygenase with dual catalytic activities from human term placenta *Biochem. J.* **293,** 83–91.

22. Datta, K. and Kulkarni, A. P. (1994) Oxidative metabolism of aflatoxin B1 by lipoxygenase purified from human term placenta and intrauterine conceptal tissues *Teratology* **50,** 311–317.

23. Hunt, J. S., Deb, S., Faria, T. N., Wheaton, D., and Soares, M. J. (1989) Isolation of phenotypically distinct trophoblast cell lines from normal rat chorioallantoic placentas. *Placenta* **10,** 161–177.

24. Soares, M. J., Schaberg, K. D., Pinal, C. S., De, S. K., Bhatia, P., and Andrews, G. K. (1987) Establishment of a rat placental cell line expressing characteristics of extraembryonic membranes. *Dev. Biol.* **124**, 134–144.

25. Shi, F., Soares, M. J., Avery, M., Liu, F., Zhang, X., and Audus, K. L. (1997) Permeability and metabolic properties of a trophoblast cell line (HRP-1) derived from normal rat placenta. *Exp. Cell Res.* **234**, 147–155.

26. Novak, D., Quiggle, F., Artime, C., and Beveridge, M. (2001) Regulation of glutamate transport and transport proteins in a placental cell line. *Am. J. Physiol. Cell Physiol.* **281**, C1014–C1022.

27. Das, U. G., Sadiq, H. F., Soares, M. J., Hay, W. W. Jr, and Devaskar, S. U. (1998) Time-dependent physiological regulation of rodent and ovine placental glucose transporter (GLUT-1) protein. *Am. J. Physiol.* **274**, R339–R347.

28. Abumrad, N. A., Perkins, R. C., Park, J. H., and Park, C. R. (1981) Mechanism of long chain fatty acid permeation in the isolated adipocyte. *J. Biol. Chem.* **256**, 9183–9191.

29. Richieri, G. V., Anel, A., and Kleinfeld, A. M. (1993) Interactions of long-chain fatty acids and albumin: determination of free fatty acid levels using the fluorescent probe ADIFAB. *Biochemistry* **32**, 7574–7580.

30. Audus, K. L., Bartel, R. L., Hidalgo, I. J., and Borchardt, R. T. (1990) The use of cultured epithelial and endothelial cells for drug transport and metabolism studies. *Pharm. Res.* **7**, 435–451.

31. Behrens, I. and Kissel, T. (2003) Do cell culture conditions influence the carrier-mediated transport of peptides in Caco-2 cell monolayers? *Eur. J Pharm. Sci.* **19**, 433–442.

32. Wilson, G. (1990) Cell culture techniques for the study of drug transport. *Eur. J. Drug. Metab. Pharmacokinet.* **15**, 159–163.

33. Nicklin, P., Irwin, B., Hassan, I., Williamson, I., and Mackay, M. (1992) Permeable support type influences the transport of compounds across Caco-2 cells. *Int. J. Pharm.* **83**, 197–209.

34. Davenport, E. A. and Nettesheim, P. (1996) Type I collagen gel modulates extra-cellular matrix synthesis and deposition by tracheal epithelial cells. *Exp. Cell. Res.* **223**, 155–162.

35. Yu, H. and Sinko, P. J. (1997) Influence of the microporous substratum and hydrodynamics on resistances to drug transport in cell culture systems: calculation of intrinsic transport parameters. *J. Pharm. Sci.* **86**, 1448–1455.

36. Anderle, P., Niederer, E., Rubas, W., et al. (1998) P-Glycoprotein (P-gp) mediated efflux in Caco-2 cell monolayers: the influence of culturing conditions and drug exposure on P-gp expression levels. *J. Pharm. Sci.* **87**, 757–762.

37. Basson, M. D., Turowski, G., and Emenaker, N. J. (1996) Regulation of human (Caco-2) intestinal epithelial cell differentiation by extracellular matrix proteins. *Exp. Cell. Res.* **225**, 301–305.

38. Innis, S. M. (2000) Essential fatty acids in infant nutrition: lessons and limitations from animal studies in relation to studies on infant fatty acid required. *Am. J. Clin. Nutr.* **71(Suppl)**, S238–S244.

39. Kuhn, D. C. and Crawford, M. (1986) Placental essential fatty acid transport and prostaglandin synthesis. *Prog. Lipid Res.* **25,** 345–353.
40. Shand, J. H. and Noble, R. C. (1979) The role of maternal triglycerides in the supply of lipids to the ovine fetus. *Biol. Neonate* **26,** 117–123.
41. Elphick, M. C., Edson, H. C., Lawler, J., and Hull, D. (1978) Source of fetal-stored lipids during maternal starvation in rabbits. *Biol. Neonate* **34,** 146–149.
42. Benassayag, C., Mignot, T. M., Haourigui, M., et al. (1997) High polyunsaturated fatty acid, thromboxane A2, and alpha-fetoprotein concentrations at the human feto-maternal interface. *J. Lipid Res.* **38,** 276–286.
43. Borchardt, R. T., Hidalgo, I. J., Hillgren, K. M., and Hu, M. (1989) Pharmaceutical applications of cell and tissue culture to drug transport. (Wilson, G., Davis, S. S., IIIum, L., and Zweibaum, A., ed.) Plenum, New York: pp. 1-14.
44. Krishna, G., Chen, K., Lin, C., and Nomeir, A. A. (2001) Permeability of lipophilic compounds in drug discovery using in vitro human absorption model, Caco-1. *Int. J. Pharm.* **222,** 77–89.
45. Youdim, K. A., Avdeef, A., and Abbott, N. J. (2003) In vitro trans-monolayer permeability calculations: often forgotten assumptions. *Drug Discov. Today* **8,** 997–1003.
46. Guzzetta, A. (2001) Reverse Phase HPLC Basics for LC/MS—Ionsource Tutorial. http://www.ionsource.com/tutorial/chromatography/rphplc.htm#Introduction
47. Haggarty, P. (2002) Placental regulation of fatty acid delivery and its effect on fetal growth—a review. *Placenta* 23(Suppl A), **S28–S38.**

17

Heterologous Expression Systems for Studying Placental Transporters

Vadivel Ganapathy, You-Jun Fei, and Puttur D. Prasad

Summary

We use two different heterologous expression systems to characterize the functional features of plasma membrane transporters cloned from placenta. The first is the vaccinia virus expression system that utilizes a recombinant vaccinia virus carrying a transgene for T7 RNA polymerase. Mammalian cells, when infected with this virus, are able to produce T7 RNA polymerase. If these cells are then transfected with a transporter cDNA which is under the control of T7 promoter in the plasmid, the T7 RNA polymerase will transcribe the cDNA and the cellular machinery will synthesize the transporter protein from the resultant mRNA and target it to the plasma membrane. The transport function of the heterologously expressed transporter can then be monitored by uptake of suitable substrates in these cells. The second is the *Xenopus laevis* oocyte expression system in which any transporter can be expressed heterologously by injection of the oocytes with corresponding cRNA. The functional features of the expressed transporter can then be monitored either by uptake of suitable substrates or by electrophysiological means if the transporter function is electrogenic. Both methods are complementary to each other and together provide an effective means to delineate the functional features of various transporters, irrespective of their independent transport mechanisms.

Key Words: Heterologous expression; transporter cDNA; mammalian cells; vaccinia virus; transfection; uptake measurements; *Xenopus laevis*; oocyte; cRNA injection; electrophysiology; substrate-induced current.

1. Introduction

To study the transport function of any cloned transporter, we need a suitable heterologous expression system. The placental transporters can be cloned by various methods, but the functional identity of these transporters cannot be established without appropriate functional expression systems. We employ two different heterologous expression systems to analyze the transport function of cloned transporters. The first system involves the expression of the cloned transporter in mammalian cells using a recombinant vaccinia virus (*1,2*). The

From: *Methods in Molecular Medicine, Vol. 122: Placenta and Trophoblast: Methods and Protocols, Vol. 2*
Edited by: M. J. Soares and J. S. Hunt © Humana Press Inc., Totowa, NJ

cDNA encoding the transporter protein is engineered into a plasmid such that its transcription is under the control of T7 promoter. The recombinant vaccinia virus carries the gene for T7 RNA polymerase (3). This method is suitable for any mammalian cell line. In this method, the mammalian cells are first infected with the recombinant vaccinia virus, which enables the mammalian cells to express T7 RNA polymerase. Subsequently, the cells are transfected with the plasmid carrying the transporter cDNA using Lipofectin. Because the cDNA in the plasmid is present downstream of the T7 promoter, the viral genome-encoded T7 RNA polymerase mediates the transcription of the transporter cDNA in these cells. The rest of the steps involved in the generation of the transporter protein and subsequent processing and insertion of the protein into the plasma membrane are mediated by the constitutive elements present in the mammalian cells. Cells treated in a similar manner but transfected with empty plasmid instead of the plasmid carrying the transporter cDNA serve as the control. The transport function of the heterologously expressed transporter is then monitored by comparing the uptake of appropriate radiolabeled substrates under suitable conditions in cDNA-transfected cells with that in cells transfected with vector alone (4–12). The transporter-specific uptake is deduced by subtracting the uptake in vector-transfected cells from the uptake in cDNA-transfected cells. As it is readily apparent, the availability of the transporter substrate in radiolabeled form markedly facilitates this method. Unlabeled substrates can be used, but analytical methods need to be standardized first to quantify the amount of substrates taken up into the cells. If such methods are available, the vaccinia virus expression technique can be employed to characterize the heterologously expressed transporter even when the transporter substrate is not available in radiolabeled form (13).

The second system involves the expression of the cloned transporter in *Xenopus laevis* oocytes (14,15). This is done by injection of corresponding cRNA into the cytoplasm of oocytes. cRNA is prepared from the plasmid carrying the transporter cDNA by using appropriate RNA polymerase. For example, if the cDNA in the plasmid is downstream of T7 promoter, T7 RNA polymerase is used to synthesize the transporter cRNA in vitro. The injected cRNA is then translated in the oocyte to generate the transporter protein, which is processed and inserted into the plasma membrane. Oocytes injected with an equal volume of water or uninjected oocytes serve as the control. The widespread use of this expression system is based on the fact that oocytes are able not only to translate exogenous RNA efficiently but also to carry out posttranslational modifications such as precursor processing, glycosylation, complex subunit assembly, intracellular trafficking, and targeting to the plasma membrane. The transport function of the heterologously expressed transporter in these oocytes can be monitored either by uptake of appropriate radiolabeled substrates (16–

18) or by electrophysiological methods if the transporter is known to be electrogenic *(7,18–21)*. When radiolabeled substrates are used, uptake is compared between the oocytes injected with the transporter cRNA and the oocytes injected with water or uninjected oocytes. The difference in uptake between these two sets of oocytes represents transport mediated by the heterologously expressed transporter. If the transport function of the transporter is associated with transfer of charge across the membrane (i.e., electrogenic), the transport function can be monitored in cRNA-injected oocytes by eletrophysiological methods. Again, either water-injected or uninjected oocytes are used as controls. This electrophysiological method involves the use of the two-microelectrode voltage-clamp technique *(22,23)*. In this technique, two microelectrodes are inserted into the oocyte and the membrane potential is clamped at a given value, usually at –50 mV. The oocyte is then exposed to an appropriate substrate under suitable conditions. If the transporter is electrogenic, its transport function is expected to be associated with the transfer of charge (positive or negative depending on the nature of the transporter function) across the plasma membrane of the oocyte. The transfer of charge leads to a change in membrane potential, but because the membrane potential is clamped with electrodes, the magnitude and the direction of the current that is necessary to clamp the membrane potential describe the transporter function. If the transport function is associated with the entry of positive charge into the oocyte, this is detected in the form of inward currents. On the other hand, if the transport function is associated with the entry of negative charge into the oocyte, this is detected in the form of outward currents. Again, by comparing the magnitude of the substrate-dependent currents between water-injected or uninjected oocytes and cRNA-injected oocytes, the activity that is specific for the heterologously expressed transporter can be deduced.

2. Materials

2.1. Mammalian Cell Expression System

1. Human retinal pigment epithelial cell line HRPE.
2. Recombinant vaccinia virus (vTF7-3) carrying the gene for T7 RNA polymerase (American Type Culture Collection [ATCC], Manassas, VA, cat. no. VR-2153).
3. Cell culture medium Dulbecco's modified Eagle's medium (DMEM)-F12 (Cellgro, Herndon, VA, cat. no. 15-090-CV).
4. L-Glutamine, 250 mM in 8.5 g/L NaCl (Cellgro, cat. no. 25-005-CI).
5. Penicillin (10,000 IU/mL)/Streptomycin (10,000 µg/mL) (Cellgro, cat. no. 30-002-CI).
6. Fetal bovine serum (FBS; Atlanta Biologicals).
7. Trypsin (2.5%) (Invitrogen, Carlsbad, CA, cat. no. 15090-046).
8. 2-Mercaptoethanol.

 9. OPTI-MEM I medium (Invitrogen, cat. no. 31985-070).
10. Lipofectin reagent (Invitrogen, cat. no. 18292-011).
11. Plasmid containing the transporter cDNA under the control of T7 promoter.
12. Plasmid without the cDNA insert.
13. Phosphate-buffered saline (PBS).
14. Uptake buffer containing NaCl: 25 mM HEPES/Tris, pH 7.5, 140 mM NaCl, 5.4 mM KCl, 1.8 mM CaCl$_2$, 0.8 mM MgSO$_4$, and 5 mM D-glucose.
15. Appropriate radiolabeled substrate depending on the function of the transporter.
16. 1% sodium dodecyl sulfate (SDS) in 0.2 N NaOH.
17. Scintillation cocktail (Scintiverse BD, Fisher Scientific, Pittsburgh, PA).

2.2. Xenopus laevis Oocyte Expression System

 1. We routinely buy the frogs from Nasco (Fort Atkinson, WI).
 2. Ethyl 3-aminobenzoate methanesulfonate (also called tricaine or MS222).
 3. Modified Barth's solution: 88 mM NaCl, 1 mM KCl, 0.3 mM Ca(NO$_3$)$_2$, 0.41 mM CaCl$_2$, 0.82 mM MgSO$_4$, 2.4 mM NaHCO$_3$, and 15 mM HEPES, pH adjusted to 7.4 with Tris.
 4. Collagenase A (Roche, Basel, Switzerland, cat. no. 1-088-785).
 5. Buffer for collagenase digestion: 96 mM NaCl, 2 mM KCl, 1 mM MgCl$_2$, 5 mM HEPES, pH adjusted to 7.5 with Tris.
 6. Defolliculation buffer: 110 mM NaCl, 1 mM ethylenediamine tetraacetic acid (EDTA), 10 mM HEPES, pH 7.6 adjusted with Tris.
 7. Watchmaker's forceps, No. 5 biology grade (Biomedical Research Instruments, Inc. Malden, MA, Dumostar, cat. no. 10-530).
 8. Nylon mesh (Spectra/Mesh N; Fisher Scientific).
 9. 10-µL microdispenser (Drummond Scientific Co., Broomall, PA).
10. Mineral oil (Sigma).
11. Sigmacote (Sigma).
12. Micropipet puller (Model P-97, Sutter Instrument Co., Novato, CA).
13. Microscope with an eyepiece graticule calibrated with a stage micrometer (Olympus, Melville, NY).
14. Micromanipulator (Tritech Research Inc., Los Angeles, CA).
15. cRNA synthesis kit (mMESSAGE mMACHINE kit from Ambion, Austin, TX).
16. Restriction enzymes.
17. Incubator for temperature maintenance at 18°C.
18. Uptake buffer: 100 mM NaCl, 2 mM KCl, 1 mM MgCl$_2$, 1 mM CaCl$_2$, 5 mM HEPES, pH adjusted to 7.4 with Tris.
19. 0.1% SDS.
20. Oocyte perifusion buffer: ND96, 96 mM NaCl, 2 mM KCl, 1 mM MgCl$_2$, 1.8 mM CaCl$_2$, 3 mM HEPES, 3 mM Mes, and 3 mM Tris, pH 7.5.
21. Electrophysiology apparatus consisting of an amplifier (GeneClamp 500 amplifier from Axon Instruments, Inc., Union City, CA), data acquisition and data analysis software, chart recorder, and software for two-microelectrode voltage-clamp configuration (Clampex computer program of pClamp software, Axon Instruments, Inc.).

3. Methods

3.1. Mammalian Cell Expression Technique

The methods described below outline (1) culture of HRPE cells, (2) infection of HRPE cells with the virus, (3) transfection of HRPE cells with plasmid, and (4) uptake measurements.

3.1.1. Culture of HRPE Cells

1. HRPE cells are cultured in DMEM-F12 medium, supplemented with 2 mM glutamine, 100 IU/mL penicillin, 100 µg/mL streptomysin, and 10% FBS.
2. The cells are maintained in 75-mm culture flasks at 37°C in the presence of 5% CO_2. Confluent cells are split 1:3 every 3–4 d.
3. The vaccinia virus-mediated expression technique is carried out in cells cultured in 24-well plates. The cells from 75-mm flasks with 70–80% confluency are used to seed the 24-well plates.
4. Culture medium from the 75-mm flask is removed by aspiration and the cell monolayer is washed once with 10 mL of PBS that has been prewarmed at 37°C. Then, 1.5 mL of trypsin solution (0.25% trypsin in 0.02% EDTA/phosphate-buffered saline) is added to the flask and gently adjusted to cover the cells with the trypsin solution. The cells are exposed to trypsin for about 1 min after which the flask is gently tapped with hand to release the cells. The cells should be exposed to trypsin only for the shortest time needed to release the cells. If the cells are in contact with trypsin for a long time, it will damage the cells.
5. The released cells are immediately suspended in 10 mL of DMEM-F12 culture medium and collected into a 15-mL tube. The tube is centrifuged for 3 min at 300g in a tabletop centrifuge to sediment the cells.
6. The cell pellet is then suspended in a small volume of fresh culture medium and the cells are counted.
7. Based on the cell count, the suspension is diluted with culture medium to give 0.03×10^6 cells/mL. The cells are then seeded into 24-well plates (2 mL/well). The plates are incubated for 24 h at 37°C in the presence of 5% CO_2 (*see* **Note 1**).

3.1.2. Infection of HRPE Cells With Recombinant Vaccinia Virus vTF7-3

1. The virus suspension is prepared at a volume of 100 µL/well and 10 pfu (plaque-forming units)/cell.
2. Twenty-four hours following the seeding of HRPE cells in 24-well plates, cells from one of the wells is trypsinized and the cells in the well are counted.
3. Depending on the cell number, the virus suspension is prepared to give 10 pfu/cell.
4. The stock virus suspension (10^7 pfu/µL) is taken out from the –80°C freezer and sonicated for 5 min in a water bath sonicator and then the required amount of the virus, as determined from the cell number and the number of wells to be treated with the virus, is pipeted from the stock and added to an appropriate volume of OPTI-MEM I medium containing 0.01% 2-mercaptoethanol. The volume of the medium is determined based on the number of wells (100 µL/well).

5. The virus suspension in the medium is mixed well and incubated for 15 min at 37°C prior to use.
6. The medium from the wells is removed by aspiration and the cells are washed with 2 mL of PBS that has been prewarmed at 37°C.
7. The virus suspension is then added to the wells at 100 µL/well and the plate is gently shaken to spread the virus suspension onto the cells in the wells.
8. The plate is kept in the cell culture hood for 30 min, which allows the virus to adsorb onto the cells and infect them.
9. The plaque-forming unit of the virus suspension is normally determined using the formula: $1\ OD_{260} = 3.75 \times 10^8$ pfu/µL. For this purpose, the virus suspension is diluted appropriately with 1 mM Tris/HCl buffer (pH 9.0) and the optical density (OD) of the diluted sample is measured at 260 nm. The OD_{260} is then used to calculate the plaque-forming units of the suspension. Prior to storing the virus stock at –80°C, we usually adjust the virus suspension at 10^7 pfu/µL (*see* **Note 2**).

3.1.3. Transfection of HRPE Cells With Plasmid

1. While the virus-treated cells are being incubated for 30 min in the cell culture hood, the plasmid suspension is prepared for subsequent transfection.
2. The DNA samples (vector-transporter cDNA construct and the empty vector) and Lipofectin are mixed in an appropriate volume of OPTI/MEM I medium containing 0.01% 2-mercaptoethanol such that the final suspension contains 1 µg DNA and 3 µL Lipofectin for each well in a volume of 350 µL/well.
3. The suspension is incubated at room temperature for 30 min prior to use. Once the virus-treated cells are incubated for 30 min, 350 µL of DNA suspension is then added to each well and the plate is kept in the CO_2-incubator (37°C, 5% CO_2) for 12 h (*see* **Note 3**).

3.1.4. Uptake Measurements

1. Twelve hours following transfection, the cells are used for uptake measurements.
2. Appropriate radiolabeled substrates are prepared in uptake buffer. This uptake buffer containing NaCl is suitable for most transporters. However, if the ion-dependence of the transport process needs to be investigated, the composition of the buffer can be altered without changing the osmolality. For example, NaCl is substituted isoosmotically with choline chloride or *N*-methyl-D-glucamine chloride to prepare the Na^+-free buffer. Similarly, NaCl is substituted isoosmotically with sodium gluconate to prepare the Cl^--free buffer. By comparing the rate of uptake in these three buffers, the dependence of the transport process on Na^+ and/or Cl^- can be assessed. The substrate concentration (labeled plus unlabeled) varies depending on the affinity of the transporter for that particular substrate.
3. Uptake measurements are made in parallel in cells transfected with the transporter cDNA and in cells transfected with empty vector so that the uptake activity associated with the heterologously expressed transporter can be differentiated from the endogenous uptake activity that may be present in these cells.
4. For uptake measurements, the 24-well plate is placed in a water bath at 37°C and the medium from the wells is removed by aspiration.

5. Cells in each well are then washed with 2 mL of uptake buffer that has been prewarmed to 37°C.
6. Then, 250 µL of uptake buffer containing radiolabeled substrate is added to the well and incubated for a desired time. The time of incubation is selected such that the measured uptake rate represents initial rates. This is essential to perform kinetic analyses of the transport process.
7. At the end of incubation, the solution from the well is removed by aspiration and the cell monolayer is washed twice with 2 mL of ice-cold uptake buffer.
8. 0.5 mL of 1% SDS in 0.2 N NaOH is then added to each well and the plate is agitated for 30 min to lyse the cells.
9. The lysates are transferred into scintillation vials and then mixed with 4 mL of scintillation cocktail.
10. The vials are shaken vigorously to mix the contents and the radioactivity associated with the lysates is determined by scintillation spectrometry.
11. Twenty-five microliters of the uptake buffer containing the radiolabeled substrate are taken into scintillation vials and mixed with scintillation cocktail and its radioactivity determined to serve as the standard. From the radioactivity associated with the lysates and the radioactivity of the standard, the amount of substrate taken up into the cells can be determined.
12. The uptake values are expressed as moles/unit time/10^6 cells. Because the number of cells present in a well is counted prior to infection with the virus, this information can be used to normalize the uptake per 10^6 cells (*see* **Note 4**).

3.2. Xenopus laevis Oocyte Expression Technique

The methods described below outline: (1) preparation of cRNA, (2) preparation of oocytes, (3) defolliculation of oocytes, (4) microinjection of oocytes with cRNA, (5) measurement of uptake of radiolabeled substrates in oocytes, and (6) electrophysiological analysis.

3.2.1. Preparation of cRNA

1. Template plasmid DNA should be relatively free of contaminating proteins and RNA. Clean template preparations always give superior quality of cRNA with a higher yield. Most commercially available plasmid preparation systems can be used for plasmid DNA preparation. Plasmid DNA as well as PCR products subcloned into appropriate plasmids that contain a RNA polymerase promoter site can be used as templates for in vitro transcription.
2. The plasmid must be linearized at a downstream site of the insert to be transcribed using a unique restriction enzyme. It is generally advisable to examine the linearized template DNA on a gel to ensure that digestion is complete. Since initiation of transcription is one of the limiting steps in in vitro transcription reactions, even a small amount of circular plasmid in the template would interfere with the generation of good quality cRNA. The restriction enzymes (such as *Kpn* I, *Pst* I, and so on) leaving 3' overhanging ends should be avoided, because a short stretch of the resultant 3' overhang end can be utilized as a priming site for RNA polymerase.

3. The linearized template plasmid DNA is subsequently subjected to proteinase K treatment (at a concentration of 100–200 µg/mL) and in the presence of 0.5% SDS for 30 min at 50°C, followed by a phenol/chloroform extraction (using an equal volume) and ethanol precipitation procedure, because DNA samples from some minipreparation procedures may be contaminated and restriction enzymes occasionally introduce RNase or other inhibitors of transcription.

4. After ethanol precipitation, the digested DNA will be pelleted for 15 min in a microcentrifuge at top speed.

5. The supernatant will be removed with a very fine-tipped pipet. The pellets are resuspended in deionized water at a concentration of 0.5–1 µg/µL.

6. In vitro transcription procedure is performed by mixing all four rNTPs and an appropriate quantity of T7 RNA polymerase with the linearized DNA template in an RNase-free condition. T3 RNA polymerase or SP6 RNA polymerase is used if the cDNA insert is under the control of T3 or SP6 promoter respectively. RNAase inhibitor and mRNA cap analog, 7-methyldiguanosine-triphosphate (mG[5']ppp[5']G), are also included. The cRNA capping is simultaneously achieved.

7. The DNA template in the reaction mixture is digested away with an RNase-free DNase following the in vitro transcription.

8. The synthetic cRNA is separated from free nucleotides by a double ethanol precipitation procedure.

9. Final concentration of the synthetic cRNA is adjusted by ultraviolet (UV) spectrophotometry and the integrity is verified by electrophoresis in a 1% formaldehyde denaturing agarose gel and visualization by ethidium bromide fluorescence.

10. An mMESSAGE mMACHINE kit from Ambion is routinely used in our lab for the in vitro synthesis of large amounts of capped cRNA. Capped cRNA mimics most eukaryotic mRNAs seen in vivo, because it has a 7-methyl guanosine cap structure at the 5'-end. The mMESSAGE mMACHINE reactions include cap analog in its transcription reaction. mMESSAGE mMACHINE Kit has a simplified reaction format in which all four ribonucleotides and cap analog are mixed in a single solution. The cap analog:GTP ratio of this solution is optimized for maxium capped cRNA yield. The cRNA produced is protected from degradation by contaminating RNase with RNasein (a broad spectrum RNase inhibitor) in the kit. Typically the yield for each reaction is approx 20–30 µg of RNA with T3 or T7 RNA polymerase and a little bit less (approx 15–25 µg) when using SP6 RNA polymerase. Final concentration of the in vitro synthesized cRNA should be made at approx 1.0 µg/µL.

11. The cRNA solution should be aliquoted into several tubes (approx 5.0 µL per tube) and stored at –80°C until injection (*see* **Notes 5** and **6**).

3.2.2. Preparation of Oocytes

1. Female *Xenopus laevis* frogs are available from a number of commercial suppliers. These are human chorionic gonadotropin-treated frogs. We specifically request shipment of largest frogs available.

2. Oocytes are collected from frogs by a surgical procedure under anesthesia. The animals are anesthetized by immersion for 15–30 min in a 0.1% solution of MS222 in deionized water kept in a stainless steel container. The volume of the anesthetic solution in the container is adjusted such that the nostrils of the frog are above the level of the solution to avoid drowning of the animal. Hand gloves should be worn throughout these procedures because MS222 is a potential carcinogen. When fully anesthetized, the frog is no longer responsive to poking and its muscles become relaxed.

3. The anesthetized frog is thoroughly washed with deionized water to remove the residual anesthetic from the skin, and then placed on a flat surface of a sterile Petri dish with the animal's abdomen facing upward.

4. The area on the posterior ventral side of the abdomen where the incision is to be made is sanitized by applying a cotton swab soaked with 70% ethanol followed by gentle wiping with another cotton swab soaked in autoclaved deionized water to remove the residual ethanol.

5. A small (approx 0.3 cm) incision through the skin and muscle is made using a sterile surgical blade.

6. The ovary, which usually consists of multiple lobes, is partially exposed through the incision.

7. Forceps are used to carefully tease out one lobe of the ovary and it is ligated at its base.

8. The lobe of the ovary is then excised using scissors and transferred to a small petri dish containing the modified Barth's solution with approx 10 µg/mL gentamicin sulfate.

9. The incision site on the abdomen is closed by suture and an antibiotic solution is applied on the sutured site to prevent infection.

10. The frog is placed on a slope partially immersed in shallow water supplemented by 0.5% NaCl in a stainless-steel container. Again, the head of the frog is kept above the surface of the water to prevent the frog from drowning. It takes approx 1–2 h for the animal to regain its consciousness, and during this period the skin of the animal is constantly kept moist by intermittently applying a wet cloth or tissue to prevent dehydration. Once the frog regains consciousness, it is returned to the aquarium tank (*see* **Note 7**).

3.2.3. Defolliculation of Oocytes

1. The ovarian lobe in the Petri dish is teased out carefully into smaller pieces without harming the oocytes.

2. These small pieces of ovarian lobes are then subjected to partial digestion at room temperature for 60 min with collagenase A (2 mg/mL) in 96 mM NaCl, 2 mM KCl, 1 mM MgCl$_2$, 5 mM HEPES, pH adjusted to 7.5 with Tris. Most of the commercially available collagenases are not pure and often contain some impurities, which are harmful to the oocytes' survival.

3. The collagenase-digested oocytes are then thoroughly washed with the above-mentioned buffer but without collagenase and transferred to a 20 mL vial con-

taining the modified Barth's solution. Treatment of oocytes with collagenase for longer than the optimal time affects their viability.

4. The oocytes are then manually defolliculated. Defolliculation is carried out in the defolliculation buffer. This buffer has higher osmolality than the buffer used for collagenase treatment. The oocytes in this buffer are expected to shrink slightly and this facilitates manual defolliculation. Only mature oocytes (developmental stage V-VI) with a prominent light-colored "equator" between the animal pole and the vegetal pole are selected for defolliculation.

5. A pair of watchmaker's forceps is ideal for this purpose. Defolliculation is done under a stereo-microscope with a light shining on the oocytes. The oocytes are never exposed to the defolliculation buffer for more than 20 min because the oocytes are prone to osmotic damage.

6. Defolliculated mature oocytes are selected and maintained at 18°C in modified Barth's medium with 10 µg/mL gentamicin sulfate.

7. Oocytes are injected with cRNA the next day, which allows the oocytes to recover from the defolliculation procedure.

3.2.4. Microinjection of Oocytes With cRNA

1. Defolliculated oocytes are subjected to a second selection after overnight incubation at 18°C because some of the oocytes are no longer viable as a result of physical damage during defolliculation and manipulation or because of excess collagenase treatment.

2. A total of approx 80 oocytes (this is a manageable number for a single injection) are evenly dispersed into a Petri dish with a piece of nylon mesh (Spectra/Mesh N) glued to the bottom. The Petri dish is half-filled with modified Barth's solution and the oocytes to be injected are submerg in the solution. The hole-size and the thickness of the nylon mesh should be selected to fit the average size of the oocytes. Each individual oocyte should be sitting in a separate hole and held in original position by gravity during the entire injection process.

3. The oocytes are then sequentially injected by a column/row fashion on the mesh.

4. A 10-µL microdispenser Drummond Scientific Co. has been used satisfactorily for oocyte injection in our laboratory for several years. The Drummond Scientific Co. also provides suitable glass capillaries to fit the microdispenser.

   a. Homemade needles are fabricated from these capillaries by a micropipette puller. We routinely make these microinjection needles with a long shaft, which can be easily cut at their tips under a microscope with an eyepiece graticule calibrated with a stage micrometer.

   b. The needle tips should be cut such that the diameter is approx 20 µm.

   c. The needles are usually siliconized with a drop of Sigmacote and then baked in an oven at 250°C for 2 h to destroy RNase that might be present as contamination due to handling of the needles.

   d. Prior to fitting the injection needle to the microinjector, the entire needle is back-filled with mineral oil.

5. The in vitro synthesized cRNA solution (approx 1.0 µg/µL) is gradually front-filled into the needle by turning the plunger knob in the microinjector. Care must be taken to avoid sucking of any air bubbles.

6. A micromanipulator attached to a magnetic stand is set up by the microscope and the microdispenser is fitted to the micromanipulator at approx 45°. In this arrangement, the microdispenser can be freely moved in a stereotaxic manner (three-dimensional directions, i.e., x-, y-, and z-orientation).

7. For each oocyte, we generally inject approx 50 nL of cRNA solution which equals to 50 ng of cRNA. The preferred injection site is toward the unpigmented vegetal pole of the oocyte because the oocyte nucleus is located just underneath the animal pole. This results in the delivery of the injected cRNA into the cytoplasm.

8. After injection, the oocytes are transferred with a plastic Pasteur pipet to a glass vial half-filled with modified Barth's solution and incubated at 18°C until the uptake measurements or electrophysiological experiments are performed. The vial caps should be closed loose to ensure sufficient oxygen supply to the oocytes. Because dead oocytes affect their neighbors' survival, the injected oocytes are inspected under a microscope everyday, dead or dying oocytes are removed, and the culture medium is replaced with fresh medium.

3.2.5. Measurement of Uptake of Radiolabeled Substrates in Oocytes

The expression levels of the injected exogenous cRNA in oocytes increase in a time-dependent manner following microinjection and reach maximal levels 4–6 d postinjection. Therefore, functional assays for the heterologously expressed transporter are normally performed within this period. One week after the injection, the oocytes start to deteriorate and are no longer viable for functional studies.

1. Uptake assays with radiolabeled substrates are carried out in a 24-well microtiter plate.

2. Each well is filled with a suitable uptake buffer whose composition would vary depending on the functional features of the transporter, and 8–10 cRNA-injected oocytes are placed in the wells.

3. The incubation time for uptake measurements is 1 h at room temperature, but this time period would vary from transporter to transporter depending on the rate of uptake. If kinetic analysis needs to be performed, it is imperative that the time period chosen for uptake measurements represents initial uptake rate.

4. Ion dependence of the uptake process is analyzed by isoosmotic substitution of NaCl in the uptake buffer with sodium gluconate (chloride-free condition), or choline chloride (sodium-free condition).

5. At the end of incubation, the oocytes are thoroughly washed with ice-cold uptake buffer without the radiolabeled substrate at least five times, transferred individually to counting vials, and lysed by adding 200 µL of 0.1% SDS.

6. The radioactivity associated with individual oocytes is then measured to quantify the amount of uptake.

7. Uninjected oocytes are used in parallel to determine the endogenous uptake activity. This endogenous activity is subtracted from uptake in cRNA-injected oocytes to determine the uptake activity that is due specifically to the injected cRNA.

3.2.6. Electrophysiologcal Analysis

The transport function of the heterologously expressed transporter in oocytes can also be monitored using an electrophysiological approach, provided the transport process is electrogenic (i.e., the transport process results in a change in oocyte membrane potential). If the transport process is electrogenic, this approach offers several advantages over the previous method utilizing radiolabeled substrates. Because the number of commercially available radiolabeled substrates is limited, the electrophysiological approach is preferable because the system employs unlabeled substrates. Transport function is monitored through studying the substrate-induced current using a two-microelectrode voltage-clamp technique. If the transport process causes depolarization of the oocyte membrane, exposure of the oocytes to substrates of the transporter will induce inward currents. On the other hand, if the transport process causes hyperpolarization of the oocyte membrane, exposure of the oocytes to substrates of the transporter will induce outward currents. If the induced current is entirely coupled to the transport of the substrate, the substrate induced-current is quantitatively proportional to the amount of the substrate transferred into the oocyte via the transporter. However, if there are uncoupled currents, the amount of substrate transferred into the oocyte via the transporter may not correlate with the substrate-induced current. There are additional advantages with this system. A single oocyte can be used repeatedly to measure transport activity under different experimental conditions. The use of a single oocyte would drastically reduce variations among the oocytes. The oocyte system is also suitable to study the influence of membrane potential on the transport activity because the membrane potential of the oocyte can be changed as desired by a computer program through the amplifier. The versatility of the system makes it possible to conduct a variety of electrophysiological studies with the cloned transporter cDNAs.

For the conventional two-microelectrode voltage-clamp technique, three components are essential: an amplifier, a software package for data acquisition and data analysis, and a chart recorder. We use a GeneClamp 500 amplifier from Axon Instruments, Inc. The membrane potential is clamped to a desired value (usually –50 mV). In this procedure, one intracellular electrode is used to record the actual membrane potential and the second electrode is used to inject current into the oocyte so as to keep the potential at the clamped value. The magnitude of this current is taken as the measure of transport activity. The two microelectrodes are fabricated by a micropipette puller and their resistance is controlled to a range of approx 1.5–2.5 mΩ.

1. The oocyte is placed in a Lucite chamber filled with desired uptake buffer.
2. The electrodes are then introduced into the oocyte under the microscope and the initial membrane potential is recorded. Then the potential is clamped at –50 mV.
3. The oocyte is then perfused with the buffer using a peristaltic pump.
4. The oocyte is then exposed to a suitable substrate by perfusing the Lucite chamber with the substrate solution (substrate solutions are made in the same uptake buffer).
5. The currents are continuously recorded during this procedure. This allows detection of the current that is induced by exposure of the oocyte to the substrate.
6. The oocytes are subjected to thorough washing with the perfusing buffer prior to exposure to a different substrate.
7. Between experiments, when the oocytes are not exposed to substrates, the oocytes are perfused with ND96 buffer. The electrophysiological method can be used to assess the substrate specificity of the transporter and also to perform kinetic analysis of the transport process.
8. Uninjected oocytes are used in a similar manner to determine if there are substrate-induced currents in these oocytes, which might indicate the presence of endogenous transport activity.
9. To investigate the dependence of the transporter activity on membrane potential, step changes to the testing potentials (V_t) from the holding potential (V_h) is achieved by a voltage clamp amplifier (GeneClamp 500, Axon Instruments, Inc.). The amplifier is controlled by the Clampex computer program of pClamp software (Axon Instruments, Inc.). Step changes in testing membrane potential are made, each for a duration of 100 ms (from +50 mV to –150 mV in 20-mV increments). The voltage-jumping protocol is applied to the oocyte first in the absence of substrate in the perfusion buffer and then in the presence of substrate after exposing the oocyte to substrate for adequate amount of time to yield the maximal substrate-induced current. The substrate-induced current at each testing potential is taken as the difference between the steady-state currents, recorded at the end of each voltage pulse, in the presence and absence of the substrate. The currents are low pass filtered at 500 Hz by a built-in Bessel filter in the amplifier, digitized at 50 μs/point, and are averaged from three sweeps.

4. Notes

1. For the vaccinia virus expression system, any mammalian cell line can be used for heterologous expression of the cloned transporters. However, we routinely use the human retinal pigment epithelial cell line HRPE for this purpose in our laboratory. Infection of the cells with vaccinia virus changes the morphology of the cells and, if the cells are not attached firmly in the 24-well plates, infection with the virus would result in the release of the cells from the plastic surface. Uptake measurements cannot be made if the cells are released because the procedure described above is suitable for measurement of uptake only with monolayer

cultures. We have used HeLa cells and COS-7 cells for vaccinia virus-mediated expression of transporter cDNAs and found that these cells are inferior to HRPE cells in terms of adherence to the plastic support. However, with careful and gentle handling, even HeLa cells and COS-7 cells can be used for uptake measurements.

2. The recombinant vaccinia virus is supposed to be non-pathogenic; however, it is advised that the individuals who handle the virus be vaccinated for small pox because the handling of the virus carries a small, however negligible, risk for infection in individuals who have not had the small pox vaccination.

3. Vaccinia virus is a lytic virus. This means that the mammalian cells infected with the virus will lyse eventually. This takes usually approx 15–20 h. If the cells lyse, they are no longer useful for uptake measurements. Therefore, uptake measurements should be made within 12–15 h following infection of the cells with the virus.

4. While performing the uptake measurements, the procedure involves washing of the cell monolayers several times with buffers. Care must be taken to perform these steps quick without letting the cells dry between the washes. If the cells are allowed to dry, this reduces the uptake activity because the cells are no longer healthy.

5. The transporter cDNAs are not always expressed with comparable efficiency in the two expression systems described previously. Most transporters are expressed well with the vaccinia virus expression system as well as with the *Xenopus laevis* oocyte expression system. However, we have found that some transporters, which are expressed well with the vaccinia virus expression system, are not expressed in oocytes. Similarly, some transporters that are expressed well in oocytes do not work in the vaccinia virus expression system. We do not know the reasons for this.

6. Even though we routinely use transporter cDNAs cloned into the pSPORT1 vector in the *Xenopus laevis* oocyte expression system, the levels of expression can sometimes be increased markedly by changing the vector. There are several designer vectors available for use in the *Xenopus laevis* expression system, and these vectors carry the 5'-untranslated region (UTR) of the *Xenopus* globin gene upstream of the multiple cloning sites and the 3'-UTR of the *Xenopus* globin gene downstream of the multiple cloning sites *(15)*. The coding region of the cloned transporter cDNA can be amplified by polymerase chain reaction (PCR) and inserted into the multiple cloning sites of these designer vectors so that the transporter cDNA is flanked by the 5'-UTR and 3'-UTR of the *Xenopus* globin gene. The resultant recombinant plasmid can then be used to prepare cRNA for subsequent injection into oocytes. In many cases, this approach increases the expression levels of the transporter. In our laboratory, we use one such vector, called pGH19 *(24,25)*. This vector does enhance the expression levels for some transporters. In our experience, the enhancement of expression is not universal. It works for some transporters but not for all.

7. The ability of the oocytes to express heterologous cRNAs varies from frog to frog. Therefore, if a frog is identified as a "good expresser," the same frog can be

used several times as the source of oocytes. This however will depend on approval from the institutional Committee on Animal Use for Research and Education. The Committee at the Medical College of Georgia allows us to use frogs a maximum of four times. This might vary from institution to institution.

Acknowledgments

This work was supported by United States Public Health Service (USPHS) grants HD44404, HL64196, and AI49849 (to V. G.), and HD37150 (to P. D. P.).

References

1. Blakely, R. D., Clark, J. A., Rudnick, G., and Amara, S. G. (1991) Vaccinia-T7 RNA polymerase expression system: evaluation for the expression cloning of plasma membrane transporters. *Anal. Biochem.* **194,** 302–308.
2. Povlock, S. L. and Amara, S. G. (1998) Vaccinia virus-T7 RNA polymerase expression system for neurotransmitter transporters. *Meth. Enzymol.* **296,** 436–443.
3. Fuerst, T. R., Niles, E. G., Studier, F. W., and Moss, B. (1986) Eukaryotic transient-expression system based on recombinant vaccinia virus that synthesizes bacteriophage T7 RNA polymerase. *Proc. Natl. Acad. Sci. USA* **83,** 8122–8126.
4. Ramamoorthy, S., Leibach, F. H., Mahesh, V. B., et al. (1994) Functional characterization and chromosomal localization of a cloned taurine transporter from human placenta. *Biochem. J.* **300,** 893–900.
5. Kekuda, R., Prasad, P. D., Fei, Y. J., et al. (1996) Cloning of the sodium-dependent broad-scope neutral amino acid transporter B^0 from a human placental choriocarcinoma cell line. *J. Biol. Chem.* **271,** 18,657–18,661.
6. Prasad, P. D., Wang, H., Kekuda, R., et al. (1998) Cloning and functional expression of a cDNA encoding a mammalian sodium-dependent vitamin transporter mediating the uptake of pantothenate, biotin, and lipoate. *J. Biol. Chem.* **273,** 7501–7506.
7. Kekuda, R., Prasad, P. D., Wu, X., et al. (1998) Cloning and functional characterization of a potential-sensitive polyspecific organic cation transporter (OCT3) most abundantly expressed in placenta. *J. Biol. Chem.* **273,** 15,971–15,979.
8. Rajan, D. P., Huang, W., Dutta, B., et al. (1999) Human placental sodium-dependent vitamin C transporter (SVCT2): Molecular cloning and transport function. *Biochem. Biophys. Res. Commun.* **262,** 762–768.
9. Dutta, B., Huang, W., Molero, M., et al. (1999) Cloning of the human thiamine transporter, a member of the folate transporter family. *J. Biol. Chem.* **274,** 31,925–31,929.
10. Prasad, P. D., Wang. H., Huang, W., et al. (1999) Human LAT1, a subunit for system L amino acid transporter: molecular cloning and transport function. *Biochem. Biophys. Res. Commun.* **255,** 283–288.
11. Wang, H., Huang, W., Sugawara, M., et al. (2000) Cloning and functional expression of ATA1, a subtype of amino acid transporter A, from human placenta. *Biochem. Biophys. Res. Commun.* **273,** 1175–1179.

12. Wu, X., George, R. L., Huang, W., et al. (2000) Structural and functional characteristics and tissue distribution pattern of rat OCTN1, an organic cation transporter, cloned from placenta. *Biochim. Biophys. Acta* **1466,** 315–327.

13. Ganapathy, M. E., Huang, W., Rajan, D. P., et al. (2000) β-Lactam antibiotics as substrates for OCTN2, an organic cation/carnitine transporter. *J. Biol. Chem.* **275,** 1699–1707.

14. Goldin, A. L. (1992) Maintenance of *Xenopus laevis* and oocyte injection. *Meth. Enzymol.* **207,** 266–279.

15. Mager, S., Cao, Y., and Lester, H. A. (1998) Measurement of transient currents from neurotransmitter transporters expressed in *Xenopus* oocytes. *Meth. Enzymol.* **296,** 551–566.

16. Fei, Y. J., Prasad, P. D., Leibach, F. H., and Ganapathy, V. (1995) The amino acid transport system y+L induced in *Xenopus laevis* oocytes by human choriocarcinoma cell (JAR) mRNA is functionally related to the heavy chain of the 4F2 cell surface antigen. *Biochemistry* **34,** 8744–8751.

17. Torres-Zamorano, V., Leibach, F. H., and Ganapathy, V. (1998) Sodium-dependent homo- and hetero-exchange of neutral amino acids mediated by the amino acid transporter ATB^0. *Biochem. Biophys. Res. Commun.* **245,** 824–829.

18. Wang, H., Fei, Y. J., Kekuda, R., et al. (2000) Structure, function, and genomic organization of human Na+-dependent high-affinity dicarboxylate transporter. *Am. J. Physiol.* **278,** C1019–C1030.

19. Wu, X., Kekuda, R., Huang, W., et al. (1998) Identity of the organic cation transporter OCT3 as the extraneuronal monoamine transporter (Uptake2) and evidence for expression of the transporter in the brain. *J. Biol. Chem.* **273,** 32,776–32,786.

20. Sugawara, M., Nakanishi, T., Fei, Y. J., et al. (2000) Cloning of an amino acid transporter with functional characteristics and tissue expression pattern identical to that of system A. *J. Biol. Chem.* **275,** 16,473–16,477.

21. Hatanaka, T., Nakanishi, T., Huang, W., et al. (2001) Na$^+$- and Cl$^-$-coupled active transport of nitric oxide synthase inhibitors via the amino acid transporter ATB$^{0,+}$. *J. Clin. Invest.* **107,** 1035–1043.

22. Parent, L., Supplisson, S., Loo, D. D. F., and Wright, E. M. (1992) Electrogenic properties of the cloned Na+/glucose cotransporter. *J. Membr. Biol.* **125,** 49–62.

23. Mackenzie, B., Loo, D. D. F., Fei, Y. J., et al. (1996) Mechanisms of the human intestinal H$^+$-coupled oligopeptide transporter hPEPT1. *J. Biol. Chem.* **271,** 5430–5437.

24. Trudeau, M. C., Warmke, J. W., Ganetzky, B., and Robertson, G. A. (1995) HERG, a human inward rectifier in the voltage-gated potassium channel family. *Science* **269,** 92–95.

25. Knauf, F., Rogina, B., Jiang, Z., Aronson, P. S., and Helfand, S. L. (2002) Functional characterization and immunolocalization of the transporter encoded by the life-extending gene *Indy*. *Proc. Natl. Acad. Sci. USA* **99,** 14,315–14,319.

18

Analysis of Trophoblast Giant Cell Steroidogenesis in Primary Cultures

Noa Sher and Joseph Orly

Summary

Placental progesterone synthesis in humans prevents abortion of the fetus by maintaining uterine quiescence and low myometrial excitability. In rodents, a transient steroidogenic output is observed in the trophoblast giant cells during mid-pregnancy. Although the exact role of this locally produced progesterone is not clear, rodent trophoblast giant cells are an important cell model for studying the regulation of placental steroidogenesis. This chapter describes the methods we developed to analyze the regulation of genes involved in progesterone biosynthesis in miniature cultures of primary trophoblast cells from rodents. These genes include cholesterol side chain cleavage cytochrome P450 (P450scc) and its accessory proteins, steroidogenic acute regulatory protein (StAR) and 3β-hydroxysteroid dehydrogenase/isomerase (3βHSD). To obtain giant cells, uterine implantation sites are sliced in half, and the trophoblast giant cell layers are separated from the surrounding decidua by scraping. Cells can subsequently be separated by gentle enzymatic digestion with trypsin, or collagenase, and plated for further study in vitro. This chapter provides instructions, insights, and comments instrumental for performing *in situ* visualization of giant cell mRNA and proteins, analyzing enzyme activities, and conducting promoter analyses with a limited number of cells.

Key Words: Trophoblast primary cultures; P450scc; StAR; 3βHSD; in situ visualizations; RT-PCR; promoter analyses.

1. Introduction

Steroid hormones such as progesterone and estrogen are essential to establish and maintain pregnancy in mammals *(1–6)*. These hormones are produced at various time points during pregnancy in the placenta, the ovarian corpus luteum, and the fetal adrenal *(6,7)*. Steroid hormone synthesis begins in these steroidogenic tissues upon conversion of cholesterol into pregnenolone, the first steroid. This reaction is catalyzed in the mitochondria by cholesterol side-chain cleavage cytochrome P450 (P450scc) and the accessory proteins adrenodoxin and adrenodoxin reductase *(8–10)*. Cholesterol substrate is mobi-

From: *Methods in Molecular Medicine, Vol. 122: Placenta and Trophoblast: Methods and Protocols, Vol. 2*
Edited by: M. J. Soares and J. S. Hunt © Humana Press Inc., Totowa, NJ

lized to the P450scc complex in the inner mitochondrial cristae by steroidogenic acute regulatory protein (StAR) (11). The reaction product, pregnenolone, is further processed into active steroid hormones by endoplasmic reticulum-bound enzymes, such as 3β-hydroxysteroid dehydrogenase/isomerase (3βHSD), cytochrome P45017α, and cytochrome P450 aromatase (12–16).

In the rodent model, progesterone production by the corpus luteum is indispensable throughout pregnancy (17). However, by the time of placentation at midpregnancy, there is a sharp rise in the expression of steroidogenic genes in the trophoblast giant cells, the steroidogenic cells of the rodent placenta (14,18–20). Expression of these enzymes peaks in the murine giant cells at day 9.5 postconception (pc), after which there is a decline in expression between days 10.5 and 14.5 pc (18). A similar sequence of events occurs during rat pregnancy, with a 2-d delay relative to mouse gestation. The rodent placenta, as opposed to the human organ, barely produces steroid hormones de novo in the second half of gestation. The role of local steroid hormone production in the rodent placenta is not clear, considering the vitality of steroidogenesis in the mouse corpus luteum, and in face of the fact that pregnancy normally proceeds to term in P450scc knockout mice (21). However, it is possible that the seemingly redundant expression of steroidogenic genes in trophoblast giant cells may be related to protection of the fetus from maternal immunorejection (20,22). It has also been demonstrated that prior to the onset of giant cell steroidogenesis, the decidual cells of the mouse uterus express P450scc and 3βHSD (18,19,23), again hinting that a local uterine production of steroids may have an important physiological role at the fetal–maternal interface.

The trophoblast giant cells of the rodent placenta are one of the first cell types to undergo differentiation in the developing embryo. They undergo multiple cycles of endoreduplication, amassing up to 1000 copies of DNA and an enormous size, hence their name (24–26). At the time of mid-pregnancy, these cells surround the conceptus sac (Fig. 1) and are in direct contact with the maternal decidua, which they invade during the process of placentation. Aiming to study the unknown regulatory aspects of steroid hormone synthesis in giant cells, we adhere to primary cultures of this unique cell type, attempting to study multiple cellular functions. The major challenge in doing so is the paucity of cells available for tasks that usually consume a relatively large number of cultured cells. Others approached this limitation by establishing cell lines of differentiating trophoblast giant cells, the most well-known being the Rcho-1 trophoblast cell line, isolated by Soares and colleagues (27–30). This chapter provides our protocols, which aim to miniaturize the procedures required for analyses of a minimal number of trophoblast giant cells in culture. In our hands, the ability to isolate cultures of primary trophoblast giant cells has been invaluable for unveiling transcription factors controlling the expression of the steroidogenic genes, readily following the expression patterns of the gene products at the mRNA and protein levels, and biochemically dissecting enzyme activities by separation of their labeled steroid products *(18,19,31,32)*.

Collectively, our studies and others' suggest that, during evolution, the ephemeral placental tissue has developed unique regulatory pathways for the execution of steroidogenic and other endocrine functions also found in adult organs *(6)*.

2. Materials

2.1. Hormonal Hyperstimulation of Mice

1. C57 x Balb/c F1 mice (6–8 wk) (*see* **Note 1**).
2. Stock 50 U/mL pregnant mare serum gonadotropin (PMSG; Gestil, Organon, Oss, Holland) in sterile phosphate-buffered saline (PBS).
3. Stock 40 U/mL hCG (Gestil, Organon, Oss, Holland) in sterile PBS.

2.2. Preparation of Trophoblast Giant Cells

1. Serum-free Dulbecco's modified Eagle's medium (DMEM)-F12 medium (Life Technologies, Paisley, UK) with 2.43 g/L NaHCO$_3$.
2. Complete DMEM-F12 medium, with 10% heat-inactivated fetal bovine serum (Life Technologies, Paisley, UK), 180 U/mL penicillin, 0.25 mg/mL streptomycin, 15 mM HEPES (pH 7.9) (*see* **Note 2**).
3. Cell dissociation medium. 1.7 mg/mL trypsin and 80 µg/mL DNase (Sigma, St. Louis, MO) in PBS. We previously used an alternative, although somewhat less effective, dissociation medium including PBS with 4 mg/mL collagenase-dispase (Vibrio alginoluticus/bacillus polymyxa, Roche Molecular Biochemicals, Mannheim, Germany), 10 mg/mL bovine serum albumin and 20 µg/mL DNase I.

2.3. Hormone Assays

1. [7-^{3}H]-pregnenolone (0.5 µM; 3 µCi/mL, NET-039 22.6 Ci/mmol, NEN Life Science Products, Boston, MA).
2. TLC plates (N-HR/UV254, Polygram Sil, Macherey-Nagel, Düren, Germany).
3. Cyanoketone (5 µg/mL, Sterling-Winthrop Research Institute, Rensselaer, NY).
4. Nonlabeled authentic pregnenolone and progesterone (Sigma, pregnenelone P9129, progesterone P0130).
5. FLA-3000 Bio-Imaging Analyzer (Fuji Photo Film Co., Ltd., Tokyo, Japan) and plate; and/or scintillation counter.

2.4. Assays of Gene Expression

2.4.1. Semi-Quantitative Reverse-Transcription Polymerase Chain Reaction Analysis

1. RNAzol B (Tel-Test, Inc., Friendwood, TX).
2. FLA-3000 Bio-Imaging Analyzer
3. RX medical X-ray film (Fuji Photo Film Co., Ltd., Tokyo, Japan).

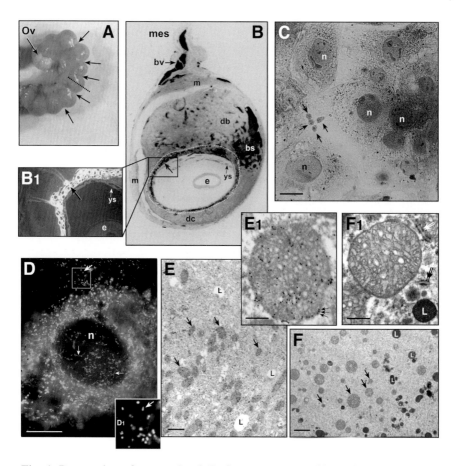

Fig. 1. Preparation of mouse day 9.5 of pregnancy steroidogenic trophoblast giant cells for primary culture. (**A**) Multiple implantation sites in a mouse uterine horn on day 9.5 of pregnancy (gonadotropin-treated animal). Individual sites are separated by scalpel knife where indicated by the arrows. A broken line depicts the plane of sectioning to obtain hemi-sites as described in **B**. Ov, ovary. (**B**) A sagittal-to-embryo/transverse-to-uterus section through one of the implantation sites. The trophoblast giant cell layers (inside the white dashed line) are immunoperoxidase stained with P450scc antiserum; note a typical false-positive staining of red blood cells in the blood sinuses (bs) of the decidua basalis (db) or mesometrial blood vessels (bv). dc, decidua capsularis; e, embryo; ys, yolk sac. **B₁** shows a high-power magnification of the giant cell layers (arrow) stained in a consecutive section collected 200 μm from section B and stained by enzyme-labeled fluorescence (ELF)-immunofluorescence using anti-3β-hydroxysteroid dehydrogenase/isomerase (3βHSD) serum. In preparation for isolation of the giant cells, the mesometrium (mes) and myometrium (m) tissues are peeled off by aid of forceps and discarded. Then each site is cut in half and the embryo

(caption continued on next page)

(Fig. 1. continued) (e) and the yolk sac (ys) are discarded. Finally, the thin tissue of the trophoblast giant cells is gently scraped with a fine spatula, and can be further processed to obtain a single cell suspension. **(C)** Trophoblast giant cells on day 2 in culture. Note the size of the giant cells and a minor contamination of much smaller nongiant placental or decidual cells (arrows). N, nucleus. Bar 50 µm. **(D)** A single giant cell immunostained with steroidogenic acute regulatory protein (StAR) antiserum. Note ample StAR-labeled mitochondria, some of which are caught underneath the nucleus (n) and are elongated (arrows), whereas most of the others are round as shown in **D$_1$** (arrow) and **E–F**. Bar = 50 µm. **(E,F)** **E–E$_1$** and **F–F$_1$** compare some characteristics of electron microscopy (EM) images depicting trophoblast giant cells prepared for immuno-electron microscopy while embedded in LR White hydophilic plastic *(34)*, or fixed and embedded in Epon plastic suitable for standard transmission EM *(44)*. **(E)** A cytoplasmic area in the giant cell with numerous mitochondria (arrows) stained with anti-StAR serum and 12 nm colloidal gold particles. A high-power mitochondrion image is shown in **E$_1$** depicting StAR-gold labeling. Some of the gold particles are localized on the mitochondrial surface (arrows), but most of the labeling associates with mature StAR localized in the gray area of the mitochondrial matrix. Note that, as a result of the mild fixation without lipid-staining osmium, the unstained cholesterol-ester lipid droplets (L) remain white and the outer and inner membranes of the mitochondria are not visible. **(F)** In contrast, micrographs **F** and **F$_1$** depict a standard Epon-embedded tissue including osmium staining, and therefore the lipid droplets (L) are stained black so that the membrane phospholipids in the endoplasmic reticulum and the mitochondrial membranes are readily visible (**F$_1$**). Note that the differentiated steroidogenic mitochondria (0.3–1.0 µm, arrows) are filled with typical tubular-vesicular cristae membranes (**F$_1$,E$_1$**). Arrows in **F$_1$** depict ribosomes on endoplasmic reticulum. Bars are 2 mm in **E** and **F**, 350 nm in **E$_1$**, and 250 nm in **F$_1$**.

4. Curix 60 film processor (Agfa, Munchen, Germany).
5. Primer sequences: rat P450scc forward 5'-AGAAGCTGGGCAACATGGA GTCAG and reverse 5'-TCACATCCCAGGCAGCTGCATGGT, rat StAR forward 5'-GCAGCAGGCAACCTGGTG and reverse 5'-TGATTGTCTTCGGCA GCC, mouse 3βHSD type I and VI forward 5'-ACTGGCAAATTCTCCA TAGCC and reverse 5'-TTCCTCCCAGCTGACAAGT, rat P45017α forward 5'-GGGGCAGGCATAGAGACAACT and reverse 5'-GCCTGAGCGCTTCTTA GATCC, rat ribosomal protein L19 forward 5'-CTGAAGGTCAAAGG GAATGTG and reverse 5'-GGACAGAGTCTTGATGATCTC. GenBank accession numbers: rat P450scc NM_017286.1, mouse StAR NM_011485.3, rat StAR NM_031558.1, mouse 3βHSD type VI NM_013821.2, rat P45017α NM_012753, ribosomal protein L19 rat NM_031103.1, and mouse L19 NM_026490.1.5.

2.4.2. Western Blot Analysis

1. Radio-immunoprecipitation assay (RIPA) lysis buffer: 150 mM NaCl, 50 mM Tris pH 7.4, 1% Triton X100, 0.1% sodium dodecyl sulfate [SDS], 0.5%

deoxycholate, containing protease-inhibitor cocktail (Sigma, cat. no. P-8340) and 10 µM Na-vanadate (Sigma). Protease inhibitors and Na-vanadate should be added immediately prior to use.

2. LumiGlo substrate for chemiluminescence detection (New England BioLabs, Beverly, MA).
3. Antibodies
   a. Polyclonal rabbit antiserum to StAR (provided by Drs. D.B. Hales and K.H. Hales, University of Illinois at Chicago, Chicago, IL) *(34,35)*.
   b. Polyclonal rabbit anti-rat P450scc antiserum *(36)*.
   c. Rabbit antiserum generated to human placental 3βHSD (provided by Dr. J. Ian Mason, University of Edinburgh, Edinburgh, Scotland).
   d. Rabbit antiserum to mouse P45017α (provided by Dr. Anita A. Payne of Stanford University, Stanford, CA).
   e. Peroxidase-conjugated AffiniPure goat anti-rabbit immunoglobulin (IgG) (H+L) (Jackson ImmunoResearch Laboratories, Inc., West Grove, PA).

2.5. Visualization of RNA and Protein Expression

2.5.1. In Situ Hybridization

1. Glass slides: SuperFrost/Plus (Menzel Glaser, Braunschweig , Germany).
2. PBST: PBS containing 0.1% Tween-20.
3. Proteinase K (Sigma, P-0390).
4. Prehybridization buffer: 50% formamide, 5X SCC, pH 4.5, 50 µg/mL yeast transfer RNA (Sigma, R-9001) and 50 µg/mL heparin.
5. Solution 1: 50% formamide 5X SSC, pH 4.5, and 0.5% SDS.
6. Solution 2: 50% formamide 2X SSC, pH 4.5.
7. Solution 3: TBST (250 mM Tris-HCl, pH 7.5, 1.3 M NaCl, 30 mM KCl, 1% Tween-20) containing 2 mM levamisole (Sigma, L-9756).
8. Enzyme-labeled fluorescence (ELF) kit, which contains a streptavidin–alkaline phosphatase conjugate that can be used to detect a biotinylated probe (Molecular Probes, Inc., Eugene, OR, E-6605).
9. 4% paraformaldehyde (pFA) in PBS, prepared as described under **Subheading 2.5.3.**
10. Tissue-Tek optimum cutting temperature (OCT) medium (Miles Scientific, Naperville, IL).
11. Available cryostat.
12. Poly-L-lysine coated glass slides.
13. 50 mM Tris-HCl pH 7.5 containing 0.125 mg/mL pronase and 2 mM ethylenediamine tetraacetic acid (EDTA).
14. 0.2% glycine in PBS, pH 7.4.
15. 0.25% acetic anhydride in 0.1 M triethanolamine, pH 8.0.
16. 10% dextran sulfate (Sigma, D8906).
17. 1X Denhardt's solution: 0.02% ficoll, 0.02% polyvinylpyrrolidone, 0.02% bovine serum albumin.
18. 5'Biotinylated, 2'-O-methyl-RNA probes (custom made by Microsynth, Balgach, Switzerland).

19. 2×10^8 cpm/mL of ^{35}S-labeled riboprobe.
20. 50% formamide/0.3 M NaCl.
21. RNase I-A.
22. NBT-2 emulsion (Eastman Kodak Company, Rochester, NY).
23. Immu-mount (Shandon, Pittsburgh, PA).
24. Nikon Labophot-2 microscope with AFX-II camera system.

2.5.2. Enzyme-Linked Immunohistochemistry

1. 4 % pFA in PBS prepared as described under **Subheading 2.5.3.**
2. Paraffin.
3. Available cryostat.
4. 3,3'-diaminobenzidine (DAB; Sigma, cat. no. D-4168) and ExtrAvidin-peroxidase (EXTRA-1) from Sigma; alternatively, ELF kit (Sigma, E-6605) from Molecular Probes, Inc. (Eugene, OR).
5. Antibodies (described previously).

2.5.3. Immunofluorescence

1. Coverslip discs No. 1, dia. 12 mm (Marienfeld, Baden-Württemberg, Germany). To reduce background fluorescence and improve cell adhesion and spreading in serum-free and serum containing media, coverslip discs are pretreated by overnight washing with sulfochromic acid (30 g $K_2Cr_2O_7$, 100 mL H_2O, and 900 mL H_2SO4), followed by numerous washes with double-distilled water (ddH_2O). It is critical all acid is removed by thorough washing, and overnight washing in ddH_2O is recommended. Discs are then washed with 70% ethanol, 100% ethanol, and are finally sterilized overnight at 180°C in a hybridization oven *(33)*.
2. 3% pFA fixative: note that properly prepared and stored fixative is critical for good immunofluorescence results. To prepare 100 mL solution, heat 75 mL (75% of final volume) ddH_2O to 50°C. Add 3 g pFA while stirring the water. Slowly add 1 N NaOH while dissolving the pFA, keeping the pH under 7.4. Continue stirring until full solubilization of pFA is achieved. Allow solution to cool at room temperature. Add 5X PBS (20% of final volume) while stirring, and adjust pH if necessary. Add, drop-by-drop, $CaCl_2$ solution to final concentration of 0.1 mM, and $MgCl_2$ to final concentration of 1 mM. The final volume is 100 mL; store in aliquots at –20°C.
3. Immu-mount (Shandon).
4. Antibodies (see above).
5. Rhodamine-conjugated AffiniPure goat anti-rabbit IgG (H+L) (Jackson ImmunoResearch Laboratories).

2.5.4. Immuno-Electron Microscopy

1. Na-cacodylate buffer: Stock 0.4 M (4X) solution contains 21.4 g Na(CH$_3$)2AsO$_2$ · 3H$_2$O in distilled water to make 250 mL.
2. LR White resin, medium grade (London Resin Co., Bassingstoke, UK).
3. Gelatin capsules, size 3 (EMS, Fort Washington, PA).

4. Ultratome 3 (LKB, Stockholm, Sweden).
5. Nickel grids (300 square mesh, Agar Scientific, Stansted, UK) coated with 1% parlodion in amyl acetate (EMS).
6. Goat serum.
7. Tris-HCl/Tween-20 buffer: Tris-HCl/Tween-20 containing 0.9% NaCl, 10 mM Tris-HCl, pH 8.2, and 0.1% Tween-20.
8. Antiserum Incubation Buffer: Tris-HCl/Tween-20, as in **step 7**.
9. 1% aqueous uranyl acetate and lead citrate.
10. Philips Technai 12 electron microscope (Eindhoven, The Netherlands) equipped with MegaView camera (Soft Imaging System GmbH, Munster, Germany), or any other transmission electron microscope available.

2.6. Promoter Analysis

1. Lipofectamine PLUS reagent (Gibco-BRL, Gaithersburg, MD).
2. Tris buffer for CAT assay cell extraction: 0.25 M Tris, pH 7.5.
3. Passive lysis buffer (PLB) (E1910, Promega, Madison, WI).
4. Dual Luciferase Assay System (Promega).
5. Buffer A: 400 mM KCl, 10 mM NaH$_2$PO$_4$ (pH 7.4), 10% glycerol, 1 mM EDTA, 1 mM dithiothreitol (DTT), 5 mM NaF, 1 mM sodium ortho-vanadate, and 1% v/v protease inhibitor cocktail (Sigma, P8340). DTT, NaF, Na vanadate, and protease inhibitor should be freshly added immediately before use.
6. Binding assay buffer: 100 mM KCl, 15 mM Tris-HCl (pH 7.5), 10 mM DTT, 1 mM EDTA, 12% glycerol, and 0.5 µg poly(dI-dC).
7. Klenow fragment (Promega Corp.).
8. [α-^{32}P] dCTP (Amersham Pharmacia Biotech, Little Chalfont, UK).
9. TBE running buffer: 50 mM Tris, 50 mM boric acid, and 10 mM EDTA (pH 8.3).
10. Econo-grind homogenizer (25–100 lambda; Radnoti, Glass Technology, Arcadia, CA, USA) or 1 mL Dounce homogenizer (Wheaton, Millville, NJ).

3. Methods

3.1. Hormonal Hyperstimulation of Mice

1. 100 µL of PMSG stock (5 U/mouse) is injected intraperitoneally (ip) at 1000–1200 h and 50 h later, 100 µL hCG (4 U/mouse) is injected ip.
2. Immediately after hCG injection, the F1 mice are placed for mating, with one male and one female per cage.
3. The following morning, mice are separated by 0700–0800 h and females exhibiting vaginal plug are considered day 0.5 of pregnancy at 1200 h.

3.2. Preparation of Trophoblast Giant Cells (Dissection and Isolation)

1. On day 9.5 pc, mice are sacrificed by CO$_2$ euthanasia and cervical dislocation.
2. Uterine horns are surgically removed from pregnant mice, and placed in prewarmed (37°C) sterile media. Implantation sites are separated by scalpel knife and the myometrial layers are removed by gentle pulling with a pair of No. 4

forceps. This is performed under a binocular microscope with uteri placed in a 60-mm Petri dish filled with complete DMEM-F12 medium.

3. Isolated implantation sites are transferred to a new Petri dish with prewarmed complete DMEM-F12 medium and are cut in half longitudinally, transverse to uterus, as shown in **Fig. 1A**. The embryo and amniotic sac are gently removed with forceps.

4. The inner layers of the trophoblast giant cells are gently scraped from the decidua with a small round-tip spatula. It is easiest to start scraping from the thicker, spongy-looking region of the labyrinthine layer toward the thinner anti-mesometrial region. Trophoblast cells are put in a new petri dish with prewarmed complete DMEM-F12 medium. At this stage, the cells can be further dissociated for culture or extracted for various assays, such as time zero analyses by electromobility shift assay (EMSAs), reverse-transcription (RT)-polymerase chain reaction (PCR), and Western blots. This cell preparation is slightly contaminated with decidual cells (10%) from the decidua capsularis or decidua basalis.

5. Trophoblast giant cells collected from 20 sites are placed in 1 mL of complete DMEM-F12 medium in a 1.5-mL Eppendorf tube. After a few min at room temperature, the medium supernatant is carefully aspirated (use of Gilson pipet is recommended) and the tissue pieces are washed once with serum-free medium.

6. Add 1 mL cell dissociation medium per Eppendorf. Place tube in 37°C for 5 min. Pipette up and down gently (approximately five to seven times) with a 1-mL Gilson pipet, mounted with a tip precut to make the hole wider (~1.5 mm). Avoid making bubbles, as bubbles indicate cellular damage and protein denaturation.

7. Repeat this protocol for an additional two to three times by incubating the tube for 5- to 7-min intervals at 37°C and pipetting with cut Gilson tips, which are gradually made narrower by cutting less of the tip end (*see* **Note 3**).

8. After most cells are dissociated, transfer the cell suspension into a 15-mL conical polypropylene tube with screw closure filled with 14 mL complete DMEM-F12 medium to stop trypsinization by the serum proteins.

9. Centrifuge cells at 200g for 2 min in a swinging rotor head (room temperature).

10. Discard supernatant and resuspend the cells in the desired volume of complete DMEM-F12 medium (*see* **Note 4**). An additional wash is possible but not necessary.

11. Plate 50–200 µL of cells in 24- or 12-well plates, precoated overnight with 0.5 or 1.0 mL complete DMEM-F12 medium, respectively. When planned for immunofluorescence studies, the cells are seeded on round coverslips (prepared as noted in Materials) placed and precoated in the same culture wells (*see* **Note 5**).

12. Maintain cells in a humidified incubator with 5% CO_2/95% air at 37°C (*see* **Note 6**).

3.3. Hormone Assays

3.3.1. Thin-Layer Chromatography

Enzyme activity is determined by measuring the conversion of [7-^{3}H]-pregnenolone to ^{3}H-progesterone by the cultured cells *(37)*.

1. Trophoblast giant cells (~100) in a single 24-well are enough and on the morning after seeding, radioactive pregnenolone (1 μM) is added to the culture medium (0.5 mL) in the absence or presence of cyanoketone (5 $\mu g/mL$).
2. One hour later, the cells are lysed by adding ethanol (final concentration 20%) and the total content of the steroids is extracted with 5 vol of ether. The duration of the incubation can be varied if the metabolism of pregnenolone >80% is too slow.
3. Thin-layer chromatography (TLC) of the extracted ^3H-steroid products is performed using nonlabeled authentic pregnenolone and progesterone (5 μg each) as internal standard markers. In the past, we used to cut each experimental lane into 50 fractions and present the radioactivity in each fraction as a percent of total cpm in the entire lane *(18)*. Alternatively, if Bio-Imaging analyzer is available with a ^3H Bio-Imaging plate, the radioactivity on the TLC plate can be quantitated with ease. Thereafter, authentic progesterone is viewed on the fluorescent TLC plate under ultraviolet (UV) light (254 nm), while pregnenolone is located after spraying with 40% H_2SO_4 in water containing 5% potassium dichromate and heating 1 min on a hot plate *(38)*.

3.3.2. Immunoassays

Steroid accumulation can also be measured from the conditioned medium or cell extracts by immunoassays. A variety of immunoassays for steroids are commercially available.

3.4. Assays of Gene Expression

3.4.1. Semi-Quantitative RT-PCR (mRNA Levels)

1. Total RNA from a single well or duplicate wells of a 24-well plate is extracted in 0.15 mL of RNAzol B according to the manufacturer's instructions. Note that if carrying out a time-dependent experiment, remnants of RNAzol in the well must be washed very carefully; otherwise, upon replacing the plate for further incubation at 37°C, the vapors of the remaining RNAzol in the formerly harvested wells can lyse the cells in neighboring wells. Alternatively, a different culture plate can be used for each time point planned. Approximately 1–1.5 μg of RNA can be obtained from a typical giant cell culture (approx 100–150 cells in a 24-well well).
2. Semiquantitative radioactive RT-PCR analysis of total RNA extracts is performed as described in detail elsewhere *(34,39)*. Primer sequences for RT-PCR determination of rat P450scc, mouse/rat StAR, mouse 3βHSD type VI, mouse P45017α and ribosomal protein L19 (internal control) mRNAs have been previously described *(18,39)*. The PCR reaction is carried out for 20 cycles, and dried gels can be quantified using a PhosphorImager. The radioactivity in each PCR band is normalized to the radioactivity of the L19 band. Gels can also be exposed to *RX* medical X-ray film for 2–16 h at –70°C and developed by a Curix 60 film processor.

3.4.2. Western Blotting (Protein Levels)

Cells are extracted by RIPA lysis buffer and analyzed by SDS-polyacrylamide gel electrophoresis (PAGE) (5–10 µg protein/lane) and electroblotting procedures as previously described *(34)*. Specific signals can be detected by chemiluminescence using the LumiGlo substrate. Enhanced chemiluminescence (ECL) signals recorded on x-ray film can be scanned and analyzed by a relative semi-quantitative approach using National Institutes of Health (NIH) Image Program (available on the Internet at http://rsb.info.nih.gov/nih-image/).

3.5. Visualization of RNA and Protein Expression

3.5.1. In Situ Hybridization

3.5.1.1. ANALYSIS USING PARAFFIN SECTIONS

1. Uteri are removed and fixed for 12 h at room temperature in freshly prepared 4% pFA solution.
2. Following embedding in paraffin, 7-µm sections are cut and mounted on microscope slides.
3. After air-drying for 1 h at 37°C, slides are stored at –20°C until further use.
4. Slides are deparaffinized by heating to 60°C for 1 h, followed by two changes of xylenes (10 min each), two washes in ethanol, and rehydration by consecutive 2 min immersions in ethanol solutions in PBST (100%, 75%, 50%, 25%, and 0%).
5. Thereafter, slides are treated at room temperature with 10 µg/mL proteinase K in PBST for 15 min, followed by one wash in 2 mg/mL glycine PBST and two washes with PBST (5 min).
6. Prehybridization is performed by incubation with prehybridization buffer (200 µL/slide). Slides are incubated for 1 h at 60°C.
7. Hybridization is performed by overnight incubation at 60°C in prehybridization buffer containing 10 µg/mL probe (5' biotinylated, 2'-*O*-methyl-RNA probe).
8. Posthybridization washes (30 min) are performed as follows: first, two room-temperature washes in Solution 1, and then two washes in Solution 2 performed at 60°C (30 min). Finally, slides are washed three times (room temperature) in Solution 3. The last wash is performed for 60 min in blocking solution (1% skim milk in Solution 3).
9. The bound probe is detected by strepavidin-alkaline phosphatase conjugate using ELF *(18)*.

3.5.1.2. ANALYSIS USING FROZEN SECTIONS

We have also successfully used frozen sections and a ^{35}S-labeled riboprobe approach *(19)*. *In situ* hybridization is performed, with modifications, according to the procedure by Hogan et al. *(40)*.

1. Tissues are removed and fixed in 4% pFA in PBS overnight at 4°C. Fixed tissue is incubated overnight in 0.5 *M* sucrose in PBS and embedded in Tissue-Tek OCT.

2. Cryostat 10μm sections are cut at –20°C using a Reichert Jung Frigocut 2000 cryostat. Sections are collected onto poly-L-lysine coated glass slides.
3. Sections are air dried, fixed in 4% pFA for 20 min, dehydrated in serial ethanol solutions (30–100%) and stored in vacuum at –20°C until hybridization.
4. Prior to hybridization, sections are treated in the following solutions: 20 min in 0.2 M HCl, 5 min in ddH$_2$O, 30 min in 2X SCC at 70°C, 5 min in ddH$_2$O, 10 min in 50 mM Tris-HCl, pH 7.5 containing 0.125 mg/mL pronase and 2 mM EDTA, 10 min in 0.2% glycine in PBS, 20 min in 4% pFA, 10 min in 0.25% acetic anhydride in 0.1 M triethanolamine pH 8.0, and finally dehydrated in graded ethanol solutions in PBST (25%, 50%, 75%, 100%).
5. Hybridization is performed in a humidified box at 50°C for 18 h in the following solution: 50% formamide, 0.3 M NaCl, 10% dextran sulfate, 1X Denhardt's solution, 1 mg/mL tRNA, 10 mM DTT, 5 mM EDTA, and 2×10^8 cpm/mL of ^{35}S-labeled riboprobe.
6. Hybridization sections are washed under stringent conditions including 50% formamide/0.3 M NaCl, treated for 30 min in 20 μg/mL RNase I-A at 37°C, and dehydrated through serial concentrations of ethanol.
7. Autoradiography is performed using NTB-2 emulsion at 4°C for 3 d. Toluidine blue (0.05% in water) is used for counterstaining. Thereafter, a glass coverslip is mounted with Immu-mount.
8. Photography is performed using Nikon Labophot-2 microscope equipped with AFX-II camera system. Kodak T-max 400 ASA film is used.

3.5.2. Enzyme-Linked Immunohistochemistry

1. Uterine horns are removed, trimmed free of fat, and fixed overnight at 4°C in 4% pFA in PBS.
2. Paraffin embedding and sectioning (6 μm) is performed according to standard procedures.
3. Sections are deparaffinized by heating to 58°C for 15 min, followed by an immediate immersion into xylene and two changes of the organic solvent (5 min each).
4. Rehydration is performed by washing in ethanol (twice) and consecutive 2-min immersions in 100%, 90%, and 80% ethanol, followed by a 30-s rinse in running water.
5. Finally, slides are transferred to PBST and washed twice.
6. A drop of 1:50 dilution of the first antibody (anti-P450scc or anti-3βHSD) in PBST is overlayed upon each section for 30 min incubation, followed by three washes in PBST (5 min each).
7. The biotinylated second antibody is similarly incubated and washed as above.
8. Finally, detection of the antigen can be based on either streptavidin-alkaline phosphatase conjugate using ELF kit, or based on ExtrAvidin-peroxidase using DAB as a substrate *(18)*.

3.5.3. Immunofluorescence

1. After 1–4 d in culture, monolayers plated onto glass disc coverslips are washed with PBS, fixed in 3% pFA PBS solution (20 min) and washed twice with PBS.

2. Neutralization of aldehyde residues is recommended by treating the fixed cells with 0.1 *M* glycine in PBS (10 min).
3. For visualization of intra-mitochondrial antigens (P450scc, StAR), cells are permeabilized in 1% Triton X-100 (4 min, room temperature), and washed with PBS (three times for 5 min). For visualization of cytoplasmic antigens (3βHSD), 0.1% Triton X-100 is sufficient.
4. Cells are immunofluorescently stained by incubation with primary antibody in PBST (30 min), washes with PBST (three times for 5 min), incubated with second antibody (30 min), and finally washed in PBST (three times for 5 min).
5. Repeated washings by changing PBST in the wells with discs are serially done with aid of an automatic pipet. Note to never let the cell monolayer dry in between the repeated PBST suction and refill. Never dispense the liquid directly on the cells, but rather on the well wall. Substantial savings of antiserum can be achieved by placing a 20- to 30 µL drop of primary or secondary diluted antiserum (1:50 and 1:20, respectively) on a sheet of parafilm stretched over a petri dish or cell culture plate lid, and setting the culture disc face down onto the antibody solution.
6. At the end of the incubation, the disc is returned to the culture well for further washing. Shearing damage can be avoided by gently injecting 100 µL of PBST underneath the glass disc, thus floating the disc on the aqueous cushion and then picking it up with forceps to return it to the dish for further washings.
7. Following the staining procedure, discs are then mounted (in Immu-mount™ or 90% glycerol in PBS) onto slides for microscopic analysis.

3.5.4. Immuno-Electron Microscopy

1. Intact uteri, trimmed free of fat and cut in small fragments (1 mm^3), are fixed in freshly prepared PBS, or 0.1 *M* Na-cacodylate buffer, containing 0.1–1.0% EM-grade glutaraldehyde and 3% pFA. If immuno-electron microscopy is performed using cultured cells, it is not recommended to exceed 0.05% glutaraldehyde.
2. After overnight incubation at 4°C, preparation of the tissue blocks in LR White resin is performed as follows: tissue is washed in PBS and dehydrated in a graded series of alcohols (10%, 25%, 50% 70%). Then, the nonosmicated (*see* **Note 7**) fragments are infiltrated with LR white resin and then placed in gelatin capsules for polymerization at 50°C for 24 h.
3. Thin, 70-nm sections are cut with an Ultratome 3 and collected on coated nickel grids.
4. Prior to incubation with antiserum, nonspecific antigenic sites are blocked by incubation for 5 min at room temperature with normal goat serum (1:100 dilution) in antiserum incubation buffer.
5. The sections are incubated overnight (4°C) with 1:20 dilution of rabbit anti-P450scc serum in antiserum incubation buffer, followed by incubation with 1:10 dilution of gold-labeled goat anti-rabbit IgG.
6. The size of the gold particles can vary between 5 and 18 nm, as required.
7. Finally, the sections are stained with 1.0% aqueous uranyl acetate and lead citrate and counter-examined by transmission electron microscope.

3.6. Promoter Analysis

3.6.1. Transfection

1. On the morning after seeding of cells, each well in 24-well plate is transfected with 250 ng DNA using Lipofectamine PLUS reagent (*see* **Note 8**) in serum-free medium according to the manufacturer's instructions.
2. Three hours after the onset of transfection, the cells are placed into the equivalent of complete DMEM-F12 medium, by adding medium with twice the concentration of serum and antibiotics.
3. On the next morning, the cells are washed, and fresh complete DMEM-F12 medium is added. Cells are left for another 24 h, and then collected for assay (*see* **Note 9**).

3.6.2. Assay

1. For CAT assays, 2 wells of a 24-well plate, containing the equivalent of two implantation sites, are necessary. Cells are extracted in 30 μL Tris CAT assay extraction buffer per well. For luciferase assays, one well of a 24-well plate is sufficient. The cells are extracted in 60 μL PLB by active scraping and one freeze–thaw cycle. The protein extract is usually sufficient for one CAT assay or for three to five luciferase assays.
2. CAT assay results are normalized by protein quantification by the Bradford method *(32,41)*. Luciferase results are normalized by Renilla luciferase readings (50 ng pRL3-null, Promega, DNA is included in each transfected well), and assays are performed according to the manufacturer's protocol (Dual Luciferase Assay System, Promega).

3.7. Electromobility Shift Assay Analysis

3.7.1. Lysate Preparation

Because the isolated giant cells provide relatively small amounts of tissue material, we recommend preparation of whole cell lysates, which we have successfully adopted for EMSA studies *(32,42,43)*, instead of nuclear extracts (*see* **Note 10**).

1. Cells are homogenized using a miniature Econo-Grind or Dounce homogenizer in 3–4 vol of buffer A, transferred into an Eppendorf tube, and the protein slurry is freeze–thawed three times in liquid nitrogen and a 37°C bath.
2. Cell lysates are then centrifuged for 3 min at 14,000g, and the protein content in the supernatants is determined by a modified Bradford assay *(41)*. Extracts can be kept at –70°C until use.

3.7.2. Assay

1. Protein extracts (10–30 μg) are incubated with 2–5 ng of double-stranded DNA previously labeled by a fill-in reaction using Klenow fragment and [α-^{32}P]-dCTP.

2. The binding assay is performed using a final volume of 30 µL containing binding assay buffer.
3. After incubation for 35 min at room temperature, the binding products are resolved on a native prerun polyacrylamide gel (5%) using 0.5X TBE running buffer.
4. When competition experiments are conducted, the protein extract should be added last to the reaction mixture. When antibodies are used for detection of a given protein–DNA complex, the reaction cocktail without the probe is preincubated with 2–8 µg of the antibody for 25 min at room temperature before addition of the labeled DNA.
5. The dried gels can be analyzed using a Bio-Imaging analyzer. Gels can also be exposed to X-ray film for 2–24 h at –70°C and subsequently developed.

4. Notes

1. Normally, over 80% of hyperstimulated females become pregnant in each treatment cycle. However, during some times of the year, we have noticed periods of low fecundity, the cause of which is unknown. Therefore, it is also possible to use timed pregnant female mice without hormonal hyperstimulation. Timed pregnant mice can be ordered from the local animal breeder. These mice have a reduced number of implantation sites per uterine horn. On the other hand, hormone hyperstimulation frequently yields smaller, and often degenerate, sites. In other words, inherent imperfections are typical of each of the mating protocols, but we have not noticed any apparent differences in the giant cell function.
2. It is also possible to use regular DMEM medium without F12. In this case, no HEPES buffer is added to the serum-containing medium.
3. The dissociation of trophoblast giant cells must be performed extremely gently. Allow enough time for trypsinization (two to three 5-min rounds at 37°C) before attempting to pass cells up and down through the uncut 1-mL pipet tip. Giant cells are very large and, therefore, fragile and can be damaged upon harsh shearing force. When most of the cells seem to have dissociated, proceed to the next step.
4. We usually resuspend so as to add 100 µL per well, and calculate the plating ratio to be about one implantation site per well of a 24-well plate.
5. Approximately one implantation site is needed per 24 wells to ensure a sufficient population of giant cells. One well yields approx 30 µg protein in RIPA extract for Western, 1–1.5 µg RNA, 10 µg cell extract in buffer A for EMSA, 0.2–0.5 µg protein in Tris extract for CAT analysis, and 0.5–1.0 µg PLB extract for luciferase analysis. Pooling of two to three wells is recommended to ensure enough extract, if needed.
6. If the affect of cAMP is to be monitored, cells should be washed and placed in serum-free medium, and 8-Br-cAMP (0.5 m*M*) is added 5 h later.
7. To maximally preserve antigenicity during processing of the tissue for immuno-electron microscopy, high pFA and low glutaraldehyde are used during fixation. For tissue pieces, 0.1–1.0% glutaraldehyde is used; higher concentrations result in better preservation of the ultrastructural details, but a loss of antigenicity. Cell

monolayers tolerate no more than 0.05% of glutaraldehyde. Also, postfixation in osmium tetroxide fixation and staining is omitted and the infiltrated plastic is hydrophilic LR White, or LR Gold, which polymerizes at a relatively low temperature (70°C). Consequently, lipid droplets and membrane phospholipids are not visible in this procedure *(18,36)*, as demonstrated in **Fig. 1E,E₁**. Because of these procedural considerations, immuno-electron microscopic analysis generally does not yield as high a resolution of ultrastructural details as standard electron microscopy.

8. We have tried several transfection methods (Lipofectamine, Lipofectamine PLUS, calcium phosphate, PEI) and have found Lipofectamine PLUS to be by far the most efficient.

9. In our experience, the trophoblast giant cell culture seems to represent a rather heterogeneous population of cells in both their expression of differentiated functions and their responses to treatments. This reflects a limitation in the culture system along with a limited amount of tissue material. For example, we have received high variability in transfection efficiency, so a high number of replicates must be performed to achieve statistical significance. This is true regardless of transfection vector (CAT, luciferase) or normalization (protein concentration, Renilla luciferase). The variability in transfection efficiency probably reflects cell-specific differences in expression of the genes under study. For example, we have previously shown that the levels of StAR vary tremendously in a cluster of giant cells, regardless of their size and the expected differences in their DNA content *(31)*. In addition, trophoblast giant cells in culture undergo time-dependent changes in gene expression. For example, P450scc expression is reduced over several days in culture. We could not tell whether this reflects a timed loss of their steroidogenic capacities, as occurs in vivo beyond day 10.5 of mouse pregnancy *(18,19)*, or results from the removal of cells from their physiological milieu. Altogether, these variations in the expression of differentiated functions suggest that care must be taken in the interpretation of results obtained from ex vivo giant cell cultures.

10. Preparation of cellular extracts instead of nuclear extracts is practically required for EMSA studies when only 100–200 giant cells are available for each treatment. We found the cellular extract protocol much easier to perform, highly reliable, and free of any unwanted artifacts related to degradation of the DNA probes, degradation of the transcription factors, or any irregular pattern of protein–DNA complex separation on the native PAGE gels.

Acknowledgments

We thank Drs. D. B. Hales and K. H. Hales for the anti-StAR serum. The authors would like to thank the following people for their contribution in the development of the procedures associated with the analyses of steroidogenic rodent trophoblast giant cells: Rachel Schiff, Jonathan Arensburg, Micha Ben-Zimra, Moriah Koler, Rina Timberg, and Naomi Melamed-Book. This work was supported by the Israel Science Foundation grant 592/03.

References

1. Csapo, A. I., Pulkkinen, M. O. and Wiest, W. G. (1973) Effects of luteectomy and progesterone replacement therapy in early pregnant patients. *Am. J. Obstet. Gynecol.* **115,** 759–765.
2. Finn, C. A. and Martin, L. (1974) The control of implantation. *J. Reprod. Fertil.* **39,** 195–206.
3. Pepe, G. J. and Albrecht, E. D. (1995) Actions of placental and fetal adrenal steroid hormones in primate pregnancy. *Endocr. Rev.* **16,** 608–648.
4. Pepe, G. J. and Rothchild, I. (1973) Metabolic clearance rate of progesterone: comparison between ovariectomized, pregnant, pseudopregnant and deciduoma-bearing pseudopregnant rats. *Endocrinology* **93,** 1200–1205.
5. Psychoyos, A. (1973) Hormonal control of ovoimplantation. *Vitam. Horm.* **31,** 201–256.
6. Strauss, J. F., 3rd., Martinez, F., and Kiriakidou, M. (1996) Placental steroid hormone synthesis: unique features and unanswered questions. *Biol. Reprod.* **54,** 303–311.
7. Albrecht, E. D. and Pepe, G. J. (1990) Placental steroid hormone biosynthesis in primate pregnancy. *Endocr. Rev.* **11,** 124–150.
8. Goldring, N. B., Durica, J. M., Lifka, J., et al. (1987) Cholesterol side-chain cleavage P450 messenger ribonucleic acid: evidence for hormonal regulation in rat ovarian follicles and constitutive expression in corpora lutea. *Endocrinology* **120,** 1942–1950.
9. Hall, P. F. (1984) Cellular organization for steroidogenesis. *Int. Rev. Cytol.* **86,** 53–95.
10. Miller, W. L. (1988) Molecular biology of steroid hormone synthesis. *Endocrine Rev.* **9,** 295–317.
11. Stocco, D. M. (2001) Tracking the role of a star in the sky of the new millennium. *Mol. Endocrinol.* **15,** 1245–1254.
12. Yamamoto, T., Chapman, B. M., Johnson, D. C., Givens, C. R., Mellon, S. H., and Soares, M. J. (1996) Cytochrome P450 17 alpha-hydroxylase gene expression in differentiating rat trophoblast cells. *J. Endocrinol.* **150,** 161–168.
13. Simpson, E. R. and Davis, S. R. (2001) Minireview: aromatase and the regulation of estrogen biosynthesis-some new perspectives. *Endocrinology* **142,** 4589–4594.
14. Durkee, T. J., McLean, M. P., Hales, D. B., et al. (1992) P450$17\alpha$ and P450scc gene expression and regulation in the rat placenta. *Endocrinology* **130,** 1309–1317.
15. Carlone, D. L. and Richards, J. S. (1997) Functional interactions, phosphorylation, and levels of 3',5'-cyclic adenosine monophosphate-regulatory element binding protein and steroidogenic factor-1 mediate hormone-regulated and constitutive expression of aromatase in gonadal cells. *Mol. Endocrinol.* **11,** 292–304.
16. Bain, P. A., Yoo, M., Clarke, T., Hammond, S. H., and Payne, A. H. (1991) Multiple forms of mouse 3β-hydroxysteroid dehydrogenase/Δ5-Δ4 isomerase and differential expression in gonads, adrenal glands, liver, and kidneys of both sexes. *Proc. Natl. Acad. Sci. USA* **88,** 8870–8874.
17. Csapo, A. I. and Wiest, W. G. (1969) An examination of the quantitative relationship between progesterone and the maintenance of pregnancy. *Endocrinology* **85,** 735–746.

18. Arensburg, J., Payne, A. H., and Orly, J. (1999) Expression of steroidogenic genes in maternal and extraembryonic cells during early pregnancy in mice. *Endocrinology* **140,** 5220–5232.

19. Schiff, R., Arensburg, J., Itin, A., Keshet, E., and Orly, J. (1993) Expression and cellular localization of uterine side-chain cleavage cytochrome P450 messenger ribonucleic acid during early pregnancy in mice. *Endocrinology* **133,** 529–537.

20. Sherman, M. I. (1983) in *Biology of Trophoblast* (Loke, Y. W. and Whyte, A., eds.). Elsevier Science Publishers B. V., Amsterdam: pp. 401–467.

21. Hu, M. C., Hsu, N. C., El Hadj, N. B., et al. (2002) Steroid deficiency syndromes in mice with targeted disruption of Cyp11a1. *Mol. Endocrinol.* **16,** 1943–1950.

22. Siiteri, P. K., Febres, F., Clemens, L. E., Chang, R. J., Gondos, B., and Stites, D. (1977) Progesterone and maintenance of pregnancy: is progesterone nature's immunosuppressant? *Ann. N.Y. Acad. Sci.* **286,** 384–397.

23. Abbaszade, I. G., Arensburg, J., Park, C. H., Kasa, V. J., Orly, J., and Payne, A. H. (1997) Isolation of a new mouse 3β-hydroxysteroid dehydrogenase isoform, 3β-HSD VI, expressed during early pregnancy. *Endocrinology* **138,** 1392–1399.

24. Nakayama, H., Scott, I. C., and Cross, J. C. (1998) The transition to endoreduplication in trophoblast giant cells is regulated by the mSNA zinc finger transcription factor. *Dev. Biol.* **199,** 150–163.

25. Zybina, E. V., Zybina, T. G., and Stein, G. I. (2000) Trophoblast cell invasiveness and capability for the cell and genome reproduction in rat placenta. *Early Pregnancy* **4,** 39–57.

26. Varmuza, S., Prideaux, V., Kothary, R., and Rossant, J. (1988) Polytene chromosomes in mouse trophoblast giant cells. *Development* **102,** 127–134.

27. Yamamoto, T., Chapman, B. M., Clemens, J. W., Richards, J. S., and Soares, M. J. (1995) Analysis of cytochrome P-450 side-chain cleavage gene promoter activation during trophoblast cell differentiation. *Mol. Cell. Endocrinol.* **113,** 183–194.

28. Peters, T. J., Chapman, B. M., Wolfe, M. W., and Soares, M. J. (2000) Placental lactogen-I gene activation in differentiating trophoblast cells: extrinsic and intrinsic regulation involving mitogen-activated protein kinase signaling pathways. *J. Endocrinol.* **165,** 443–456.

29. Hamlin, G. P., Lu, X. J., Roby, K. F., and Soares, M. J. (1994) Recapitulation of the pathway for trophoblast giant cell differentiation in vitro: stage-specific expression of members of the prolactin gene family. *Endocrinology* **134,** 2390–2396.

30. Faria, T. N. and Soares, M. J. (1991) Trophoblast cell differentiation: establishment, characterization, and modulation of a rat trophoblast cell line expressing members of the placental prolactin family. *Endocrinology* **129,** 2895–2906.

31. Ben-Zimra, M., Koler, M., Melamed-Book, N., Arensburg, J., Payne, A. H., and Orly, J. (2002) Uterine and placental expression of steroidogenic genes during rodent pregnancy. *Mol. Cell. Endocrinol.* **187,** 223–231.

32. Ben-Zimra, M., Koler, M., and Orly, J. (2002) Transcription of cholesterol side-chain cleavage cytochrome P450 in the placenta: activating protein-2 assumes the role of steroidogenic factor-1 by binding to an overlapping promoter element. *Mol. Endocrinol.* **16,** 1864–1880.

33. Orly, J., Clemens, J. W., Singer, O., and Richards, J .S. (1996) Effects of hormones and protein kinase inhibitors on expression of steroidogenic enzyme promoters in electroporated primary rat granulosa cells. *Biol. Reprod.* **54,** 208–218.

34. Ronen-Fuhrmann, T., Timberg, R., King, S. R., et al. (1998) Spatio-temporal expression patterns of steroidogenic acute regulatory protein (StAR) during follicular development in the rat ovary. *Endocrinology* **139,** 303–315.

35. Hales, K. H., Diemer, T., Ginde, S., et al. (2000) Diametric effects of bacterial endotoxin lipopolysaccharide on adrenal and Leydig cell steroidogenic acute regulatory protein. *Endocrinology* **141,** 4000–4012.

36. Farkash, Y., Timberg, R., and Orly, J. (1986) Preparation of antiserum to rat cytochrome P-450 cholesterol side chain cleavage, and its use for ultrastructural localization of the immunoreactive enzyme by protein A-gold technique. *Endocrinology* **118,** 1353–1365.

37. Bitzur, S. and Orly, J. (1989) Microanalysis of hormone responsive ovarian interstitial gland cells in miniature culture. *Endocrinology* **124,** 1471–1484.

38. Goldring, N. B. and Orly, J. (1985) Concerted metabolism of steroid hormones produced by cocultured ovarian cell types. *J. Biol. Chem.* **260,** 913–921.

39. Orly, J., Rei, Z., Greenberg, N. M., and Richards, J. S. (1994) Tyrosine kinase inhibitor AG18 arrests follicle-stimulating hormone-induced granulosa cell differentiation: use of reverse transcriptase-polymerase chain reaction assay for multiple messenger ribonucleic acids. *Endocrinology* **134,** 2336–2346.

40. Hogan, B., Constantini, F., and Lacy, E. (1986) *Manipulating the Mouse Embryo— A Laboratory Manual* Cold Spring Harbor, NY.

41. Zor, T. and Selinger, Z. (1996) Linearization of the Bradford protein assay increases its sensitivity: theoretical and experimental studies. *Anal. Biochem.* **236,** 302–308.

42. Welte, T., Garimorth, K., Philipp, S., and Doppler, W. (1994) Prolactin-dependent activation of a tyrosine phosphorylated DNA binding factor in mouse mammary epithelial cells. *Mol. Endocrinol.* **8,** 1091–1102.

43. Silverman, E., Eimerl, S., and Orly, J. (1999) CCAAT enhancer-binding protein beta and GATA-4 binding regions within the promoter of the steroidogenic acute regulatory protein (StAR) gene are required for transcription in rat ovarian cells. *J. Biol. Chem.* **274,** 17,987–17,996.

44. Ishii, T., Hasegawa, T., Pai, C., et al. (2002) The roles of circulating high-density lipoproteins and trophic hormones in the phenotype of knockout mice lacking the steroidogenic acute regulatory protein. *Mol. Endocrinol.* **16,** 2297–2309.

19

Establishment of an ELISA for the Detection of Native Bovine Pregnancy-Associated Glycoproteins Secreted by Trophoblast Binucleate Cells

Jonathan A. Green and R. Michael Roberts

Summary

The pregnancy-associated glycoproteins (PAGs) are a large gene family expressed in trophoblast cells of ruminant ungulates. The detection of PAGs in maternal serum has served as the basis for pregnancy detection in ruminant ungulates and also for use as markers of trophoblast development and placental viability. The methods described provide a means for the rapid purification of bovine PAGs by affinity chromatography and the establishment of an enzyme-linked immunosorbent assay (ELISA) to measure PAG concentrations in maternal blood plasma and other biological fluids.

Key Words: Placenta; trophoblast; pregnancy; pregnancy detection; cattle.

1. Introduction

In ruminant ungulates, there are two morphologically distinct trophoblast cell types—mononucleate and binucleate trophoblasts. Binucleate cells (BNC) are a secretory cell type that can first be noted at about the time of definitive cell-to-cell attachment of the trophoblast to the uterine wall (*1*). The BNCs comprise a population of granulated cells that can migrate from the trophecto-derm to fuse with maternal uterine epithelial cells (*2*). Exocytosis of granules occurs from these fused cells toward the underlying maternal capillary beds, allowing BNC products to reach the maternal blood supply (*2–7*). One such product, placental lactogen, is synthesized exclusively by binucleate cells (*5*) as is another protein, pregnancy-associated glycoprotein (PAG)-1 (*8,9*), known also as pregnancy-specific protein B (PSPB) (*10*) and "pregnancy serum protein of M_r 60 kDa" (PSP60) (*11*). Because of its expression by binucleate cells and because it enters the maternal circulation, the detection of PAG-1 has been used as the basis for a useful pregnancy test and as a marker for trophoblast viability and proliferation in ruminant ungulate species (*11–22*).

From: *Methods in Molecular Medicine, Vol. 122: Placenta and Trophoblast: Methods and Protocols, Vol. 2*
Edited by: M. J. Soares and J. S. Hunt © Humana Press Inc., Totowa, NJ

Recent molecular cloning has revealed that PAG-1 actually belongs to a group of related proteins and that the PAGs comprise a rather large gene family expressed in bovine, ovine, and caprine placentas *(23–25)*. To date, 21 distinct full-length cDNA representing bovine (bo) PAG members have been cloned from cattle, but in all likelihood, there are many more *(24,25)*.

The PAGs belong to the aspartic proteinase family *(8)*. However, molecular modeling suggested that some PAGs are unable to act as proteinases as a result of unusual amino acid substitutions around the catalytic center *(24–26)*. Possibly, these PAGs are not functional proteinases, but instead have another role, such as peptide binding. Many PAGs, for example, are able to bind the aspartic proteinase inhibitor, pepstatin, and preliminary data from our laboratories have indicated that they do so with differing affinities *(27)*.

Phylogenetic analysis demonstrated that the PAGs of cattle, sheep, and goats can be subdivided into ones of ancient origin (arising >87 MYA) and ones that duplicated more recently (≤52 MYA) *(24,28)*. *In situ* hybridization studies indicated that the recently evolved PAGs, those related to PAG-1, were expressed only in binucleate cells of the cotyledonary trophoblast, whereas members of the ancient group, typified by boPAG-2, were expressed by both mononucleate and binucleate trophoblasts *(24)*. Interestingly, the bovine PAG family can be rapidly fractionated into ancient and BNC-specific PAGs based on their differential affinities for pepstatin. This observation was used to purify a mixture of BNC-PAGs and to establish a simple enzyme-linked immunosorbent assay (ELISA) for the detection of these proteins in the maternal sera of pregnant cows and heifers.

The methods section in this chapter describes: (1) The rapid isolation of bovine BNC-specific PAGs from cotyledonary extracts or from conditioned medium by using pepstatin affinity chromatography, and (2) the biotinylation of anti-PAG antibodies and their use in the establishment of a simple ELISA for the detection of PAGs in maternal serum, allantoic fluid, trophoblast cell culture media, and so on. The ELISA design described here employs a rabbit polyclonal antibody to trap PAGs in the wells of a 96-well ELISA plate. Biotinylated anti-PAG polyclonal rabbit antibody is then bound to the immobilized PAG. The entire complex is then detected by using alkaline phosphatase (AP)-conjugated avidin (or an avidin derivative) in conjunction with the AP substrate, para-nitrophenyl phosphate.

2. Materials

2.1. Purification of Pregnancy-Associated Glycoproteins

2.1.1. Cotyledon Extract Production

1. Cotyledon homogenization buffer: 10 mM phosphate, pH 7.0, 150 mM NaCl, 5 mM ethylenediamine tetraacetic acid (EDTA), 0.2 mM phenylmethylsulfonylfluoride (PMSF), 0.02% w/v NaN$_3$.

2. Dialysis buffer A: 20 mM Tris-HCl, pH 8.3, 1 M NaCl, 1 mM EDTA, 0.2 mM PMSF, 0.02% NaN$_3$, and 0.1 mM 2-mercaptoethanol.
3. Dialysis buffer B: 20 mM Tris, pH 7.0, 0.15 M NaCl, 1 mM EDTA, 0.2 mM PMSF, 0.02% NaN$_3$, 0.1 mM 2-mercaptoethanol.

2.1.2. Production of Cotyledon-Conditioned Medium

1. Cotyledon culture medium: Dulbecco's modified Eagle's medium (DMEM) containing penicillin (100 U/mL), streptomycin (100 µg/mL), and fungizone (0.5 µg/mL).
2. Dialysis Buffer A (see above).
3. Dialysis Buffer B (see above).

2.1.3. Pepstatin-Affinity Purification of PAGs

1. Pepstatin A-Agarose (Sigma Chemical Company, St. Louis, MO).
2. Pepstatin A-Agarose equilibration buffer: 20 mM Tris-HCl, pH 7.0, 0.15 M NaCl, 1 mM EDTA, 0.2 mM PMSF, 0.02% NaN$_3$, 0.1 mM 2-mercaptoethanol.
3. Wash buffer: 20 mM Tris-HCl, pH 7.0, 1 M NaCl, 1 mM EDTA, 0.2 mM PMSF, 0.02% NaN$_3$, 0.1 mM 2-mercaptoethanol, 1% Triton X-100.
4. Elution buffer: 20 mM Tris-HCl, pH 9.5, 1 M NaCl, 1 mM EDTA, 0.2 mM PMSF, 0.02% NaN$_3$, 0.1 mM 2-mercaptoethanol, 1% Triton X-100.
5. Dialysis buffer C: 20 mM citrate, pH 5.0, 0.15 M NaCl, 1 mM EDTA, 0.2 mM PMSF, 0.02% NaN$_3$, and 0.1 mM 2-mercaptoethanol.
6. High salt/detergent wash buffer: 20 mM citrate, pH 5.0, 1 M NaCl, 1 mM EDTA, 0.2 mM PMSF, 0.02% NaN$_3$, 0.1 mM 2-mercaptoethanol, 1% Triton X-100.
7. Elution Buffer A: 20 mM Tris-HCl, pH 7.0, 1 M NaCl, 1 mM EDTA, 0.2 mM PMSF,0.02% NaN$_3$, 0.1 mM 2-mercaptoethanol, 1% Triton X-100.
8. Elution buffer B: 20 mM Tris-HCl, pH 9.5, 1 M NaCl, 1 mM EDTA, 0.2 mM PMSF, 0.02% NaN$_3$, 0.1 mM 2-mercaptoethanol, 1% Triton X-100.

2.2. An ELISA for the Detection of PAGs

2.2.1. Production of Anti-PAG Antibodies Purified PAGs.

2.2.2. Purification and Biotinylation of Anti-PAG Antibodies

1. NHS-biotin, neutravidin, and Protein A sepharose were obtained from Pierce (Rockford, IL).
2. Dialysis buffer for rabbit serum: 1.5 M NaCl, 100 mM glycine, pH 9.5.
3. Protein A-Sepharose elution buffer: 100 mM sodium citrate, pH 3.0.
4. Dialysis buffer for purified immunoglobulin: 50 mM sodium phosphate, pH 7.5, 100 mM NaCl.
5. Ethanolamine.
6. Dialysis buffer for biotinylated Anti-PAG: 50 mM sodium phosphate, pH 7.5, 100 mM NaCl, 1 mM EDTA, 0.2 mM PMSF, 0.02% NaN$_3$.

2.2.3. ELISA

1. Purified rabbit anti-PAG IgG.
2. Purified PAG.

3. Flat-bottomed 96-well high binding ELISA plates were obtained from Fisher Scientific (Pittsburgh, PA).
4. Blocking solution: 2% ovine serum albumin, 1% nonfat dry milk.
5. ELISA wash buffer: 0.15 M NaCl, 0.05% Tween-20.
6. Alkaline Phosphatase (AP)-conjugated neutravidin (Pierce).
7. P-nitrophenyl phosphate (PNPP; Sigma).
8. 96-well plate washer (e.g., ELx405, BioTek, Winooski, VT).
9. Spectrophotometric plate reader (e.g., EL808 plate reader; Bio-Tek).

3. Methods

3.1. Purification of Pregnancy-Associated Glycoproteins (see Note 1)

3.1.1. Cotyledon Extract Production

1. Homogenize cotyledons in cotyledon extraction buffer.
2. Centrifuge the extract at 2000–5000g to remove insoluble debris and place the extract inside a 50K molecular weight cut-off (MWCO) membrane and dialyze it two times against approx 40 vol of dialysis buffer A (*see* **Note 2**).
3. Dialyze the extract two times against approx 40 vol of dialysis buffer B to decrease the amount of salt in the extract and to decrease the pH in preparation for binding to pepstatin.
4. Filter the supernatant through a 0.45- or 0.8-μm filter to remove debris and proceed to the affinity purification steps.

3.1.2. Production of Cotyledon-Conditioned Medium

1. Gently separate the cotyledons from the uterine caruncles and the rest of the extra-embryonic membranes as cleanly as possible. Cut the cotyledons into approx 2-mm^3 pieces, rinse them three times in cotyledon culture medium and place them in a humidified incubator at 37°C in 5% CO_2:95% air for 12 h. After the incubation, collect the medium by centrifugation.
2. Dialyze the media as described above for the cotyledonary extracts.

3.1.3. Pepstatin-Affinity Purification of PAGs (see Note 3)

1. Equilibrate 50 mL of pepstatin-agarose in Pepstatin A-Agarose equilibration buffer.
2. Pass the extract through the column two or three times. Wash the column extensively (10–20 column volumes) with the Pepstatin A-Agarose equilibration buffer and then wash the column with approx 10 vol of wash buffer (*see* **Note 4**).
3. Elute the neutral pH-binding PAGs with elution buffer possessing a higher pH to regenerate the matrix (*see* **Note 5**).
4. Isolation of the acidic pH-binding PAGs involves dialysis of the *flow-through* from the pH 7.0 pepstatin column two times against approx 40 vol of dialysis buffer C. Remove precipitated proteins by centrifugation and filtration and check the pH of the solution to confirm that it is 5.0 ± 0.1.

5. Equilibrate the pepstatin–agarose matrix in the same buffer as the protein extract/ media (*see* **Note 6**) and pass the protein solution through the column two to three times, then wash the column extensively (10–20 column volumes) with the equilibration buffer followed by a high salt/detergent wash buffer.
6. Elute the bound PAG by increasing the pH of the buffer in a stepwise fashion. Collect 5- to 8-mL fractions during the first three column volumes of each step (*see* **Note 7**). Wash the column with elution buffer A and elution buffer B for 10 column volumes each.
7. Analyze the fractions by protein quantitation and sodium dodecyl sulfate (SDS)-polyacrylamide gel electrophoresis (PAGE), to identify those fractions containing PAG (*see* **Note 8**).

3.2. An ELISA for the Detection of PAGs

3.2.1. Production of Anti-PAG Antibodies

The PAGs affinity purified as described above can be used as antigens for the production of antibodies in rabbits and use as reagents in a PAG ELISA. These approaches are standard and will not be described here. The interested reader can obtain protocols for antibody production in the manual written by Harlow and Lane *(29)*.

3.2.2. Purification and Biotinylation of Anti-PAG Antibodies (see **Note 9**)

1. Dialyze serum obtained from immunized rabbits against 100 vol of dialysis buffer for rabbit serum in 100,000 MWCO tubing overnight at 4°C.
2. Apply the dialyzed serum to a 25-mL protein A-Sepharose column equilibrated in the same buffer and wash the column with 5 to 10 vol of loading buffer.
3. Elute the bound immunoglobulin with three column volumes of Protein A-Sepharose elution buffer and collect approx 5-mL fractions. Include 100 µL of 1 *M* Tris, pH 8.5, in each fraction tube to neutralize the protein solution as it exits the column. The immunoglobulin present in the eluted fractions can be quantified by Bradford assay with rabbit IgG as the standard.
4. Dialyze the purified immunoglobulin five times against 100 vol of dialysis buffer for purified immunoglobulins (*see* **Note 10**).
5. Solubilize 1 mg of NHS-LC-LC-biotin in dimethylsulfoxide and mix this reagent in a 20:1 molar ratio with the purified dialyzed immunoglobulin and allow it to incubate at room temperature for 2 h. Terminate the reaction by adding ethanolamine to a final concentration of 10 m*M* and dialyze the reaction against dialysis buffer for biotinylated anti-PAG (*see* **Note 11**).

3.2.3. ELISA Design

1. Incubate 2 µg (in 100 µL) of purified rabbit anti-PAG IgG in the wells of a 96-well ELISA plate in the presence of 0.1 *M* sodium bicarbonate, pH 9.5 overnight at 4°C. Remove the antibody by inverting the plate and tapping it on a

clean paper towel. Fill the wells with blocking solution and incubate at room temperature for at least 1 h on a rocking platform.

2. Remove the blocking solution and add 100 μL of either bovine sera from pregnant animals or serially diluted PAG standards (in nonpregnant heifer serum) to each duplicate well (*see* **Note 12**). Nonpregnant heifer serum alone should be included in at least a couple wells as a blank. Incubate the plates overnight at 4°C.

3. The following day, remove the serum and wash the wells five times with ELISA wash buffer with a 96-well plate washer. Add 1 μg (in 100 μL) of the biotinylated IgG diluted in blocking solution to each well at room temperature for 1 h.

4. Wash the plate and add 100 μL of AP-conjugated neutravidin diluted 1:2000 in 0.1X blocking solution and incubate the plate at room temperature for 20–30 min. Wash the plate three times with ELISA Wash Buffer and add 100 μL of 1 mg/mL PNPP to each well. After 15–30 min, measure the absorbance at 405 nm in the wells with a spectrophotometric plate reader.

5. Determine the concentration of PAG in the biological sample by comparison with the standard curve.

4. Notes

1. Native PAGs are most easily purified from bovine cotyledons. The source that yields the most protein is cotyledonary extracts. Generally, one can expect approximately 0.5 mg of PAG for each gram of total protein in the cotyledonary extract. Another excellent source of native PAGs can be obtained from explant culture of cotyledons from a mid- to late-stage pregnant uterus. The yield is much less than that from cotyledonary extracts, but the purified PAGs probably more closely resemble those present in the maternal circulation.

2. Dialysis at slightly alkaline pH and high salt was determined empirically to increase binding to pepstatin.

3. The affinity purification scheme shown is a two-step process—binding of PAGs first at neutral pH, elution of the matrix and then binding of PAGs at acidic pH followed by elution. As mentioned in the Introduction, bovine PAGs can be separated into the ancient grouping and the BNC-specific grouping based on the differential binding of bovine PAGs to pepstatin. The ancient PAGs bind predominantly at neutral pH whereas the BNC-specific PAGs predominantly bind under acidic conditions. Most of the PAGs that are detectable in maternal serum are those expressed exclusively in BNCs. Exposing the cotyledonary extracts/media to pepstatin at neutral pH permits the selective removal of ancient PAGs from the final purified PAG preparation, thereby increasing the specificity and utility of the PAG ELISA produced from these reagents. However, this differential binding of PAGs to pepstatin appears to be a feature of *bovine* PAGs. Although different ovine PAG populations also bind to pepstatin under neutral and acidic conditions, the purified PAGs are not as easily segregated into ancient and BNC-specific PAGs as is the case for the bovine PAGs.

4. Washing of the matrix with high salt (1 M NaCl) and detergent 1% Triton X-100 permits the removal of many nonspecifically bound proteins. Some PAGs with only a weak affinity for pepstatin will be eluted by this wash. This material can be collected if these PAGs are of interest to the researcher. However, additional purification work will be required.

5. If the investigator is interested in obtaining those bovine PAGs bound at neutral pH (predominantly ancient PAGs), they can be eluted by increasing the pH in a stepwise fashion or by using a gradient and collecting fractions of the eluted material.

6. It is often a good idea to repack the matrix between the neutral-binding and acidic-binding PAG isolations. The changes in pH can cause the matrix beads to shrink and swell, thereby creating channels through which the buffer preferentially flows. When this occurs, the flow dynamics of the column will become altered and the column will also suffer a decrease in apparent binding capacity.

7. For the high-pH elution buffer (elution buffer B), place 0.2 mL of 1 M Tris, pH 7.0 in each collection tube to neutralize the solution as it is collected so that the purified proteins are exposed to the high pH for as short a time as possible.

8. The protein in each fraction can be determined by measurement of absorbance at 280 nm. The protein present in each elution step can be visualized by staining of SDS-PAGE gels by Coomassie dye. Numerous PAGs will be present in each elution series and will range in M_r between 50,000 and 90,000, with the majority of the proteins migrating at approx 65,000 M_r. Furthermore, in a typical purification scheme, distinct PAG populations will be apparent under each elution condition. Evidence for such different populations will be apparent by the distinct mobilities of each set of proteins by SDS-PAGE.

9. The particular ELISA design described here is a "sandwich" type of assay in which anti-PAG immunoglobulin is used to coat the wells of an ELISA plate. The immunoglobulin binds PAG present within a biological sample and sequesters it in the well. The bound PAG is then reacted with a biotinylated aliquot of the same anti-PAG immunoglobulin and the amount of PAG in each well is determined indirectly by detecting the biotinylated immunoglobulin by using alkaline phosphatase-conjugated neutravidin. The alkaline phosphatase converts the substrate PNPP into the compound, p-nitrophenol, which absorbs strongly at 405 nm.

10. It is critical to remove the Tris buffer and any other compounds containing free amine groups. If not removed, these groups will interfere with the biotinylation reaction, which uses a NHS-ester to conjugate biotin to free amine groups (mainly from lysine residues) on the immunoglobulin.

11. This ratio of NHS-biotin to immunoglobulin generally produces approximately four biotin molecules bound to each IgG molecule—an incorporation rate that works well in this assay design. However, the optimal biotinylation ratio must be determined empirically for each antibody in order to produce a biotinylated reagent that has the greatest possible signal to noise ratio. The specific number of biotins cross-linked to each immunoglobulin can be calculated by using

the 4-hydroxyazobenzene-2-carboxylic acid (HABA) assay marketed by Pierce (Rockford, IL).

12. A standard curve should be generated by using the native bovine PAG isolated by pepstatin affinity chromatography as described previously. The authors use diluted PAG standards that provide a range from 0.039 ng to 40 ng. A line equation can be generated by nonlinear regression of a LOG(ng PAG) vs absorbance plot with software such as Graphpad Prism. Alternatively, a straight line equation can be generated in a spreadsheet such as Excel by graphing the results as LOG(ng PAG std) versus LOG(absorbance). A PAG standard curve should be included on every ELISA plate if space permits.

Acknowledgments

The authors thank Tina Parks, Mary Avalle, and April McLain for their participation in the development of the procedures used to purify PAGs by affinity chromatography and in the establishment of the ELISA for the detection of PAGs. This work was supported by United States Department of Agriculture (USDA) grant 96-35203-3257 and funding from Monsanto Co. and the Missouri Agriculture Experiment Station.

References

1. Wooding, F. B. P. (1983) Frequency and localization of binucleate cells in the placentomes of ruminants. *Placenta* **4,** 527–540.
2. Wooding, F. B. (1992) Current topic: the synepitheliochorial placenta of ruminants: binucleate cell fusions and hormone production. *Placenta* **13,** 101–113.
3. Wooding, F. B., Morgan G., Brandon M. R., and Camous S. (1994) Membrane dynamics during migration of placental cells through trophectodermal tight junctions in sheep and goats. *Cell Tissue Res.* **276,** 387–397.
4. Wooding, F. B., Morgan, G., and Adam, C. L. (1997) Structure and function in the ruminant synepitheliochorial placenta: central role of the trophoblast binucleate cell in deer. *Microsc. Res. Tech.* **38,** 88–99.
5. Wooding, F. B. (1981) Localization of ovine placental lactogen in sheep placentomes by electron microscope immunocytochemistry. *J. Reprod. Fertil.* **62,** 15–19.
6. King, G. J., Atkinson, B. A., and Robertson, H. A. (1982) Implantation and early placentation in domestic ungulates. *J. Reprod. Fertil. Suppl.* **31,** 17–30.
7. King, G. J., Atkinson, B. A., and Robertson, H. A. (1980) Development of the bovine placentome from days 20 to 29 of gestation. *J. Reprod. Fertil.* **59,** 95–100.
8. Xie, S. C., Low, B. G., Nagel, R. J., et al. (1991) Identification of the major pregnancy-specific antigens of cattle and sheep as inactive members of the aspartic proteinase family. *Proc. Natl. Acad. Sci. USA* **88,** 10,247–10,251.
9. Zoli, A. P., Demez, P., Beckers, J.-F., Reznik, M., and Beckers, A. (1992) Light and electron microscopic immunolocalization of bovine pregnancy-associated glycoprotein in the bovine placentome. *Biol. Reprod.* **46,** 623–629.

10. Sasser, R. G., Crock, J., and Ruder-Montgomery, C. A. (1989) Characteristics of pregnancy-specific protein B in cattle. *J. Reprod. Fertil. Suppl.* **37,** 109–113.
11. Mialon, M. M., Renand, G., Camous, S., Martal, J., and Menissier, F. (1994) Detection of pregnancy by radioimmunoassay of a pregnancy serum protein (PSP60) in cattle. *Reprod. Nutr. Dev.* **34,** 65–72.
12. Zoli, A. P., Guilbault, L. A., Delahaut, P., Ortiz, W. B., and Beckers, J.-F. (1992) Radioimmunoassay of a bovine pregnancy-associated glycoprotein in serum: its application for pregnancy diagnosis. *Biol. Reprod.* **46,** 83–92.
13. Sasser, R. G., Ruder, C. A., Ivani, K. A., Butler, J. E., and Hamilton, W. C. (1986) Detection of pregnancy by radioimmunoassay of a novel pregnancy-specific protein in serum of cows and a profile of serum concentrations during gestation. *Biol. Reprod.* **35,** 936–942.
14. Wood, A. K., Short, R. E., Darling, A. E., Dusek, G. L., Sasser, R. G., and Ruder, C. A. (1986) Serum assays for detecting pregnancy in mule and white-tailed deer. *J. Wild Manag.* **50,** 684–687.
15. Willard, S. T., Sasser, R. G., Jaques, J. T., White, D. R., Neuendorff, D. A., and Randel, R. D. (1998) Early pregnancy detection and the hormonal characterization of embryonic-fetal mortality in fallow deer (*Dama dama*). *Theriogenology* **49,** 861–869.
16. Willard, J. M., White, D. R., Wesson, C. A., Stellflug, J., and Sasser, R. G. (1995) Detection of fetal twins in sheep using a radioimmunoassay for pregnancy-specific protein B. *J. Anim. Sci.* **73,** 960–966.
17. Ropstad, E., Johansen, O., King, C., et al. (1999) Comparison of plasma progesterone, transrectal ultrasound and pregnancy specific proteins (PSPB) used for pregnancy diagnosis in reindeer. *Acta Vet. Scand.* **40,** 151–162.
18. Houston, D., Robbins, C., Ruder, C., and Sasser, R. (1986) Pregnancy detection in mountain goats by assay for pregnancy-specific protein B. *J. Wildlife Management* **50,** 740–742.
19. Haigh, J., Gates, C., Ruder, C., and Sasser, R. (1991) Diagnosis of pregnancy in wood bison using a bovine assay for pregnancy-specific protein B. *Theriogeneology* **40,** 905–3911.
20. Haigh, J., Dalton, W., Ruder, C., and Sasser, R. (1993) Diagnosis of pregnancy in moose using a bovine assay for PSPB. *Theriogeneology* **40,** 905–911.
21. Ranilla, M., Sulon, J., Carro, M., Mantecon, A., and Beckers, J.-F. (1994) Plasmatic profiles of pregnancy-associated glycoprotein and progesterone levels during gestation in Churra and Merino sheep. *Theriogenology* **42,** 537–545.
22. Melo de Sousa, N., Zongo, M., Pitala, W., et al. (2002) Pregnancy-associated glycoprotein concentrations during pregnancy and the postpartum period in azawak zebu cattle. *Theriogenology* **59,** 1131–42.
23. Garbayo, J. M., Green, J. A., Mannekin, M., et al. (2000) Caprine pregnancy-associated glycoproteins (PAG): their cloning, expression and evolutionary relationship to other PAG. *Mol. Reprod. Dev.* **57,** 311–322.
24. Green, J.A., Xie, S., Quan, X., et al. (2000) Pregnancy-associated bovine and ovine glycoproteins exhibit spatially and temporally distinct expression patterns during pregnancy. *Biol. Reprod.* **62,** 1624–1631.

25. Xie, S., Green, J., Bixby, J. B., et al. (1997) The diversity and evolutionary relationships of the pregnancy-associated glycoproteins, an aspartic proteinase subfamily consisting of many trophoblast-expressed genes. *Proc. Natl. Acad. Sci. USA* **94,** 12,809–12,816.

26. Guruprasad, K., Blundell, T. L., Xie, S., et al. (1996) Comparative modeling and analysis of amino acid substitutions suggests that the family of pregnancy-associated glycoproteins includes both active and inactive aspartic proteinases. *Protein Eng.* **9,** 849–856.

27. Landon, L. A., McLain, A., Roberts, R. M., and Green, J. A. (1999) Rapid fractionation of pregnancy-associated glycoproteins in placental extracts. *Biol. Reprod.* **60,** 492.

28. Hughes, A. L., Green, J. A., Garbayo, J. M., and Roberts, R. M. (2000) Adaptive diversification within a large family of recently duplicated, placentally-expressed genes. *Proc. Natl. Acad. Sci. USA* **97,** 3319–3323.

29. Harlow, E. and Lane, D. (eds.) (1988) *Antibodies: A laboratory manual.* Cold Spring Harbor Laboratory, Cold Spring Harbor, NY.

20

Alkaline Phosphatase Fusion Proteins as Tags for Identifying Targets for Placental Ligands

Heiner Müller and Michael J. Soares

Summary

In this chapter, we describe protocols for the generation and characterization of alkaline phosphatase–ligand fusion proteins and their use as tools for the identification of specific ligand–receptor interactions.

Key Words: Alkaline phosphatase fusion protein; SEAP; protein tags; placenta; ligand–receptor interactions.

1. Introduction

Human placental alkaline phosphatase (PLAP) cDNA encodes 530 aa (17 aa signal peptide, 513 aa mature peptide). The C-terminus confers membrane binding. In an attempt to generate a new reporter gene with superior sensitivity and ease of use, Berger and coworkers *(1)* inserted a stop codon in front of the sequence that codes for membrane binding of the human PLAP. This translational terminator, which also generated an Hpa I site, truncated PLAP by 24 aa at the C-terminus. The resulting protein is secreted, consists of 506 aa (17 aa signal peptide, 489 aa mature peptide), and is referred to as the secreted form of human placental alkaline phosphatase (SEAP). Unlike the other AP isozymic forms (termed intestinal- and tissue-unspecific AP), PLAP and SEAP are unaffected by the presence of 10 mM homoarginine and extremely heat stable. The latter feature is very useful, because background AP activity can be virtually eliminated by simply heating the sample at 65°C for 30 min.

Typically, the tissue distribution of receptors for various ligands has been studied by radiolabeled ligand autoradiography or, when reagents are available, by immunocytochemical or *in situ* hybridization procedures. Flanagan and Brennan and their colleagues have utilized an alternative approach involving the generation of SEAP–ligand fusion proteins that has proven particularly

From: *Methods in Molecular Medicine, Vol. 122: Placenta and Trophoblast: Methods and Protocols, Vol. 2*
Edited by: M. J. Soares and J. S. Hunt © Humana Press Inc., Totowa, NJ

useful for identifying components of receptor tyrosine kinase signaling pathways, including ligands and receptors *(2–9)*. Other groups utilized similar approaches, e.g., for the identification of the leptin receptor *(10)*, a novel chemokine *(11)*, and the monitoring of interactions between endothelial cells and leukocytes *(12)*. The question arose whether this approach could be used to identify specific targets of placental proteins.

Rodent placentas prominently express an expanded family of genes that are structurally related to prolactin (PRL). The nomenclature for members of the PRL family reflects biological activities (placental lactogens [PLs]), structural relationships with PRL (PRL-like proteins [PLPs], PRL-related proteins [PRPs]), or associations with proliferation (proliferin). Those members of the PRL family that effectively mimic PRL action have been referred to as classical members of the PRL family. However, most members of the PRL family do not activate the PRL receptor and are referred to as nonclassical members. Before the application of the SEAP-tagging strategy, target tissues and physiological roles for most nonclassical members of the PRL family were unknown.

As a first step, the use of the AP tag for monitoring the behavior of a classical PRL family member was evaluated *(13)*. Rat PL-I was chosen because (a) it is secreted by the developing placenta in a temporally and spatially specific pattern, (b) the recombinant protein was available, (c) targets with high expression of PRL receptors (PRL-R) were well known, (d) PL-I had been shown to bind the PRL-R, and (e) it possesses a number of actions previously attributed to pituitary PRL. Thus, the AP-PL-I model could be used to demonstrate that SEAP-tagging does not interfere with ligand binding and biological activities.

Using polymerase chain reaction (PCR)-cloning techniques, the cDNA for mature rat PL-I was inserted into the cytomegalovirus promoter (pCMV)-SEAP vector generating a probe that consisted of a fusion protein between human placental AP and rat PL-I (AP-PL-I). This construct was transfected into 293 cells. After a 2-wk selection with G418, single clones were isolated by limiting dilution and screened for AP expression. AP activity was monitored in the untreated, conditioned medium from transfected cells using a simple colorimetric assay. The unmodified AP vector was similarly transfected and selected and served as a control. Immunoreactivity was investigated by Western blotting. In vitro, AP-PL-I specifically bound to liver membranes, known to express high levels of PRL-R. The binding was specific because excess ovine PRL competed with AP-PL-I. PRL-like biological activities of the AP-PL-I fusion protein were successfully demonstrated using the rat Nb2 lymphoma cell proliferation assay. Binding of AP-PL-I to tissue sections was also specific and could compete with ovine PRL. Subsequently, the technique has been successfully applied to other members of the rodent PRL-gene family leading to the detection of their specific targets. The specific binding of PLP-A to natural killer (NK) cells *(14)* and of decidual PRL-related protein (dPRP) to heparin and eosinophils *(15)* were identified with the help of SEAP-tagging. Other groups in the field adopted the technique and identified the binding of PLP-E and PLP-F to megakaryocytes *(16,17)* and of ovine PL to sheep uterine endometrial glands *(18)*. Thus, the generation of SEAP–ligand fusion proteins provides a useful tool for the identification of specific ligand–receptor interactions.

2. Materials

1. The 293 human fetal kidney cells (American Type Culture Collection [ATCC], Manassas, VA or LGC Promochem, Teddington, UK).
2. 293 cell culture medium. Minimum essential medium (MEM) culture medium supplemented with 20 mM HEPES, 100 U/mL penicillin, 100 mg/mL streptomycin, and 10% fetal bovine serum (FBS).
3. pCMV-SEAP vector (Tropix, Inc., Bedford, MA).
4. Mouse monoclonal anti-human placental alkaline phosphatase (clone 8B6)-agarose (Sigma Chemical Co., St. Louis, MO, cat. no. A-2080).
5. Coplin jars (50 mL) (Fisher Scientific, Pittsburgh, PA).
6. HBS buffer: 20 mM HEPES, 150 mM NaCl, pH 7.0.
7. HBHA buffer: Hank's balanced salt solution with 0.5 mg/mL bovine serum albumin (BSA), 0.1% NaN$_3$, 20 mM HEPES, pH 7.0.
8. Acetone/formaldehyde fixative: 60% acetone, 3% formaldehyde in 20 mM HEPES, pH 7.0.
9. AP buffer: 100 mM Tris-HCl, pH 9.5, 100 mM NaCl, 5 mM MgCl$_2$.
10. AP stain: AP buffer containing 0.17 mg/mL 5-bromo,4-chloro,3-indolylphosphate (BCIP) and 0.33 mg/mL nitroblue tetrazolium (NBT).
11. Disposable vinyl specimen molds (e.g., 25 × 25 × 5 mm, Tissue-Tek, Ted Pella Inc., Redding, CA, cat. no. 4557).
12. Tissue freezing medium (Triangle Biomedical Sciences, Durham, NC or Fisher Scientific, cat. no. 15-183-13).
13. Coated slides (Fisher Scientific, e.g., Superfrost Plus, precleaned, cat. no. 12-550-15).
14. Hydrophobic marker (Pap Pen, Kiyota, Japan or Ted Pella Inc., cat. no. 22303).

3. Methods

We have used the AP-tagging strategy for investigating the biology of a number of members of the PRL family. The techniques described below are based on our experiences.

3.1. Generation of AP–Ligand Fusion Protein

1. A vector containing ampicillin and neomycin resistance genes and SEAP situated downstream of a CMV promoter (pCMV-SEAP) is commercially available.
2. A nucleotide region representing the mature ligand is then amplified using primers with Xba I sites (*see* **Note 1**) and ligated into the pCMV-SEAP vector linear-

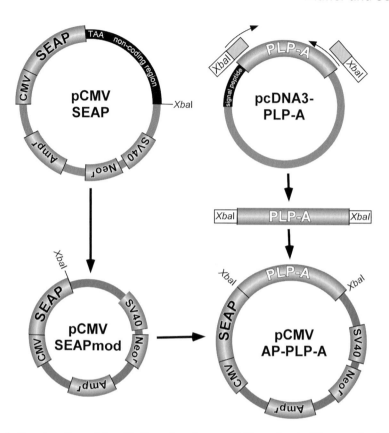

Fig. 1. Construction of the alkaline phosphatase (AP)-prolactin-like protein A (PLP-A) expression vector. A fusion protein consisting of a modified human placental AP and rat PLP-A was generated and used to monitor PLP-A target cell interactions. SEAP is situated downstream of the cytomegalovirus promoter (pCMV) in a vector containing ampicillin and neomycin resistance genes (pCMV-SEAP). From another vector, a nucleotide region representing the mature rat PLP-A was amplified and ligated into the modified pCMV-SEAP vector using the Xba1-site. Ligation with the PLP-A insert resulted in a CMV promoter-driven vector containing the ligated cDNAs encoding a secreted human placental AP (SEAP)-PLP-A fusion protein (AP-PLP-A).

ized at its unique Xba I site (**Fig. 1**). Ligation with the cDNA results in a CMV promoter driven vector containing the SEAP–ligand fusion gene. DNA sequencing of the insert is necessary to verify the orientation and the accuracy of the PCR amplification.

3. After linearization, the AP–ligand construct is electroporated into 293 human fetal kidney cells.

4. After a 2- to 3-wk selection with 500 mg/mL G418, single clones are isolated by limiting dilution and screened for AP expression.

5. An unmodified pCMV-SEAP vector (AP) should be similarly transfected, selected, and will serve as a negative control.
6. Transfected 293 cells are cultured in 293 cell culture medium in an atmosphere of 5% CO_2-95% air at 37°C in a humidified incubator.
7. After the cells reach confluence, the medium is changed to serum-free 293 cell culture medium, further conditioned for 72 h, collected and clarified by centrifugation, and filter sterilized (0.22 µm).
8. The achieved protein concentration can be determined by measuring AP-activity (*see* **Subheading 3.2.**). If needed, serum-free conditioned medium can be concentrated using membranes with a suitable molecular-weight cut-off. In our investigation, Amicon spiral cartridge concentrators were used at 4°C to prevent protein degradation. For small samples, spin columns with similar membranes work equally well. All conditioned media should be stored at −20°C until used.

3.2. AP Fusion Protein Characterization

AP activity can be measured from conditioned medium via a colorimetric assay. The AP tag can also be used to enrich the fusion protein.

3.2.1. AP Assay

1. Initially, samples are heated for 30 min in a 65°C water bath in order to inactivate endogenous heat labile AP.
2. Samples are then incubated at room temperature in a glycine buffer (50 mM glycine, pH 10.4, 0.5 mM $MgCl_2$, 0.5 mM $ZnCl_2$) containing nitrophenylphosphate (0.5 mg/mL) in a total reaction volume of 200 µL.
3. Following a 5-min incubation, absorbance is measured at 405 nm.
4. One unit of AP activity is defined as the amount of enzyme that hydrolyzes 1 µmol of *p*-nitrophenylphosphate to *p*-nitrophenol in 1 min at 37°C in a volume of 1 mL.

3.2.2. AP–Ligand Isolation

AP–ligand preparations can be isolated from conditioned medium using immunoprecipitation or immunoaffinity chromatography with a monoclonal antibody to human PLAP (clone 8B6) conjugated to agarose *(14)*.

3.2.3. Immunological Characterization

The AP–ligand fusion protein can be characterized by polyacrylamide gel electrophoresis and Western blotting with antibodies to human PLAP or with antibodies to the ligand *(13,14)*.

3.2.4. Other Types of Biological Characterization

If in vitro bioassays are available for the ligand, then the AP fusion protein can be tested to determine whether the addition of the AP tag influences ligand biological activities. The Nb2 lymphoma cell proliferation assay represents a highly sensitive in vitro assay for assessing classical PRL-like biological activities *(19)* (*see* **Note 2**).

3.3. Analysis of AP-PLP-A Binding to Tissues and Cells (see Note 3)

3.3.1. Tissue Preparation

1. A container is filled with enough liquid nitrogen to cover all samples. Sealable plastic bags and cryomolds are labeled. The cryomolds are filled with tissue freezing medium.
2. After the animal is sacrificed, target tissue is prepared as quickly as possible. The tissue is placed in the cryomold with the interesting side either up or down (sections will be transverse). Samples must be covered with tissue freezing medium.
3. With long forceps, cryomolds are placed onto liquid nitrogen and allowed to freeze from the bottom up while floating. Samples will sink when completely frozen.
4. When all the samples are frozen, they are taken out of the liquid nitrogen, wrapped in aluminum foil, put in sealable plastic bags, and placed in containers with dry-ice until finished. All samples are stored at –80°C until processed.
5. Alternatively, samples can be frozen directly in dry-ice-cooled heptane. Once frozen, the samples are transferred to suitable containers and stored at –80°C until processed.

3.3.2. Preparation of Frozen Sections

1. Tissue samples are equilibrated to temperature in the cryostat (e.g., –18 to –13°C).
2. Sections are cut 6–10 µm thick and, if necessary, flattened with a small brush.
3. Coated slides that will attract tissue sections electrostatically are used to pick up the tissue section by simply touching them.
4. Cytospins can be prepared to look for binding to cells in suspension.
5. All slides are frozen at –80°C until performance of the binding assay.

3.3.3. AP In Situ Binding Assay (see **Fig. 2**)

1. A 50-mL Coplin jar is filled with HBS buffer, covered with a lid, and placed in a 65°C water bath in preparation for the heat-inactivation step (*see* **Note 4**).
2. The AP or AP–ligand fusion protein solutions are prepared and stored on ice. Even for small sections, at least 200 µL is needed. To cover the entire surface of the slide, 1 mL is usually sufficient (*see* **Notes 5–7**).
3. Frozen sections or cytospins are taken out of the freezer. The white frost should dry out (this is not very time-critical, but allow to dry no longer than 1 h) (*see* **Note 8**).
4. Slides are labeled with a xylene-resistant marker or pencil and then soaked once for approx 5 min in HBHA Buffer.
5. Slides are drained and their backs, as well as their front edges, are wiped dry with gauze.

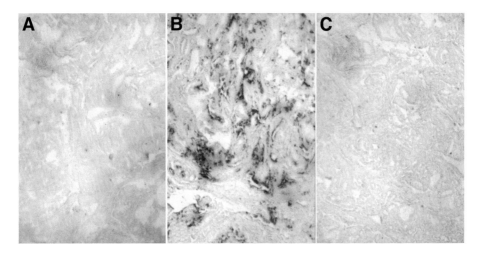

Fig. 2. *In situ* analysis of alkaline phosphatase (AP)-PL-I binding to tissue sections. Tissue sections were prepared with the aid of a cryostat. Sections were mounted on glass slides, washed, and incubated with AP **(A)**, AP-PL-I **(B)**, or AP-PL-I + prolactin (PRL) **(C)** for 75 min at room temperature. After incubation the sections were washed, fixed, washed, heated at 65°C for 30 min to inactivate endogenous tissue AP activity, and processed for detection of the heat-stable AP activity. The specificity of binding was further assessed by the addition of ovine PRL (5 μg/mL) to the tissue section **(C)**. **(A–C)** Mouse mammary tumor from pseudopregnant mice of the DDD strain of *Mus musculus* carrying the mouse mammary tumor virus (MMTV), 40× magnification.

6. Samples are overlayed with fusion protein supernatant for 75 min at room temperature in a humidified chamber (moist and level). Sections should not be allowed to become dry.
7. Samples are washed six times for 5 min in HBHA buffer + 0.1% Tween 20. The slides are drained by tapping on paper towels, rinsed briefly in the first wash, and placed in the second wash. They are agitated at the beginning, middle, and end of each wash.
8. Tissue sections are fixed with acetone/formaldehyde fixative for 2 min.
9. Slides are washed three times for 5 min with HBS buffer.
10. To heat-inactivate endogenous AP, slides are transferred into a Coplin jar filled with HBS buffer and then to a water bath already adjusted to 65°C.
11. After 30 min, slides are transferred to another Coplin jar containing AP buffer to be cooled and rinsed in order to pre-adjust pH and temperature.
12. Slides are drained and their backs and front edges wiped dry with gauze. Sections should not be allowed to become dry.
13. Sections are overlayed with AP Stain for 2 h in a humidified chamber.

14. The process of staining is monitored on a white background (e.g., wet white filter paper). The required staining time can vary between 10 min and 16 h. When staining is sufficient, stain is drained off onto a paper towel (*see* **Note 9**).
15. Slides are rinsed five times in distilled water and then air-dried for 30 min. Ethanol/xylene dehydration should be avoided because the precipitated stained material will wash out.
16. Immediately before coverslipping, slides are rinsed briefly (<1 min) in xylene.
17. Following coverslipping with Permount (aqueous mounting medium), the slides are air-dried (usually approx 3 d at room temperature).

4. Notes

1. The cDNA insert (corresponding to the protein of interest) must be subcloned in-frame with the SEAP-coding sequence and without its signal peptide. Glycine may serve as a linker.
2. AP-tagged PL-I retains its PRL-like biological activities *(13)*. This need not be the case for all AP-tagged ligands. In some cases, the AP tag may disrupt and/or modify ligand–receptor interactions.
3. Others have successfully adopted the SEAP-tagging strategy for the identification of targets for placental ligands *(17,18)*. There are also examples of using the AP–ligand fusion proteins as a screening tool in expression cloning strategies for identification of the ligand's receptor *(10)*.
4. The exact temperature is critical for effective heat-inactivation of background AP activity. Therefore, the waterbath should adjust to 65°C for at least 1 h before using.
5. Two different negative controls should be used: the serum-free cell culture medium for 293 cells to check for successful heat inactivation of endogenous AP in the tissue, and SEAP containing conditioned medium, to check for binding related to SEAP itself. The specificity of binding can be assessed by incubation with the AP control or addition of various peptide hormones.
6. To achieve good staining, 100–500 mU/mL of fusion protein are needed. To calculate the amounts of tagged protein, the following estimation could be useful: SEAP: 1000 mU = 1 µg, SEAP-PRL family ligand: 600 mU approx 1 µg. The enzymatic activity per mass of SEAP fusion protein depends on the molecular weight ratio between SEAP and the tagged protein.
7. The application of the technique to another nonclassical member of the PRL family, dPRP, turned out to be more difficult as a result of the heparin-binding of dPRP. Wang et al. *(15)* demonstrated that AP–dPRP fusion protein bound readily to heparan sulfate-containing wild-type Chinese hamster ovary (CHO) cells but not to heparan sulfate-deficient CHO-pgsD-677 cells. Using heparan sulfate-deficient CHO cells transiently transfected with the long form of the rat PRL-R, it could be shown that AP–dPRP failed to bind the PRL-R. In contrast, AP–PL-I, a known ligand of the PRL receptor, effectively bound to these PRL receptor-transfected cells. Binding assays showed that AP–dPRP bound to virtually all components of the uterus. The challenge was to overcome the strong affinity to heparin

and to show heparin-independent binding. By pretreatment with heparitinase and/ or heparin, dPRP binding to tissues was dramatically affected. A population of non-heparin binding sites was identified by consecutively incubating tissue sections with AP–d/tPRP followed by excess heparin (250 μg/mL to 10 mg/mL). This strategy finally led to the identification of discrete d/tPRP target cells within the endometrium and myometrium of the nonpregnant rat.

8. Circling the tissue sections with a hydrophobic marker helps to save reagents.
9. Both reagents used in the AP histochemical assay, NBT and BCIP, are toxic (especially the dust). Wearing gloves and careful handling is mandatory. A stock solution should be prepared and stored at 4°C. Tubes should be covered with aluminum foil because both AP substrates are light-sensitive.

Acknowledgments

The authors would like to thank Belinda M. Chapman, Christopher B. Cohick, Bing Liu, and Guoli Dai for their participation in the development of the procedures and techniques. This work was supported by grants from the Deutsche Forschungsgemeinschaft (DFG) of Germany (Mu 1183 1-1, Mu 1183 3-1), the National Institutes of Health (NIH) (HD20676, HD39878), and the Hall Family Foundation.

References

1. Berger, J., Hauber, J., Hauber, R., Geiger, R., and Cullen, B. R. (1988) Secreted placental alkaline phosphatase: a powerful new quantitative indicator of gene expression in eukaryotic cells. *Gene* **66,** 1–10.
2. Brennan, C., Monschau, B., Lindberg, R., et al. (1997) Two Eph receptor tyrosine kinase ligands control axon growth and may be involved in the creation of the retinotectal map in the zebrafish. *Development* **124,** 655–664.
3. Brennan, C. and Fabes, J. (2003) Alkaline phosphatase fusion proteins as affinity probes for protein localization studies. *Sci STKE* **2003(168),** PL2.
4. Cheng, H. J. and Flanagan, J. G. (1994) Identification and cloning of ELF-1, a developmentally expressed ligand for the Mek4 and Sek receptor tyrosine kinases. *Cell* **79,** 157–168.
5. Cheng, H. J., Nakamoto, M., Bergemann, A. D., and Flanagan, J. G. (1995) Complementary gradients in expression and binding of ELF-1 and Mek4 in development of the topographic retinotectal projection map. *Cell* **82,** 371–381.
6. Chiang, M. K. and Flanagan, J. G. (1995) Interactions between the Flk-1 receptor, vascular endothelial growth factor, and cell surface proteoglycan identified with a soluble receptor reagent. *Growth Factors* **12,** 1–10.
7. Chiang, M. K. and Flanagan, J. G. (1996) PTP NP, a new member of the receptor protein tyrosine phosphatase family, implicated in development of nervous system and pancreatic endocrine cells. *Development* **122,** 2239–32250.
8. Flanagan, J. G. and Leder, P. (1990) The kit ligand: a cell surface molecule altered in steel mutant fibroblasts. *Cell* **63,** 185–194.

9. Flanagan, J. G. and Cheng, H. J. (2000) Alkaline phosphatase fusion proteins for molecular characterization and cloning of receptors and their ligands. *Methods Enzymol.* **327,** 198–210.

10. Tartaglia, L. A., Dembski, M., Weng, X., et al. (1995) Identification and expression cloning of a leptin receptor, OB-R. *Cell* **83,** 1263–1271.

11. Nagira, M., Imai, T., Hieshima, K., et al. (1997) Molecular cloning of a novel human CC chemokine secondary lymphoid- tissue chemokine that is a potent chemoattractant for lymphocytes and mapped to chromosome 9p13. *J. Biol. Chem.* **272,** 19,518–19,524.

12. Fong, A. M., Erickson, H. P., Zachariah, J. P., et al. (2000) Ultrastructure and function of the fractalkine mucin domain in CX(3)C chemokine domain presentation. *J. Biol. Chem.* **275,** 3781–3786.

13. Müller, H., Dai, G., and Soares, M. J. (1998) Placental lactogen-I (PL-I) target tissues identified with an alkaline phosphatase-PL-I fusion protein. *J. Histochem. Cytochem.* **46,** 737–743.

14. Müller, H., Liu, B., Croy, B. A., et al. (1999) Uterine natural killer cells are targets for a trophoblast cell-specific cytokine, prolactin-like protein-A. *Endocrinology* **140,** 2711–2720.

15. Wang, D., Ishimura, R., Walia, D. S., et al. (2000) Eosinophils are cellular targets of the novel uteroplacental heparin-binding cytokine decidual/trophoblast prolactin-related protein. *J. Endocrinol.* **167,** 15–28.

16. Lin, J. and Linzer, D. I. (1999) Induction of megakaryocyte differentiation by a novel pregnancy- specific hormone. *J. Biol. Chem.* **274,** 21,485–21,489.

17. Zhou, B., Lum, H. E., Lin, J., and Linzer, D. I. (2002) Two placental hormones are agonists in stimulating megakaryocyte growth and differentiation. *Endocrinology* **143,** 4281–4286.

18. Noel, S., Herman, A., Johnson, G. A., et al. (2003) Ovine placental lactogen specifically binds to endometrial glands of the ovine uterus. *Biol. Reprod.* **68,** 772–780.

19. Tanaka, T., Shiu, R. P. C., Gout, P. W., Beer, C. T., Noble, R. L., and Friesen, H. G. (1980) A new sensitive and specific bioassay for lactogenic hormones: measurement of prolactin and growth hormone in human serum. *J. Clin. Endocrinol. Metab.* **51,** 1058–1063.

21

Bacterial Expression of Prolactin Family Proteins

Arieh Gertler

Summary

Complementary DNAs of three recombinant proteins related to the prolactin family: ovine placental lactogen (oPL), ovine prolactin (oPRL), and rabbit soluble extracellular domain of prolactin receptor (rbPRLR-ECD) were subcloned by different methods and inserted into prokaryotic expression plasmids. *Escherichia coli* cells transformed with those plasmids overexpressed the respective proteins either by induction or constitutively, resulting in accumulation of the recombinant proteins in insoluble inclusion bodies, which were subsequently purified, used for refolding and purifying of the proteins by one-step chromatography. The isolated oPL, oPRL, and rbPRLR-ECD were biologically active over >95% pure monomers. Ten-liter bacterial culture yielded hundreds of milligrams or more than gram quantities of recombinant proteins. The methodology described in the present chapter allows large-scale preparation of pure, monomeric, biologically active oPL, oPRL, and rbPRLR-ECD suitable for performing in vitro and in vivo experiments.

Key Words: Recombinant proteins; ovine prolactin; ovine placental lactogen; rabbit prolactin receptor; extracellular domain.

1. Introduction

Recombinant protein methodology is a major method for preparation of animal, plant, and bacterial proteins for research and therapy purposes. So far, the cheapest, fastest, and most efficient method of obtaining large amounts of recombinant proteins is overexpression of bacterial plasmids carrying the target gene in various strains of *Escherichia coli*. Efficient expression leads to accumulation of the recombinant proteins in insoluble inclusion bodies (IBs) that may consist of up to 50–80% of total cell proteins. Upon isolation, IBs may contain up to 80–90% of pure denatured recombinant protein as evidenced by sodium dodecyl sulfate (SDS)-polyacrylamide gel electrophoresis (PAGE) under denaturing conditions. Proper refolding followed by chromatography is required to obtain pure, monomeric, biologically active protein. The method suffers from two main disadvantages: (a) no universal protocol of

From: *Methods in Molecular Medicine, Vol. 122: Placenta and Trophoblast: Methods and Protocols, Vol. 2*
Edited by: M. J. Soares and J. S. Hunt © Humana Press Inc., Totowa, NJ

refolding proteins is available and a specific protocol has to be adjusted for each protein and (b) no glycosylation or other posttranslational modifications occur in *E. coli*. Preparation of recombinant ovine placental lactogen (oPL) *(1)*, ovine prolactin (oPRL) *(2)*, and rabbit prolactin receptor extracellular domain (rbPRLR-ECD) *(3)* in up to gram quantities exemplifies application of this methodology to preparation of three proteins (two hormones and one soluble receptor) related to the prolactin family.

2. Materials

1. pET8 (Novagen, Inc. Milwaukee, WI), pTrc99A (Pharmacia LKB Biotechnology AB, Uppsala) and pMON3401 (received from Mr. Nick Staten, Monsanto Co. St. Louis, MO) prokaryotic vectors.
2. cDNA encoding oPL, oPRL, and rbPRLR-ECD.
3. *E. coli* strains JM-109 , BL21 (DE3), W3110, and MON-105.
4. Oligonucleotide primers.
5. Restriction enzymes, T7 polymerase, and T4 DNA ligase.
6. Stratagene Quickchange(tm) mutagenesis kit (Stratagene, La Jolla, CA).
7. Agarose gels.
8. DNA sequencer.
9. Luria broth (LB) and terrific broth (TB) media.
10. Ampicillin and spectinomycin.
11. Isopropyl-β-ᴅ-thio-galactopyranoside (IPTG) and nalidixic acid.
12. Sonicator.
13. SDS-PAGE equipment.
14. Chromatography equipment (high-performance liquid chromatography [HPLC] or fast protein liquid chromatography [FPLC]).
15. Fast-flow Q-Sepharose (Amersham Biosciences Europe GmbH, Freiburg, Germany).
16. TN buffer: 25 mM Tris-HCl, pH 8.0 containing 150 mM NaCl.
17. Sorvall or other refrigerated high-speed centrifuge equipped with GSA or similar rotor.
18. Analytical Superdex(tm)75 HR 10/30 and preparative Hi-Load Superdex 75 (120 or 300 mL bead volume) columns (Amersham Biosciences Europe GmbH, Freiburg, Germany).
19. Tissue culture facilities.
20. T cell–derived Nb2-11C *(4)* and FPC-P1 3B9 *(5)* cell lines.
21. 96-well plates suitable for cell growth and reading in enzyme-linked immunosorbent assay (ELISA) reader.
22. 3-[4,5-Dimethylthiazol-2-yl-2,5-diphenyltetrazolium bromide], (MTT; Thiazol Blue).
23. Ultra pure water filtered through 5 kDa filter to remove endotoxin.
24. BIAcore 2000 instrument (Pharmacia Biosensor AB, Uppsala, Sweden).
25. pCH110, a plasmid encoding β-galactosidase (β-gal) activity (Pharmacia, Uppsala, Sweden).

3. Methods

The methods described below outline: (1) preparation of cDNA and construction of the respective plasmids, (2) protein expression, (3) preparation of IBs, (4) refolding and purification of recombinant proteins, (5) characterization of physical and chemical properties, and (6) determination of its biological activity in tissue culture and/or binding assays. Ultra pure water filtered through 5 kDa filter is used in all buffers (*see* **Note 1**).

3.1. Preparation of the cDNA and Expression Plasmids

Three different methods for preparation of the respective prokaryotic expression plasmids are described below (*see* **Note 2**). In all cases, the prepared DNA was analyzed to verify the proper sequence and the bacteria were stored at –80°C as glycerol cultures (*see* **Note 3**).

3.1.1. Ovine PL

The cDNA encoding oPL was prepared by reverse-transcription (RT)-polymerase chain reaction (PCR) using 1 μg sheep placental cotelydon total RNA as a source *(1)*. The insert having the respective *Nco*I and *Pst*I restriction sites was first subcloned into pTrc99A vector, but after finding that this plasmid gave very poor expression in *E. coli* W3110 strain, the *Pst*I site was changed into a *BamH*1 site and the oPL encoding insert was subcloned into pET8 vector, propagated in JM-109 *E. coli*, and finally passaged to *E. coli* strain BL21 (DE) and the isolated colonies expressed oPL upon induction by 1 mM IPTG *(1)* (*see* **Note 4**).

3.1.1 Ovine PRL

The pMON3839 plasmid containing the mature bPRL-encoding sequence was used as the starting material for preparation of oPRL. To facilitate the mutagenesis, the bPRL-encoding DNA was excised with *Xba*I and *Hind*III and ligated into a pTRC vector. Subsequently, the pTRC plasmid containing the bPRL sequence was modified with the Stratagene Quickchange mutagenesis kit according to the manufacturer's instructions resulting in four mutations (N10D, D31N, A108V, and Y165H) that converted the bPRL to oPRL *(2)*. Then the XbaI/HindIII insert was removed from the pTRC plasmid and ligated to pMON3401 vector linearized with the same enzymes. This construct was transfected into *E. coli* strain MON 105 and the isolated colonies expressed oPRLR either constitutively or upon induction with nalidixic acid.

3.1.3 Rabbit PRLR-ECD

The cDNA of rbPRLR-ECD encoding the G29 (i.e., the fifth amino acid downstream to the signal peptide cleavage site) to D235 (the last amino acid before the transmembrane domain) was prepared by PCR reaction using 100 pg of the cloned rbPRLR cDNA *(6)* as a template and the respective 5' primer with *Nco*I sites and the 3' primer possessing the stop codon and downstream *Xba*I restriction site. The DNA fragment amplified between these amino acids was isolated and inserted between the *Nco*I and *Xba*I sites of the prokaryotic expression vector pTrc99A *(3)*. This construct was subsequently transfected into *E. coli* strain W3310 and the isolated colonies were tested for expression of rbPRLR-ECD upon induction by IPTG. The bacterial clone expressing the highest level of rbPRLR-ECD (W5) was used for further studies.

3.2. Protein Expression

1. Starter bacterial cultures are grown overnight at 37°C at 200 rpm in 100 mL in LB supplemented with the respective antibiotics (ampicillin for BL21 or spectinomycin for Mon105 cells) in a 500-mL flask.
2. The cultures are then mixed with 2400 mL LB or TB (without antibiotics) and grown in 2-L flasks (500 mL/flask) at 37°C at 200 rpm until the A_{600} reaches 0.8–0.9.
3. Then IPTG, in the case of oPL and rbPRLR-ECD, is added respectively to 0.4 and 1 mM.
4. The incubation is continued for an additional 4 h and the cells are harvested by centrifugation (10 min at 8000g) at 4°C and frozen at –20°C.
5. In the case of oPRL, preliminary experiments have shown that induction with nalidixic acid (50 µg/mL) is not necessary because the expression of oPRL is constitutive. Therefore the bacteria (500 mL in 2-L flasks) are incubated for 12–14 h (37°C at 200 rpm), then harvested by 10-min centrifugation at 8000g and frozen at –20°C.
6. In all cases, more than 95% of the respective recombinant protein is found in the inclusion bodies.

3.3. Preparation of IBs

1. Bacterial pellets obtained from 10 L of bacterial culture are thawed and suspended in 600 mL 10 mM ethylenediamine tetraacetic acid (EDTA), pH 8.0 containing 100–300 mg lysosyme, and mixed gently on ice for 30 min.
2. The suspension is then sonicated on ice, and the inclusion bodies (IBs) are precipitated at 15,000g for 15 min and washed by sonication with H_2O, 0.1% Triton X-100 and, finally, with H_2O five times. During the washing procedure the volume is gradually descreased to 100–200 mL.
3. The final precipitate can be stored at –20°C for at least 1 yr.
4. The protein content of the isolated IBs can be semiquantitaively determined by SDS-PAGE in presence of reducing agent. The expressed protein should represent at least 50 to 80 % of the total protein (*see* **Note 5**). A typical example of IBs containing rbPRLR-ECD obtained after induction with IPTG is presented in **Fig. 1**.

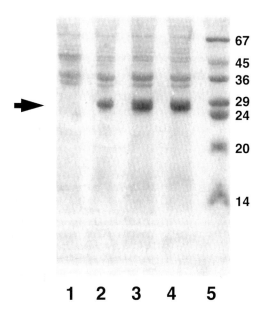

Fig. 1. Sodium dodecyl sulfate-polyacrylamide gel electrophoresis (15% gel run in presence of β-mercaptoethanol) analysis of the insoluble fraction prepared from clone W5 of *Eshcerichia coli* transformed with plasmid expressing rabbit prolactin receptor extracellular domain prior (**lane 1**) and 2, 4, and 8 h after induction with isopropyl-β-D-thio-galactopyranoside. **Lane 5**, molecular mass markers. The gel was stained with Coomassie Brilliant Blue R-250.

3.4. Refolding and Purification of the Recombinant Protein

A general procedure for solubilization and refolding the expressed proteins is described as follows, and the differences among the protocols for the three proteins are outlined.

1. The IB pellet obtained from 5- to 10-L fermentation cultures is thawed, briefly sonicated in water, and solubilized in 500 mL of 4.5 *M* urea buffered with 10 m*M* Tris base, pH 11.3, containing 0.1 m*M* cysteine (oPL and rbPRLR-ECD) or 1 m*M* cysteine (oPRL).
2. The clear, yellowish solution is gently stirred at 4°C for 1 h, diluted with 2 vol of cold water, and dialyzed for 48 h against 5 × 10 L of 10 m*M* Tris-HCl, pH 9.0 (oPL and oPRL) or pH 8.6 (rbPRLR-ECD).
3. Any turbidity formed during the dialysis is removed by centrifugation prior to column chromatography.
4. The resultant solution is loaded at 120–500 mL/h onto a Q-Sepharose column (2.6 × 7 cm) pre-equilibrated with 10 m*M* Tris-HCl, pH 9.0 or pH 8.6, respectively (*see* **Note 6**).

5. Elution is carried out using a discontinuous NaCl gradient in the same buffer at a rate of 120–500 mL/h, and 10- to 50-mL fractions are collected.
6. All procedures are carried out at at 4°C.
7. Protein concentrations are determined by absorbance at 280 nm and monomer content is monitored in aliquots by gel filtration chromatography using analytical Superdex75 HR 10/30 column equilibrated with TN buffer (see **Note 7**).
8. The recombinant proteins (expected representation of monomers to dimers/oligomers is 95% and <5%, respectively) are eluted with 50 mM NaCl (oPL), 100 mM NaCl (rbPRLR-ECD), or is found in both the breakthrough fraction and the 50 mM NaCl eluate (oPRL). Both eluates of oPRL are equally potent. In general, fractions eluted with higher salt concentrations contain increasing amounts of dimers and oligomers.
9. Tubes containing the monomeric protein are pooled, dialyzed against $NaHCO_3$ at 4:1 or 3:1 (w/w) protein/salt ratio, and freeze-dried.
10. The freeze-dried proteins are stored at –20°C (oPL and oPRL) or –70°C (rbPRLR-ECD) for at least 1 yr without formation of dimers or oligomers.
11. To obtain proteins containing 100% of monomers, further purification could be achieved using preparative Hi-Load Superdex 75 16/60 or 26/60 columns equilibrated with TN buffer.
12. The yield of the purified protein (from 10 L of fermentation cultures) varies between 500 and 1000 mg for oPL, 1000 and 1500 mg for oPRL, and 150 and 300 mg for rbPRLR-ECD.

3.5. Physical and Chemical Properties of the Isolated Proteins

Several methods can be used to characterize the purified proteins. The comparative results of those studies are summarized in **Table 1**.

1. The purity and molecular mass of the proteins can be tested by SDS-PAGE in presence or absence of reducing agent (7) and by gel filtration on analytical Superdex 75 column in TN buffer. The accurate molecular mass can also be determined in some cases by mass spectroscopy analysis using matrix-assisted laser desorption/ionization time-of-flight (MALDI-TOF) (2E, Micromass UK).
2. The amino terminal sequence is determined utilizing an automated Edman degradation technique.
3. The proper refolding of the protein is verified by of circular dichroism (CD) spectra as described previously (8). For the secondary structure determination, the CD data are expressed in degree cm^2dmol^{-1} per mean residue, based on a respective molecular mass calculated for each protein from its amino acids composition. The secondary structure of protein is calculated by applying the procedure and computer program CONTIN developed by Provencher and Glöckner (9). This program determines α-helices, β-strands, and β-turns as percentage of amino acid residues involved in these ordered forms. Unordered conformation is determined as unity minus the sum of all elements of the secondary structure (10). The use of CD is particularly important in the case of oPL and oPRL which have a characteristic four bundle of α-helices.

Table 1
**Physical and Chemical Characterization of Recombinant Ovine Placental
Lactogen (oPL), Ovine Prolactin (oPRL), and Rabbit Prolactin Receptor
Extracellular Domain (rbPRLR-ECD)**

Parameter tested	oPL	oPRL	rbPRLR-ECD
Monomer content (%)	>98	>95	>97
Molecular mass[a]	23 kDa	23 kDa	25 kDa
Molar extinction coefficint[b]	20690	23670	66515
Amino terminal sequence[c]	AQAQHPP-Y	ATPV-PN	GKPFI
CD spectra:α-helix (%)	48	52	ND
β sheet (%)	3	5	ND
β turn (%)	18	17	ND
random coil (%)	31	26	ND

[a]Determined by sodium dodecyl sulfate-polyacrylamide gel electrophoresis; more accurate values can be obtained by matrix-assisted laser desorption/ionization time-of-flight mass spectrometry.
[b]Calculated according to **ref. 11**.
[c]The N-terminal methionine was processed in the *Escherichia coli* to >80–90% extent so that the sequence represents the major product. The minor products have an additional Met at their terminus. The missing amino acids at positions 5 and 8 in the case of oPRL and oPL, respectively are likely cysteines, which are destroyed in Edman procedure.
ND, not determined

4. Protein concentrations are determined using extinction coefficients calculated from theoretical amino acid composition according to Pace et al. *(11)* (*see* **Note 8**).

3.6. Biological Activity of the Isolated Proteins

The biological activity of the recombinant proteins can be determined by binding experiments using the classic radio-receptor assays (RRA), measuring the ability of the hormones of forming complexes with the respective soluble receptors (or with hormone in the case of rbPRLR-ECD), and real-time kinetic measurements of the interactions between macromolecules, based on surface plasmon resonance (SPR). This technique enables determination of kinetic association (k_{on}) and dissociation (k_{off}) constants and the stoichiometry of interaction of a complex in which one component is immobilized on a flexible dextran matrix (oPL or oPRL), whereas the other (rbPRLR-ECD) is free in solution. In addition, the biological activity of oPL and oPRL is determined in vitro using rat lymphoma Nb2-11C cells possessing intermediate form of rat PRLR, FDC-P1-3B9 cells stably transfected with rbGH receptor (for oPL only), and in human embryonic kidney (HEK) 393T cells transiently transfected with oPRLR. The two hormones can also be tested in additional in vitro or in vivo bioassays *(2,12)*, not reported here.

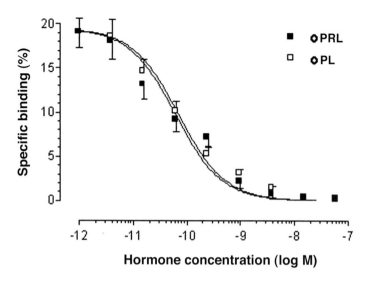

Fig. 2. Competition of unlabeled ovine prolactin (oPRL) (full squares) or oPRL (empty squares) with ^{125}I-oPRL, for binding to rabbit prolactin receptor extracellular domain. The specific binding was 19%. Full lines were calculated using the PRIZMA curve-fitting program.

3.6.1. RRA

The binding assays are carried out in 25 mM Tris-HCl, pH 8.0 buffer containing 10 mM MgCl$_2$ and radioimmunoassay grade bovine serum albumin (BSA) (1 mg/mL) (*see* **Note 9**) as described previously, using goat α-rbPRLR antiserum 46 for immunoprecipitation of the rbPRLR-ECD: hormone complex *(3,13)*. Radioiodinated hGH is used as a ligand. Results of a typical RRA are presented in **Fig. 2**.

3.6.2. Complex Formation

Complexes between rbPRLR-ECD and oPL or oPRL are prepared at various molar ratios in TN buffer. After a 20- to 30-min incubation at room temperature, 200-µL aliquots are applied to a Superdex75 HR 10/30 column. To determine the molecular mass of the complex, the column is calibrated with several pure proteins. Results of a typical experiment are presented in **Fig. 3**.

3.6.3. Biacore Experiments

Kinetic measurements of R-ECD:Hormone interactions are determined using the BIAcore 2000 instrument.

1. The hormone being tested is covalently immobilized through amino-group coupling.

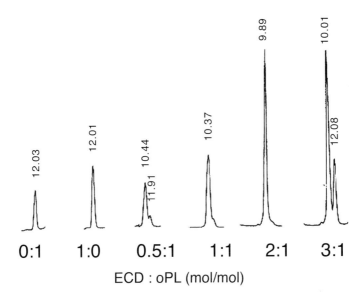

Fig. 3. Gel filtration of ovine placental lactogen (oPL) complexes with rabbit pro-lactin receptor extracellular domain (rbGHR-ECD) on a Superdex(tm)75 HR 10/30 column. Complex formation was carried out during 20 to 30 min of incubation at room temperature in TN buffer using various ECD:oPL ratios. The initial hormone con-centration was constant (1.6 μ*M*). Aliquots (200 μL) of the incubation mixture were applied to the column, pre-equilibrated with the same buffer. Complex formation was monitored by absorbance at 280 nm. The column was developed at 1 mL/min.

2. Serial dilutions of each R-ECD are injected for 480 s and then washed with HBS for 720 s prior to regeneration *(14)*.
3. Because the recombinant rbPRLR-ECDs was lyophilized with Na-bicarbonate, bulk refractive indexes varied with sample dilution, and these variations were corrected by injecting the same dilutions into flow cells in which unrelated ligands had been immobilized.
4. Data analysis and calculation of kinetic constants are performed using BIAcore incorporated software (BIA Evaluation and BIA Simulation, Version 2.1) that allows us to fit experimental curves with 1:1 or 1:2 association/dissociation mod-els and calculate the probabilities of each being the most accurate representation of reality and to calculate kinetic constants with standard deviations *(14)*. Kinetic and thermodynamic constants for interaction of rbPRLR-ECD with oPL and oPRL are summarized in **Table 2**.

3.6.4. In Vitro Bioassays in Stably Transfected FDC Cells

In vitro bioassay of oPL in which the signal is transduced through somato-genic receptors is based on the proliferation of FDC-P1 cells transfected with

Table 2
Calculation of Kinetic and Thermodynamic Constants
of Sites I and II for the Interaction of Rabbit Prolact
in Receptor Extracellular Domain (rbPRLR-ECD)
With Ovine Placental Lactogen (oPL) and Ovine Prolactin (oPRL)

Hormone (sites I and II)	k_{on} (mol$^{-1} \times$ s^{-1})	k_{off} (s$^{-1} \times 10^{-4}$)	K_d (nM)	ECD:hormone (molar ratio)[a]	Half-life (min) $\times 10^4$
oPL site I	2.0	1.9	9.5	2:1	61.0
oPL site II	6.4	61	94		1.9
oPRL site I	16	1.5	0.9	1:1	77.0
oPRL site II	3.5	546	1580		0.2

[a]Apparent stoichiometry as determined by surface plasmon resonance. The 1:1 apparent stoichiometry of rbPRLR-ECD-oPRL complex results most likely from the extremely short half-life of the putative 2:1 complex.

rbGHR (clone FDC-P1-3B9) *(5)* as described previously *(15)*, except that cell growth is not determined in 96-well plates using the MTT method *(16)*. The somatogenic activity of oPL in this system is similar to that of ovine growth hormone yielding the respective EC$_{50}$ values (mean ± SEM) of $2.5 \pm 0.7 \times 10^{-11}$ M and $2.7 \pm 0.3 \times 10^{-11}$ M.

3.6.5. In Vitro Bioassays in Nb2 Cells

An in vitro bioassay, in which the signal is transduced through lactogenic receptors, is performed in rat Nb$_2$-11C lymphoma-cell-proliferation bioassay as described previously *(17)*, but modified for use of 96-well plates and MTT method *(16)*. Lactogenic activity of recombinant oPRL in an Nb$_2$ cell proliferation bioassay is as potent as that of oPL *(2)*, yielding the respective EC$_{50}$ values (mean ± SEM) of $3.9 \pm 0.7 \times 10^{-12}$ M and $2.7 \pm 0.3 \times 10^{-12}$ M.

3.6.6. In Vitro Bioassays in Transiently Transfected 293 Cells

An additional bioassay can be carried out in a in HEK 293T cell line transiently transfected with oPRLR and co-transfected with a plasmid that carries the luciferase reporter gene *(18)*.

1. The HEK 293 cells are seeded in six-well plates.
2. After 4–8 h, the cells are transfected with oPRLR-pcDNA3 (100 ng/well). In parallel, cells are transfected with LHRE-TK-luc, a plasmid bearing six repeats of the rat β-casein STAT5-responsive sequence upstream of a thymidine kinase minimal promoter linked to a luciferase reporter gene *(19)* and pCH110, a plasmid encoding β-gal activity. Transfection is carried out using the calcium-phosphate procedure described elsewhere *(20)*.

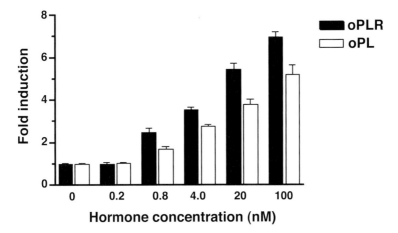

Fig. 4. Stimulation of luciferase (LUC) activity in human embryonic kidney (HEK) 293 cells transiently transfected with full-size ovine prolactin (oPRL) receptor by oPRL (full squares) and ovine placental lactogen (empty squares). The results are given as mean ± SD. For other details, see text.

3. After 24 h, the cells are transferred to serum-free medium, recombinant oPRL or oPL are added, and cells are incubated for an additional 18 h.
4. Luciferase enzymatic activity is measured as described elsewhere *(21)*.
5. The results are expressed as fold induction, and the ratio of stimulated to nonstimulated cells following normalization for β-gal activity, to take into account the efficiency of transfection.
6. An example of the effects of oPRL actions on HEK 293 cells transiently transfected with the homologous full-size oPRLR is shown in **Fig. 4**. In this bioassay, the activity of oPRL is significantly higher than that of oPL, and the respective EC_{50} values (mean ± SEM) are $5.4 \pm 1 \times 10^{-9}\,M$ vs $9.7 \pm 11 \times 10^{-9}\,M$. The concentrations of both oPRL and oPL required for half-maximal activity are three orders of magnitude higher than in the Nb_2 cell proliferation bioassay.

4. Notes

1. We have observed that the vast majority of endotoxin found in the purified recombinant protein results not from the bacteria but rather from the water used for purification process. This can be dramatically lowered to an accepted level by using ultra pure water filtered through a 5-kDa filter. Many instruments for preparation of ultra pure water are equipped with such filters. This procedure is much cheaper than purchasing commercially available endotoxin-free water.
2. It should be noted that the recent developments in preparation of synthetic DNA enable ordering the requested cDNA at relatively low price ($2–3 per basepair in 2004). Availability of this methodology, along with the existing information of

the amino acid sequence of target proteins, makes it possible to skip the laborious cloning or subcloning procedures and allows planning of the requested cDNA with an optimal bacterial codon usage and selected restriction enzymes sites. This procedure is very fast and the ordered cDNA can be obtained in 2–3 wk.

3. Storage of bacteria expressing recombinant proteins as glycerol culture is a common procedure. However, we have observed that within a year or more, the level of expression tends to decrease. Plating the bacteria and selecting clones giving the highest expression is therefore recommended.

4. In some cases, overnight incubation of starter cultures of BL21 cells carrying pET expression plasmids may lead to lower level of expression. In such cases, we recommend growing the bacteria to $A_{600} = 0.4$–0.5, storing overnight at 4°C, and continuing the growth of the starter cultures the next morning, followed by expression in large flasks as described previously.

5. We have found that efficient removal of the nonrelated bacterial proteins improves the proper refolding of the recombinant proteins. In the present paper, we describe the method used in our laboratory, but other related methods are likely similarly efficient.

6. In our initial publications we have reported flow rates of 120–150 mL/h. Recently, we have found the flow rate can be increased up to 500–600 mL/h without affecting the resolution or the yield of the purified proteins.

7. Monitoring the molecular mass of the purified protein by gel filtration is extremely important because, unlike SDS-PAGE, it is performed under nondenaturing conditions and thus enables identification of dimers and oligomers resulting from hydrophobic interactions that are overlooked in SDS-PAGE. From our extensive experience with over 200 proteins and their mutants, monomeric proteins are almost always indicative of proper refolding.

8. To calculate the accurate extinction coefficient at 280 nm, it is absolutely necessary to centrifuge the protein solution at high speed to avoid light scattering.

9. We prefer using the RIA grade BSA from Sigma Chemical Company. If other sources of BSA are used, it is important to determine prior to RRA that they do not contain traces of lactogenic hormones.

Acknowledgments

I wish to acknowledge the help and advice of my colleague Dr. Jean Djiane from the Institut National de la Recherche Agronomique, Jouy-en-Josas, France; Dr. Jeanne Grosclaude from the same Institute for performing the SPR experiments; Ms. Nava Chapnik-Cohen from my group for her help in the Nb$_2$ and FDC-P1 bioassays; and my postgraduate students listed in cited publications. We also thank Prof. Michael Waters from University of Queensland, Australia for providing the FDC-P1 3B9 cells. This work was supported by research grant no. US-2643-95 from The United States-Israel Binational Agricultural Research and Development Fund (BARD) and by grant no. 4425-1-92 from the Ministry of Science and Technology, Israel and French Ministry of Research and Technology.

References

1. Sakal, E., Bignon, Ch., Kantor, A., et al. (1997) Large-scale preparation of recombinant ovine placental lactogen. *J. Endocrinol.* **152,** 317–327.
2. Leibovich, H., Raver, N., Herman, A., Gregoraszczuk, E.L., Gootwine, E., and Gertler, A. (2001) Large-scale preparation of recombinant ovine prolactin and determination of its in vitro and in vivo activity. *Protein. Expr. Purif.* **22,** 489–496.
3. Bignon, C., Sakal, E., Belair, L., Chapnik-Cohen, N., Djiane, J., and Gertler, A. (1994) Preparation of recombinant extracellular domain of rabbit prolactin receptor expressed in *Escherichia coli* and its interaction with lactogenic hormones. *J. Biol. Chem.* **269,** 3318–3324.
4. Tanaka, T., Shiu, R. P., Gout, P. W., Beer, C. T., Noble, R. L., and Friesen, H. G. (1980) A new sensitive and specific bioassay for lactogenic hormones: measurement of prolactin and growth hormone in human serum. *J. Clin. Endocrinol. Metab.* **51,** 1058–1063.
5. Rowlinson, S. W., Barnard, R., Bastiras, S., Robins. A.J., Brinkworth, R., and Waters, M. J. (1995) A growth hormone agonist produced by targeted mutagenesis at binding site 1. Evidence that site 1 regulates bioactivity. *J. Biol. Chem.* **270,** 16,833–16,839.
6. Edery, M., Jolicoeur, C., Levi-Meyrueis, C., et al. (1989) Identification and sequence analysis of a second form of prolactin receptor by molecular cloning of complementary DNA from rabbit mammary gland. *Proc. Natl. Acad. Sci. USA* **86,** 2112–2116.
7. Laemli, U. K. (1970) Cleavage of structural proteins during assembly of the head of bacteriophage T_4. *Nature* **227,** 680–685.
8. Venyaminov, S. Yu. and Yang J. T. (1996) Determination of secondary structure, in: *Circular Dichroism and the Conformational Analysis of Biomolecules* (Fasman, G. D., ed.). Plenum, New York: pp.69–107.
9. Provencher, S. W. and Glöckner, J. (1981) Estimation of globular protein secondary structure from circular dichroism. *Biochemistry* **20,** 33–37.
10. Sreerama, S. and Woody, R. W. (1993) A self-consistent method for the analysis of protein secondary structure from circular dichroism. *Anal. Biochem.* **209,** 32–44.
11. Pace, C. N., Vajdos. F., Fee. L., Grimsley, G., and Gray, T. (1995) How to measure and predict the molar absorption coefficient of a protein. *Protein. Sci.* **4,** 2411–2423.
12. Gertler, A. and Djiane, J. (2002) Mechanism of ruminant placental lactogen action: molecular and in vivo studies. Review. *Mol. Genet. Metab.* **75,** 189–201.
13. Cahoreau, C., Petridou, B., Cerutti, M., Djiane, J., and Devauchelle, G. (1992) Expression of the full-length rabbit prolactin receptor and its specific domains in baculovirus infected insect cells. *Biochimie* **74,** 1053–1065.
14. Gertler, A., Grosclaude, J., Strasburger, C. J., Nir, S. and Djiane, J. (1996) Real-time kinetic measurements of the interactions between lactogenic hormones and prolactin-receptor extracellular domains from several species support the model of hormone-induced transient receptor dimerization. *J. Biol. Chem.* **271,** 24,482–24,491.

15. Helman, D., Staten, N. R., Grosclaude, J., et al. (1998) Novel recombinant analogues of bovine placental lactogen. G133K and G133R provide a tool to understand the difference between the action of prolactin and growth hormone receptors. *J. Biol. Chem.* **273,** 16,067–16,074.

16. Raver, N., Gussakovsky, E. E, Keisler, D. H., Krishna, R., Mistry, J., and Gertler, A. (2000) Preparation of recombinant bovine, porcine, and porcine W4R/R5K leptins and comparison of their activity and immunoreactivity with ovine, chicken, and human leptins. *Prot. Express. Purif.* **19,** 30–40.

17. Gertler, A., Walker, A., and Friesen, H. G. (1985) Enhancement of human growth hormone-stimulated mitogenesis of Nb2 node lymphoma cells by 12-O-tetradecanoyl-phorbol-13-acetate. *Endocrinology* **116,** 1636–1644.

18. Herman, A., Bignon, C., Daniel, N., Grosclaude, J., Gertler, A. and Djiane, J. (2000) Functional heterodimerization of prolactin and growth hormone receptors by ovine placental lactogen. *J. Biol. Chem.* **275,** 6295–6301.

19. Sotiropoulos, A., Moutoussamy, S., Renaudie, F., et al. (1996) Differential activation of Stat3 and Stat5 by distinct regions of the growth hormone receptor. *Mol. Endocrinol.* **10,** 998–1009.

20. Lebrun, J. J., Ali, S., Goffin, V., Ullrich, A. and Kelly, P. A. (1995) A single phosphotyrosine residue of the prolactin receptor is responsible for activation of gene transcription. *Proc. Natl. Acad. Sci. USA* **92,** 4031–4035.

21. Bignon, C., Daniel, N., and Djiane, J. (1993) Beta-galactosidase and chloramphenicol acetyltransferase assays in 96-well plates. *Biotechniques* **15,** 243–246.

22

Analysis of Placental Regulation of Hematopoiesis

Beiyan Zhou and Daniel I. H. Linzer

Summary

Placental hormones contribute to changes in maternal physiology, especially to changes in the blood system. Methods are described to express a placental hormone from a cloned cDNA by transfection into a mammalian cell line, to purify the hormone, and to assess the activities of the hormone in primary mouse bone marrow cell cultures. The example used in this chapter is prolactin-like protein F (PLP-F), a recently discovered mouse placental hormone that acts on the myeloid lineage. This hormone has been expressed at high levels in stably transfected Chinese hamster ovary cells. The protein is secreted from these cells after cleavage of the signal sequence and the addition of N-linked carbohydrate. A series of chromatographic steps are used to purify the protein to homogeneity, which is verified by gel electrophoresis and silver staining; the identity of the purified protein is confirmed by immunoblot analysis. Purified protein is then assayed by addition to primary bone marrow cells and scoring the growth and the differentiation of the megakaryocyte progenitor, colony forming unit-megakaryocyte.

Key Words: Prolactin; placenta; hematopoiesis; megakaryocyte.

1. Introduction

In mammalian pregnancy, a significant expansion of plasma volume (30%–50%) occurs, which contributes to the efficient transport of nutrients and oxygen to the fetal compartment *(1)*. Accompanying this dramatic change is the requirement for enhanced hematopoiesis, cascades of cell proliferation, and differentiation from a limited number of pluripotent self-renewal stem cells giving rise to a variety of blood cell types. Hematopoiesis is finely regulated by a broad array of hematopoietic cytokines acting in concert. To achieve the rapid and pronounced increases in blood cell production to compensate for the expansion in plasma volume, cytokines of pregnancy, especially placental hormones, may superimpose their functions on the homeostatic array of factors operating in the nonpregnant state.

With its comparatively large size, the placenta is one of the most important endocrine organs during gestation. It secretes a large number of hormones,

From: *Methods in Molecular Medicine, Vol. 122: Placenta and Trophoblast: Methods and Protocols, Vol. 2*
Edited by: M. J. Soares and J. S. Hunt © Humana Press Inc., Totowa, NJ

affecting most if not all physiological systems. The most abundantly secreted placental proteins in the rodent are members of the prolactin (PRL)/growth hormone (GH) family. A large number of PRL-like proteins (PLP) have been identified on the basis of their sequence similarity to PRL, including PLP-A, PLP-B, PLP-E, and PLP-F *(2)*. These PLPs target various hematopoietic cell types. Investigation of the functions of these placental hematopoietic cytokines is of importance for understanding the regulation of hematopoiesis during pregnancy. PLP-F will be used to illustrate methods to express, purify, and assay a placental regulator of hematopoiesis.

2. Materials

1. pMT2 mammalian expression vector.
2. Chinese hamster ovary (CHO) cells.
3. Helper plasmid pSV2neo.
4. GenElute Minus EtBr Spin Columns (Sigma Chemical Co., St. Louis, MO).
5. Restriction enzymes and T4 DNA ligase.
6. Dulbecco's modified Eagle's medium (DMEM).
7. Iscove's modification of Dulbecco's medium (IMDM).
8. Fetal bovine serum (FBS).
9. Nutridoma (Roche Molecular Biochemicals, Indianapolis, IN).
10. L-glutamine.
11. Penicillin/streptomycin.
12. OPTI-MEM medium (GIBCO BRL, Gaithersburg, MD).
13. MegaCult C medium (Stem Cell Technology, Vancouver, Canada).
14. Superfect transfection reagent (Qiagen, Valencia, CA).
15. Plasmid DNA preparation kits (Qiagen).
16. Nitrocellulose membranes.
17. Polyclonal antiserum against PLP-F and anti-rabbit immunoglobin.
18. Trypsin (GIBCO BRL).
19. Geneticin (G418) (GIBCO BRL).
20. CHO cell culture medium: DMEM culture medium supplemented with 10% FBS, 2 mM L-glutamine, and penicillin/streptomycin.
21. Standard buffer: 2 M ZnSO$_4$ solution, 0.5 M ethylenediamine tetraacetic acid (EDTA), 50 mM Na 3-[N-morpholino]propanesulfonic acid (pH 8.0).
22. β-mercaptoethanol.
23. Bio-Rad protein assay (Bio-Rad Laboratories, Hercules, CA).
24. Sodium dodecyl sulfate-polyacrylamide gel electrophoresis (SDS-PAGE) equipment and gel transfer equipment.
25. Agarose gel electrophoresis equipment.
26. Centricon-30 mini column and ultrafiltration units (Amicon, Beverly, MA).
27. Chromatography S-200 sizing column (Amersham Pharmacia Biotech, Piscataway, NJ).
28. Chromatography ion exchange TSK DEAE column (Supleco, Bellefonte, PA).

29. Lentil lectin Sepharose matrix (Amersham Pharmacia Biotech).
30. Fast protein liquid chromatography (FPLC) equipment.
31. Silver stain plus kit (Bio-Rad Laboratories).
32. Blocking buffer: 20 m*M* Tris-HCl, pH 7.6, 150 m*M* NaCl, 0.5% Triton X-100, and 5% nonfat milk.
33. Washing buffer: 20 m*M* Tris-HCl, pH 7.6, 150 m*M* NaCl, 0.05% Triton X-100.
34. SuperSignal WestPico chemiluminescent substrate (Pierce Chemical Co., Rockford, IL).
35. Commercially available cytokines, including interleukin (IL)-3, IL-6, and thrombopoietin (TPO).
36. Graphpad Prism Software, Version 2.0a (Graph Pad Software, Inc. San Diego, CA).

3. Methods

The methods below focus on expression, purification and in vitro functional analysis of placental hematopoietic cytokine PLP-F. Procedures include: (1) expression vector construction; (2) transient or stable transfection of cell lines with DNA expression constructs; (3) protein purification by FPLC; and (4) hematopoietic functional analysis in colony formation assays.

3.1. Expression Vector Construction

The expression vector is a modified form of the pMT2 mammalian expression vector *(3)*. Transcription of a cDNA insert in this vector is controlled by the adenovirus major late promoter. DNA manipulations were performed by standard procedures *(4)*. Methods described as follows outline the construction of PLP-F expression plasmid (*see* **Note 1**).

1. Release the full-length PLP-F cDNA, including the coding region for the secretion signal sequence, from plasmid pT7T3-PLP-F by restriction enzyme digestion according to standard molecular procedures *(4)*.
2. Prepare modified pMT2 mammalian expression vector by restriction enzyme digestion.
3. Separate DNA fragments by agarose gel electrophoresis.
4. Recover DNA with GenElute Minus EtBr Spin Columns according to manufacturer's instructions.
5. Insert PLP-F cDNA fragment between the Sma I and Sal I sites of the modified pMT2 vector by incubating DNA fragments with T4 DNA ligase at 16°C overnight.
6. Transform *Escherichia coli* DH5α competent cells with ligation mixture using standard molecular biology methods *(4)*; plate cells on LB plates containing ampicillin and incubate overnight at 37°C.
7. Select single colonies and grow in LB liquid media overnight at 37°C.
8. Extract plasmid DNA from cell culture using Plasmid mini kit.
9. Screen for clones with the correct insert by restriction enzyme digestion and gel electrophoresis; confirm by polymerase chain reaction (PCR) amplification.

10. Grow in large scale the bacterial cells containing the desired construct and isolate plasmid DNA with the Qiagen plasmid maxi kit according to manufacturer's instructions.

3.2. Gene Transfection

To express PLP-F in its native form, including the co- and posttranslational modifications of signal sequence removal and *N*-linked glycosylation, the pMT2-PLP-F expression construct is transfected into CHO cells. Transient transfection is used to determine if introduction of pMT2-PLP-F into mammalian cells results in secretion of glycosylated PLP-F that is similar in size to PLP-F found in the circulation of pregnant mice. Once gel electrophoresis and Western blotting demonstrate the production of the protein then stably transfected CHO cells are generated by co-transfection of pMT2-PLP-F and pSV2neo, and selection for resistance to G418. Cell cultures are maintained in CHO cell culture medium (*see* **Subheading 2., item 20**). The steps under **Subheadings 3.2.1.** and **3.2.2.** describe the methods of transient and stable transfection of CHO cells (*see* **Note 2**).

3.2.1. Transient Transfection of CHO Cells

1. Split confluent CHO cell cultures 1:4 into six-well plates 2 d before transfection such that the dishes are 40–80% confluent.
2. Mix 4 µg plasmid DNA with 15 µL of Superfectin transfection reagent in 200 µL OPTI-MEM medium; incubate the plasmid-transfection reagent mixture at room temperature for 5–10 min.
3. Add DMEM to the DNA-transfection reagent mixture and apply to confluent cells that have been washed twice with phosphate-buffered saline (PBS); incubate cells and transfection mixture for one to three h at 37°C.
4. Feed cells with fresh medium containing 10% FBS and incubate overnight.
5. Change medium to DMEM without serum and incubate at 37°C for another 2 d.
6. Collect conditioned medium and measure protein concentrations using the Bio-Rad Protein Assay reagent.
7. Fractionate protein samples by SDS-PAGE, transfer proteins to membranes, and incubate with antiserum against PLP-F *(4)*.

3.2.2. Stable Transfection of Expression Constructs into CHO Cells

1. Mix 2 µg pMT2-PLP-F plasmid DNA with 0.5 µg pSV2neo plasmid DNA and 20 µL Superfectin transfection reagent in 400 µL OPTI-MEM medium according to the manufacturer's instructions; let the mixture stand at room temperature for 5–10 min before adding DMEM.
2. Incubate confluent cells with the DNA-transfection reagent mixture for one to 3 h at 37°C.
3. Change to fresh medium containing FBS and incubate cells overnight.

4. Split cell cultures at different ratios into fresh containers and grow cells in DMEM containing FBS for another 48 h.
5. Add fresh medium containing 400 µg/mL G418 sulfate; supplement G418 sulfate every 48 h until G418-resistant colonies emerge.
6. Pick each G418-resistant colony by trypsin treatment in glass cloning cylinders and seed in single wells in 12-well plates containing 3 mL CHO cell culture medium supplemented with 400 µg/mL G418 sulfate.
7. Collect conditioned medium and assay for PLP-F protein by Western blotting.
8. Grow producing cell lines in DMEM, and harvest cells for long-term storage; store positive cell lines in 90% FBS, 10% DMSO at –80°C for 48–72 h and transfer cell stocks into liquid nitrogen.

3.3. PLP-F Protein Purification by FPLC Chromatography

Cell lines stably transfected with the pMT2-PLP-F expression plasmid secrete products in addition to the cytokine PLP-F, and some of these other products may have activity in hematopoietic assays. Thus, the medium from these cultures ("conditioned" medium) must be put through a series of steps to isolate purified PLP-F for use in biological assays. The following steps outline the procedures for purifying native PLP-F protein by FPLC. All purification steps are performed at 4°C except for Western blot analysis (*see* **Note 3**).

1. Clarify conditioned medium by centrifugation at 12,000g for 10 min.
2. Precipitate protein from the supernatant with 100 mM ZnSO$_4$: add 2 M ZnSO$_4$ stock solution drop by drop to reach the final concentration while mixing with a low speed stir bar, and continue mixing for another 30 min.
3. Collect the protein as a pellet by centrifugation at 12,000g for 10 min.
4. Solublize the protein pellet in buffer containing 0.5 M EDTA (pH 8.0), 1 mM β-mercaptoethanol; remove insoluble substances by centrifugation at 45,000g for 10 min.
5. Concentrate protein mixture in an ultrafiltration cell.
6. Apply the protein preparation to an FPLC S-200 sizing column equilibrated with 50 mM Na 3-[N-morpholino] propanesulfonic acid (pH 8.0), 1 mM β-mercaptoethanol.
7. Identify hormone-containing fractions by Western blotting analysis.
8. Pool fractions containing PLP-F, concentrate with a Centricon-30 mini column, and apply the protein preparation to an FPLC ion exchange TSK DEAE column in 50 mM Na 3-[N-morpholino]propanesulfonic acid (pH 8.0), 1 mM β-mercaptoethanol; elute bound proteins with a gradient of sodium acetate, and identify positive fractions by Western blot analysis. We find that PLP-F elutes at 230–280 mM sodium acetate.
9. Pool positive fractions and apply to a lentil lectin Sepharose matrix and elute PLP-F with 0.2 M α-D-methylmannoside according to manufacturer's instructions.
10. Determine protein purity by silver staining after SDS-polyacrylamide gel electrophoresis (**Fig. 1**).

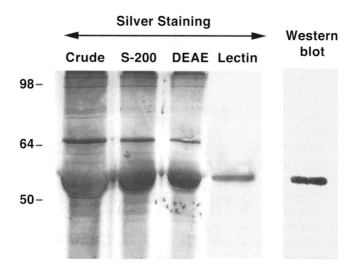

Fig. 1. Purification of prolactin-like protein (PLP)-F. Recombinant PLP-F was purified from the conditioned medium of Chinese hamster ovary cells (Crude) stably transfected with a PLP-F expression construct. Purity was monitored by sodium dodecyl
sulfate-polyacrylamide gel electrophoresis and silver staining after S-200 gel filtration, DEAE ion exchange, and lectin affinity chromatography. Total protein in each
lane is 1.2 µg (Crude), 500 ng (S-200), 430 ng (DEAE), and 18 ng (Lectin). After the
lectin purification step, a single species of 60 kD is detected, consistent with extensive
N-linked glycosylation of the PLP-F polypeptide. The presence of PLP-F after purification is confirmed by Western blot.

3.4. Colony Formation Assays

Purified native cytokine PLP-F can be tested for hematopoietic activity.
Cytokine function can be investigated in cell culture using a colony formation
assay. PLP-F binds to an unknown cell surface receptor on megakaryocytes.
Therefore, the effects of PLP-F on megakaryocytopoiesis can be studied by
measuring the number of colonies that form from the megakaryocyte progenitor population in primary bone marrow preparations. The steps below describe
the protocol to determine the effects of PLP-F on colony forming unit-megakaryocyte (CFU-MK) growth (*see* **Note 4**).

1. Flush femurs from CD1 female mice with 5 mL IMDM supplemented with 10%
   FBS.
2. Pass marrow cells through 21- and 25-gage needles sequentially to separate cells.
3. Culture marrow cells for 45 min at 37°C to remove stromal cells by attachment to
   the culture dish surface.
4. Collect nonadherent cells by centrifugation at low speed and wash with IMDM
   supplemented with 1% Nutridoma.

5. Resuspend cell pellet in IMDM, 1% Nutridoma and plate in MegaCult C semi-solid medium following instructions provided by the manufacturer.

6. Grow bone marrow cells for 7–10 d in two-well chamber slides. Typically, 10 ng/mL murine IL-3, 15 ng/mL murine IL-6, 50 ng/mL murine TPO, and 150 ng/mL PLP-F were included in the treatments. For dose–response assays, the concentration of PLP-F ranges from 50 ng/mL to 300 ng/mL.

7. Dry and fix slides according to the manufacturer's instructions, and stain the slides for acetylcholinesterase (AchE) activity.

8. Score positively stained colonies under the microscope; colonies of cells arising from a single CFU-MK cell are defined as clusters of at least three cells staining positive for AchE.

9. Measure the diameter of megakarcyotes under the microscope for megakaryocyte differentiation analysis; increased cell size can be observed in treatment with IL3+PLP-F compared with IL-3 treatment.

10. Quantitatively analyze results of CFU-MK colony numbers and megakaryocyte cell size in the various treatments (we use Prism software); statistical significance is determined by a one-way analysis of variance (ANOVA) and a *post hoc* Tukey's test (**Figs. 2** and **3**).

4. Notes

1. Bacterial produced protein may be used for cytokine activity assays, but care must be taken because this form of the hormone lacks post-translational modifications, including N-linked glycosylation. For the cytokine PLP-E, we have found that mammalian cell produced hormone is approx 100 times more active than a bacterial expressed PLP-E fusion protein; for PLP-F, bacterial fusion protein has no detectable activity. Thus, mammalian cells stably transfected with expression constructs are greatly preferred as a source of cytokines. Various mammalian expression vectors are available in addition to pMT2, such as the pcDNA series, the pSG5 vector, and the pCMVScript vectors *(3,5–7)*. Gene expression in these vectors is regulated by the adenovirus major late promoter, the early SV40 promoter or the cytomegalovirus (CMV) promoter.

2. Depending on the cell types used for DNA transient or stable transfection, alternative transfection reagents can be selected, for example, Superfect *(8)*. To generate stably transfected cells, typically a selection plasmid is co-transfected that confers antibiotic resistance; transfected cells take up both DNAs with high frequency. Nonetheless, the ratio of selection plasmid to expression construct DNA should be kept low to ensure that most antibiotic resistant colonies have integrated both the selection and the expression plasmids. After resistant colonies emerge, single colonies should be picked and cultured separately to generate clones, as individual transfectants display a wide range of expression levels due to variation in chromosomal integration sites and the number of integrated copies of the plasmid. Therefore, each colony isolated must be individually screened to determine its expression level of the desired product, and while these assays are being conducted parallel cultures should be grown to create frozen stocks for

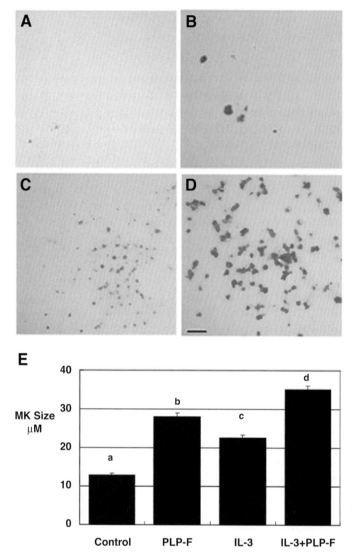

Fig. 2. Prolactin-like protein (PLP)-F and differentiation of megakaryocyte (MK) cells. Primary bone marrow cultures were grown in MegaCult C culture medium, and were either untreated (**A**), or treated with 125 ng/mL PLP-F (**B**), 10 ng/mL interleukin (IL)-3 (**C**), or 10 ng/mL IL-3 +125 ng/mL PLP-F (**D**). Cultures were fixed and stained for AchE activity after one week of growth. Large MK cells with intense AchE staining are seen in cultures treated with PLP-F. Scale bar, 100 μm. (**E**) Quantitative analysis of the various treatments. Results are mean ± SEM, $n = 150$. Statistical significance was determined by a one-way analysis of variance and a *post hoc* Tukey's test, b vs a, $p < 0.001$; c vs b, $p < 0.001$, d vs c, $p < 0.001$.

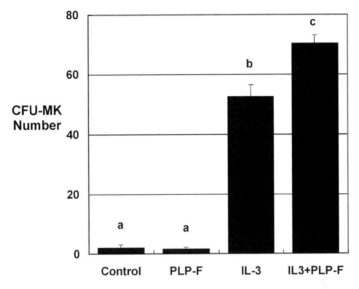

Fig. 3. Effect of prolactin-like protein (PLP)-F on colony forming unit-megakaryo-cyte (CFU-MK) growth. Primary bone marrow cultures were treated with no cytokine, 125 ng/mL PLP-F, 10 ng/mL of interleukin (IL)-3, or combinations of 10 ng/mL IL-3 and 125 ng/mL PLP-F and grown in semisolid media. After a week, clusters of at least three AchE-positive cells were scored as colonies. Data shown are the mean ± SEM and were evaluated by a one-way analysis of variance followed by a Tukey's test; a vs b, $p < 0.001$; a vs c, $p < 0.001$; b vs c, $p < 0.01$; $n = 4$.

long-term storage. By screening a sufficient number of stable transfectants to identify high producers, costs in time and materials will be minimized for the production and purification steps.

3. The medium collected for protein purification should be serum-free to eliminate many proteins present in serum. In the absence of serum, though, cultures will likely not grow or survive well. Daily collection of medium and replacement with fresh medium will ensure maximum recovery. The conditioned medium collected each day should be stored frozen to reduce protein degradation. The properties of the particular protein to be purified (molecular weight, glycosylation, and isoelectric point) dictate what purification steps would be most useful, and what binding and elution conditions should be used. Various zinc sulfate concentrations should be tested for precipitation of the desired protein before large-scale protein precipitation is performed. During salt precipitation, low-speed stirring can help maintain protein activity by avoiding denaturation by local, high salt concentrations. Immunological methods, including Western blot-ting, can be employed to detect positive fractions, but other methods may be available depending on the protein in question (e.g., an enzyme assay). Protein purification should be performed in the cold and the entire sequence of steps

should be carried out as quickly as possible to minimize protein degradation. Before freezing purified protein for storage, divide into many tubes, each with a small volume, to avoid protein damage caused by freeze–thaw cycles.

4. Collagen and methylcellulose-based semi-solid colony forming reagents are often used for assays of cytokine activity. These semi-solid culture conditions permit limited cell movement, thereby allowing determination of cell clusters (colonies) that derive from a single progenitor. The precise medium components and culture conditions vary depending on which hematopoietic precursor is under study (CFU-MK, burst forming unit-erythrocyte (BFU-E), colony forming unit-granulocyte/macrophage (CFU-GM), and colony forming unit-granulocyte/erythroid/macrophage/megakaryocyte (CFU-GEMM). Human collagens can support the growth of BFU-E, CFU-GM and CFU-GEMM, but inhibit CFU-MK growth. Mouse BFU-E colonies can be detected after 7 d incubation in collagen-based semi-solid medium, whereas mouse CFU-GM colonies require 12 d of culture to be scored *(9,10)*. Some cytokines do not show their effect individually, but instead require the presence of other cytokines to reveal synergistic activity. Various cytokine combinations may therefore need to be tested to investigate cytokine effects. When primary bone marrow cells are used in the colony-forming assay, stromal cells may be present in the cell preparation. Because of the effects of stromal cells that may secrete various growth factors regulating hematopoietic precursor cell expansion, spontaneous colonies may emerge in the absence of any cytokines. Stromal cells may also secrete negative regulatory factors which can mask the activity of an added cytokine *(11–13)*. Immunodepletion of a specific cytokine from cytokine cocktails is a useful tool to confirm that an activity is the property of that particular protein. In addition to colony formation assays, several other methods can be used to evaluate the effects of hematopoietic cytokines on cell expansion, including flow cytometric analysis *(14–17)*.

References

1. Davison, J. M. and Lindheimer, M. D. (1989) Volume homeostasis and osmoregulation in human pregnancy. *Baillieres Clin. Endocrinol. Metab.* **3**, 451–472.
2. Linzer, D. I. and Fisher, S. J. (1999) The placenta and the prolactin family of hormones: regulation of the physiology of pregnancy. *Mol. Endocrinol.* **13**, 837–840.
3. Bonthron, D. T., Handin, R. I., Kaufman, R. J., et al. (1986) Structure of pre-pro-von Willebrand factor and its expression in heterologous cells. *Nature* **324**, 270–273.
4. Sambrook, J., Fritsch, E. T., and Maniatis, T. (1989) *Molecular Cloning: A Laboratory Manual*, Second ed. Cold Spring Harbor Laboratory Press, Cold Spring Harbor, New York.
5. Hofman, K., Swinnen, J. V., Claessens, F., Verhoeven, G., and Heyns, W. (2000) Apparent coactivation due to interference of expression constructs with nuclear receptor expression. *Mol. Cell. Endocrinol.* **168**, 21–29.
6. Ornatsky, O. I., Andreucci, J. J., and McDermott, J. C. (1997) A dominant-negative form of transcription factor MEF2 inhibits myogenesis. *J. Biol. Chem.* **272**, 33,271–33,278.

7. Wong, M. J., Goldberger, G., Isenman, D. E., and Minta, J. O. (1995) Processing of human factor I in COS-1 cells co-transfected with factor I and paired basic amino acid cleaving enzyme (PACE) cDNA. *Mol. Immunol.* **32,** 379–387.

8. Tang, M. X., Redemann, C. T., and Szoka, F. C., Jr. (1996) In vitro gene delivery by degraded polyamidoamine dendrimers. *Bioconjug. Chem.* **7,** 703–714.

9. Allegraud, A., Dobo, I., and Praloran, V. (1997) Collagen gel culture of the human hematopoietic progenitors CFU-GM, CFU-E, and BFU-E. *Methods Mol. Biol.* **75,** 221–230.

10. Dobo, I., Bidet, J. M., Acquart, S., et al. (1999) Reproducible scoring of CFU-GM and BFU-E grown in collagen-based semisolid medium after a short (3 h) training. *J. Hematother.* **8,** 45–51.

11. Oehler, L., Foedinger, M., Koeller, M., et al. (1997) Interleukin-10 inhibits spontaneous colony-forming unit-granulocyte-macrophage growth from human peripheral blood mononuclear cells by suppression of endogenous granulocyte-macrophage colony-stimulating factor release. *Blood* **89,** 1147–1153.

12. Zermati, Y., Fichelson, S., Valensi, F., et al. (2000) Transforming growth factor inhibits erythropoiesis by blocking proliferation and accelerating differentiation of erythroid progenitors. *Exp. Hematol.* **28,** 885–894.

13. Calvi, L. M., Adams, G. B., Weibrecht, K. W., et al. (2003) Osteoblastic cells regulate the haematopoietic stem cell niche. *Nature* **425,** 841–846.

14. Lefebvre, P., Lin, J., Linzer, D. I., and Cohen, I. (2001) Murine prolactin-like protein E synergizes with human thrombopoietin to stimulate expansion of human megakaryocytes and their precursors. *Exp. Hematol.* **29,** 51–58.

15. Dai, C. H., Krantz, S. B., Kollar, K., and Price, J. O. (1995) Stem cell factor can overcome inhibition of highly purified human burst-forming units-erythroid by interferon gamma. *J. Cell. Physiol.* **165,** 323–332.

16. Wood, J. C. (1995) Flow cytometer performance: fluorochrome dependent sensitivity and instrument configuration. *Cytometry* **22,** 331–332.

17. van de Ven, C., Ishizawa, L., Law, P., and Cairo, M. S. (1995) IL-11 in combination with SLF and G-CSF or GM-CSF significantly increases expansion of isolated CD34+ cell population from cord blood vs. adult bone marrow. *Exp. Hematol.* **23,** 1289–1295.

23

Methods for Studying Interferon Tau Stimulated Genes

Fuller W. Bazer and Thomas E. Spencer

Summary

Interferon (IFN)τ, a Type I IFN produced by the conceptus trophectoderm, is the pregnancy recognition signal in ruminants that prevents development of the endometrial luteolytic mechanism. In addition, IFNτ acts in a paracrine manner on the ovine endometrium to induce or increase expression of type I IFN-stimulated genes (ISGs). Initially, endometrial explants were cultured with native IFNτ, and the secreted radiolabeled proteins that responded to IFNτ were identified by two-dimensional polyacrylamide gel electrophoresis and fluorography. Next, the ontogeny of putative ISGs was determined in endometrium from cyclic and pregnant ewes; ISGs were confirmed in cyclic ewes that were infused with IFNτ into the uterus. These studies found that most ISGs are increased in the endometrial stroma and glandular epithelium using signal transducer and activator of transcription 1 (Stat1)-dependent pathways. Most ISGs are not induced or increased by IFNτ in the Stat1-negative endometrial luminal epithelium. Recent experiments have used human 2fTGH and U3A (Stat1 null) cells to determine the IFNτ signaling pathway and discover ISGs regulated by IFNτ using transcriptional profiling. Given that ISGs are increased in the endometrium during pregnancy across diverse species, they may be important in establishment of uterine receptivity to implantation of the conceptus.

Key Words: Interferon; interferon stimulated gene; gene regulation; microarray; uterus; endometrium; ovine.

1. Introduction

Establishment and maintenance of pregnancy in domestic animals and humans require reciprocal biochemical signaling between the conceptus (embryo/fetus and associated extraembryonic membranes) and the maternal system (*1*). These signals abrogate the uterine luteolytic mechanism involving prostaglandin $F_{2\alpha}$ (PGF) to allow maintenance of a functional corpus luteum (CL) that produces progesterone required to support a uterine environment supportive of all phases of conceptus development. In sheep, mononuclear trophectoderm cells of the conceptus secrete the antiluteolytic signal, interferon (IFN)τ, between d 10 and 21–25 of pregnancy. Conceptus production of IFNτ is maximal on d 15–16 of pregnancy, when it produces approx 1×10^9 antiviral units of IFNτ during

From: *Methods in Molecular Medicine, Vol. 122: Placenta and Trophoblast: Methods and Protocols, Vol. 2*
Edited by: M. J. Soares and J. S. Hunt © Humana Press Inc., Totowa, NJ

a 24 h in vitro culture period. IFNτ acts in a paracrine manner on the endometrium to abrogate development of the luteolytic mechanism by silencing transcription of the estrogen receptor (ER)α gene and, indirectly, the oxytocin receptor (OTR) gene in the lumenal and superficial ductal glandular epithelia (LE and sGE, respectively), which prevents endometrial production of luteolytic PGF pulses *(2,3)*. Like other Type I IFNs (α, β, and ω), IFNτ induces or increases a number of IFN-stimulated genes (ISG) in the uterus. These ISGs appear to be important for establishment of uterine receptivity to implantation of the conceptus *(4–7)*. Given that similar ISGs are increased in endometrium of domestic animals, laboratory rodents, primates and humans during the peri-implantation period of pregnancy *(8,9)*, ISGs may be universally important in establishment of uterine receptivity to conceptus implantation given their stage-specificity in endometrium across diverse species.

The initial studies aimed at discovering IFNτ-stimulated genes in the ovine uterus were conducted using explant cultures of endometrium from d 12 cyclic ewes that were treated with IFNτ protein purified from conceptus-conditioned culture medium *(10)*. Overall, IFNτ increased the amount of radiolabeled protein released into the culture medium. Using two-dimensional polyacrylamide gel electrophoresis (2D-PAGE) and fluorography, six radiolabeled proteins were identified as selectively increased by IFNτ. However, the fluorographs did not consider incorporation of radiolabeled leucine into high molecular weight (>500,000) mucin-like components that do not enter the second dimension gel and whose synthesis may have been influenced by IFNτ. Using a double-label technique, it was determined that secretion of 11 proteins was enhanced and secretion of 6 was reduced in response to IFNτ compared with bovine serum albumin (BSA). Most of the proteins increased by IFNτ were acidic. As one example, the double-label method detected a 70 kDa protein with an isoelectric point (pI) of 4 that was increased up to fourfold by IFNτ, whereas several proteins were inhibited by IFNτ. Both the single and double label methods provided insight into the molecular size and pI of proteins, but did not inform about the actual identity or function of the proteins.

Experiments to determine ISGs have also been conducted in vivo using uteri from cyclic and early pregnant ewes and uteri from cyclic ewes injected with recombinant ovine IFNτ (roIFNτ) into the uterine lumen *(7,11–15)*. The IFNτ-stimulated genes discovered to date include signal transducer and activator of transcription (Stat)1, Stat2, IFN regulatory factor (IRF)-9, IRF-1, ISG15/17 (also known as ubiquitin cross-reactive protein or UCRP), 2',5'-oligoadenylate synthase (OAS), Mx, major histocompatibility complex (MHC) class I α chain, β2-microglobulin (β2MG), the 1-8 family (1-8U and Leu-13/9-27), IFN-inducible 56-kDa protein (IFI56), ISG12 or p27, guanylate binding protein isoform I (GBP-2), IFNγ-inducible protein 10 kDa (IP-10), and Wnt7a *(7,12–19)*. In vivo studies revealed that most ISGs, except for Wnt7a and ISG12, were only induced or increased in the endometrial stroma and GE. Expression of most ISGs is not detected in endometrial LE and sGE of pregnant ewes, and none of the classical ISGs were induced or increased in the endometrial LE. This finding was initially surprising, because all endometrial cell types express the type I interferon receptor (IFNAR)1 and IFNAR2 subunits of the common Type I IFN receptor *(20)*. However, IRF-2, a known transcriptional repressor of Type I ISGs as well as the Type I IFN genes themselves, was determined to be constitutively expressed in endometrial LE and sGE and increases during early pregnancy, consequently preventing induction or increases in their transcription by IFNτ *(14)*.

The classical Type I IFN signal transduction pathway involves activation of Janus kinases (JAK) followed by Stats and IRFs *(21,22)*. Stat1 and Stat2 are activated via phosphorylation of tyrosine residues by the JAK1 and Tyk2 tyrosine kinases. Activated Stat1 and Stat2 form two transcriptional complexes, Stat1 homodimer or γ-activated factor (GAF) and IFN-stimulated gene factor (ISGF)3 consisting of Stat1, Stat2, and IRF-9. These transcriptional complexes translocate to the nucleus and induce transcription of ISGs, including Stat1, Stat2, and IRF-9. The ISGF3 binds to IFN-stimulated response elements (ISRE) in the promoter region of target genes to regulate their transcription. The GAF regulates transcription of target genes through binding γ activation sequences (GAS) in the promoter region. One of the prototypical target genes for GAF is IRF-1, a transcriptional activator of target genes containing ISREs and IRF elements (IRFE). IRF-1 also increases IRF-2, which is a transcriptional repressor that normally attenuates the antiviral pathway *(23)*. The signaling pathway activated by IFNτ induces formation of both GAF and ISGF3 transcription factors that stimulate GAS and ISRE-containing promoters, respectively, in ISGs *(14,24–26)*. Most ISGs have multiple ISREs in their promoter DNA, whereas some genes have GAS and ISREs as well as IRFEs. The architecture of the promoter within the context of chromatin is the ultimate determinant of the complex regulation of their basal expression levels and responsiveness to Type I IFNs.

A number of studies have elucidated the IFNτ signaling pathway in ovine endometrial cell lines as well as human 2fTGH fibrosarcoma cells and their derivatives (*see* **Table 1**) *(24–27)*. In addition, the ontogeny of Stat1, Stat2, IRF-9, and IRF-1 were studied in uteri of cyclic and pregnant ewes *(14)*. Collectively, these studies found that induction and increases of most ISGs in response to Type I IFNs are mediated by an intracellular signal transduction system involving ISGF3 and GAF (*see* **Fig. 1**). During early pregnancy, the endometrial LE and sGE do not express Stat1, Stat2, or IRF-9 genes, thereby precluding IFNτ regulation of expression of genes in those cell types using the

Table 1
Characteristics of Human Fibroblast Cell Lines
Lacking Specific Interferon Signaling Components

Cell line	Missing protein	Complement
2fTGH	None	None
U1A	Tyk2	None
U2A	IRF-9 (ISGF3γ/p48)	None
U3A	Stat1	None
U4A	JAK1	None
U5A	IFNAR2c	None
U6A	Stat2	None
U3A-701	Stat1	Stat1 Tyr-701 mutant
U3A-727	Stat1	Stat1 Ser-727 mutant
U3A-SH2	Stat1	Stat1 SH2 domain mutant
U3A-p84	Stat1	Stat1β (p84)
U3A-p91	Stat1	Stat1α (p91)

IRF, interferon regulatory factor; ISGF, interferon-stimulated gene factor; Stat, signal transducer and activator of transcription; JAK, Janus kinase; IFNAR2c, type I interferon receptor 2 chain.

Fig. 1. (*opposite page*) Working hypothesis on interferon (IFN)τ signaling in endometrial epithelia and stroma of the ovine uterus. IFNτ, produced in large amounts by the developing conceptus, binds to the Type I IFN receptor (IFNAR) present on cells of the ovine endometrium. In stroma (S) and middle to deep glandular epithelium (GE), IFNτ mediates association of the IFNAR subunits to facilitate the cross-phosphorylation and activation of two Janus kinases, Tyk2 and JAK1, which in turn phosphorylate the receptor and create a docking site for signal transducer and activator of transcription (Stat)2. Stat2 is then phophorylated, thus creates a docking site for Stat 1 which is then phosphorylated. Stat1 and Stat2 are then released from the receptor and can form two transcription factor complexes. IFN-stimulated gene factor (ISGF)3, formed by assocation of the Stat1-2 heterodimer with IFN regulatory factor (IRF)-9 in the cytoplasm, translocates to the nucleus, and transactivates genes containing an IFN stimulated response elements (ISREs), such as Stat 1, Stat 2, IRF-9, IFN-stimulated gene (ISG)15, and 2',5'-oligoadenylate synthase (OAS). γ-Activated factor (GAF) is formed by binding Stat 1 homodimers, which translocate to the nucleus and transactivates genes containing a γ activation sequence (GAS) element(s), such as IRF-1. IRF-1 can also bind and transactivate ISRE-containing genes. The simultaneous induction of Stat2 and IRF-9 gene expression by IFNτ appears to shift transcription factor formation from GAF towards predominantly ISGF3. Therefore, IFNτ activation of the JAK-Stat signal transduction pathway allows for constant formation of ISGF3 and GAF transcription factor complexes and hyperactivation of ISG expression. In the

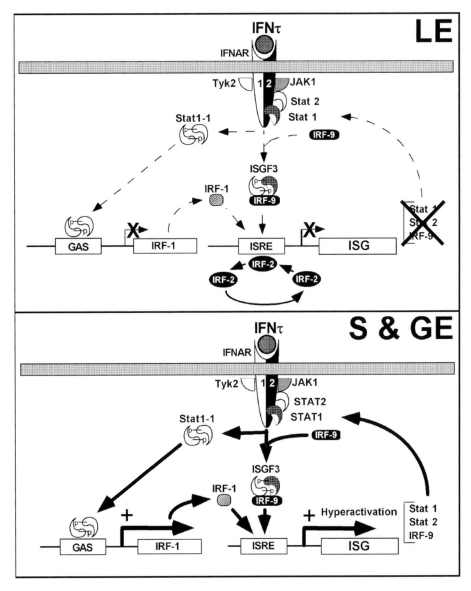

luminal epithelium (LE) and superficial ductal glandular epithelium (sGE), IFNτ is prevented from activating ISGs by IRF-2. IRF-2, a potent and stable repressor present in the nucleus, is constitutively expressed in cyclic ewes and increases in the LE and sGE in early pregnant ewes. The continual presence of IRF-2 inhibits expression of ISRE-containing target genes through direct ISRE binding and coactivator repulsion. Recent evidence indicates that IFNτ increases Wnt7a gene expression in LE in a Stat1-independent manner, suggesting that IFNτ can regulate transcription of genes in LE through a novel signaling pathway.

classical JAK-STAT pathway involving ISGF3 and GAF transcription factors. The expression of most classical ISGs, such as Stat1, Stat2, and IRF-9, are induced or increased only in endometrial stroma and GE, probably as a result of expression of IRF-2, which is a potent transcriptional repressor of many ISGs that is constitutively expressed in the endometrial LE and sGE of both cyclic and pregnant ewes *(14)*.

Transcriptional profiling of genes responsive to IFNτ in human 2fTGH and U3A fibrosarcoma cells is an effective heterologous approach to identifying genes regulated by IFNτ in the ovine endometrium *(7)*. In 2fTGH cells, IFNτ increased expression of many ISGs known to be induced or increased by IFNτ in the ovine uterus. In this example, GBP-2 and IFI56 increased in the endometrial stroma and GE in response to IFNτ and was dependent on Stat1, as is the case with most ISGs. In contrast, ISG12 mRNA increased in the endometrial LE and GE during pregnancy and in response to intrauterine administration of IFNτ, but did not increase in the stroma. Thus, ISG12 is somewhat unique in that its expression is increased in ovine LE in response to IFNτ. Although endometrial stroma and GE of the ovine uterus are Stat1-positive during early pregnancy, the LE and sGE are Stat1-negative. Therefore, IFNτ induction of ISG12 must require a signaling pathway that is independent of Stat1-containing transcription factors and not active in stroma. Also, U3A (Stat1 null 2fTGH) cells respond to IFNτ with increased expression of the Wnt7a gene, which was the first report that any IFN regulates Wnt7a gene transcription. Wnt7a expression in endometrial LE increases between days 14 and 16 of pregnancy consistent with increasing IFNτ production by the conceptus and in response to intrauterine injections of IFNτ. Thus, Wnt7a is a novel IFNτ-stimulated gene.

Therefore, ISGs regulated by IFNτ can be discovered using a variety of methods that include endometrial explant cultures, intrauterine infusion of IFNτ, and human cell lines.

2. Materials

2.1. Endometrial Explants

1. Eagle's minimum essential medium (MEM) for endometrial explant cultures *(28)*. MEM is supplemented with penicillin (200 U/mL), streptomycin (200 μg/mL), fungizone (0.5 μg/mL), insulin (0.2 U/mL), and 10% (v/v) nonessential amino acids (*see* **Note 1**). Phenol red (10 μg/mL) may be added as an indicator of pH.
2. [^{3}H]-leucine (Amersham Corp., Arlington Heights, IL).
3. Endometrium from cyclic ewes (female sheep).
4. Petri dishes (60 mm and 100 mm diameter).
5. Surgical scissors (fine).
6. Forceps.

7. Scalpel blades.
8. Controlled atmosphere chamber (Bellco Biological Glassware, Vineland, NJ).
9. Rocking platform for chamber with adjustable cycle control.
10. Special gas mixture (50% O_2, 45% N_2, 5% CO_2).
11. Incubator at 37°C.
12. Dialysis tubing (Spectrum Laboratories, Inc.).
13. Dialysis buffer: 10 m*M* Tris-HCl, pH 8.2.

2.2. Intrauterine Infusion of IFNτ to Study ISGs in the Ovine Uterus

1. Cyclic ewes.
2. Polyvinyl catheter tubing (V6 and V8, BoLab, Lake Havasu City, AZ).
3. Serum proteins from a day-6 cyclic ewe. Jugular vein blood is collected and then allowed to clot at room temperature for 1 h and then overnight at 4°C. Serum is harvested by centrifugation (3000*g* for 30 min at 4°C), filtered (0.45 μm), and stored at –20°C. The Bradford protein assay is used for protein determination.
4. roIFNτ produced in *Pichia pastoris (29)*. The roIFNτ is assayed for biological activity (antiviral units) using a standard cytopathic effect assay *(30)*.
5. roIFNτ is prepared for intrauterine injection by aliquoting 1×10^7 antiviral units into a sterile tube, adding ovine serum proteins to increase total protein to 1.5 mg, and adding sterile saline to increase the total volume to 1.0 mL.
6. A protein mixture, for injection into the uterine catheters of control ewes, is made by adding 1.5 mg of ovine serum proteins to a sterile tube and then adding sterile saline to increase the total volume to 1.0 mL.

2.3. Human 2fTGH Cells to Discover IFNτ-Regulated Genes

1. The 2fTGH parental and derivative (U1-U6) cells, which are human fibrosarcoma cells lines, are invaluable reagents to determine the precise roles of JAKs and Stats in the IFN signaling pathway (*see* **Table 1**) *(31–37)*. The 2fTGH cells and their derivatives can be obtained from George R. Stark (Lerner Research Institute, Cleveland Clinic Foundation, Ohio, USA).
2. Culture media. Dulbecco's modified Eagle's medium (DMEM)-F12 supplemented with 10% fetal bovine serum (FBS) and penicillin/streptomycin/amphotericin B solution. The U1A, U2A, U3A, U4A, U5A and U6A cells are maintained in basal medium with Hygromycin B (250 μg/mL; Sigma-Aldrich, St. Louis, MO). The U3A-701, U3A-727, U3A-SH2, U3A-p84, and U3A-p91 cells are maintained in basal medium with Hygromycin B and G418-sulfate (400 μg/ml; Geneticin, Gibco-BRL, Gaithersburg, MD).

3. Methods
3.1. Endometrial Explant Cultures (Basic)

1. Ewes are hysterectomized on day 12 of the estrous cycle (day 0 = estrus)
2. Uteri transported to a sterile laminar flow hood where endometrium is dissected from myometrium using sterile scissors and forceps.

3. Endometrium is placed into 10-mL modified MEM in a 100-mm Petri dish and cut into small pieces (2–4 mm^3) using two scalpel blades.

4. A total of 200 mg endometrium is placed in 60-mm Petri dishes containing 5 mL MEM with either BSA (5 µg/mL) or IFNτ (5 µg/mL) and [^{3}H]-leucine (10 µCi/ mL) (*see* **Note 3**).

5. Explant cultures are then placed in a controlled atmosphere chamber on a rocking platform (6 cycles/min) and maintained at 37°C for 24 h under an atmosphere of 50% O$_2$, 45% N$_2$, and 5% CO$_2$.

6. At the end of the incubation period, tissue and medium are centrifuged (12,500g for 10 min), separated, and flash-frozen. Samples should be stored at –20°C until analyzed.

7. Medium from each culture is dialyzed against three changes (4 L) of dialysis buffer (10 mM Tris-HCl [pH 8.2]).

8. Aliquots of medium are subjected to scintillation counting for radioactivity to estimate relative amounts of radiolabeled proteins synthesized *de novo* and released into the medium.

9. Aliquots of dialyzed medium are then separated by 2D-PAGE, and radiolabeled proteins visualized by fluorography (*see* **Note 4**).

3.2. Endometrial Explant Cultures (Enhanced)

A more novel approach to determining effects of IFNτ on qualitative and quantitative aspects of secreted endometrial proteins is to use a dual radioisotope technique *(38)*.

1. Ewes are hysterectomized on day 12 of the estrous cycle (day 0 = estrus).

2. Uteri transported to a sterile laminar flow hood where endometrium is dissected from myometrium using sterile scissors and forceps.

3. Endometrium is placed into modified MEM and cut into small pieces (2–4 mm^3) using two scalpel blades.

4. A total of 200 mg endometrium is placed in 60-mm Petri dishes containing 5 mL MEM with one of the following treatments: BSA with ^{35}S-Met (BSA-S-Met); BSA with ^{3}H-Met (BSA-H-Met); IFNτ with ^{3}H-Met (IFNτ-H-Met); and IFNτ with ^{35}S-Met (IFNτ-S-Met) (*see* **Note 5**).

5. Explant cultures are then placed in a controlled atmosphere chamber on a rocking platform (6 cycles/min) and maintained at 37°C for 24 h under an atmosphere of 50% O$_2$, 45% N$_2$, and 5% CO$_2$.

6. At the end of the incubation period, tissue and medium are centrifuged (12,500g for 10 min), separated, and flash-frozen. Samples should be stored at –20°C until analyzed.

7. Medium from each culture is dialyzed against three changes (4 L) of dialysis buffer.

8. Aliquots of medium are subjected to scintillation counting for radioactivity to estimate relative amounts of radiolabeled proteins synthesized *de novo* and released into the medium.

9. Dialyzed MEM samples are then mixed (1.5 mL of each culture) to obtain the following: BSA-H-Met plus BSA-S-Met; IFNτ-H-Met plus IFNτ-S-Met; BSA-H-Met plus IFNτ-S-Met; and BSA-S-Met plus IFNτ H-Met (*see* **Note 6**).
10. Mixed samples are then separated by 2D-PAGE, and radiolabeled proteins visualized by fluorography.
11. Selected radiolabeled proteins on the gels can be numbered and punched out using the appropriate size cork borer.
12. Gel punches are placed in 0.5 mL 30% H_2O_2 at 80°C until the gel is soluble.
13. Samples are the mixed with 0.5 mL 50 m*M* ascorbic acid and subjected to differential scintillation counting to determine the ^3H:^{35}S Met ratio for each selected protein spot.
14. The relative changes in proteins between IFNτ and BSA treatments can be calculated *(38)*.
15. For each protein, analysis of variance is performed on the radioisotope ratios for each mixture after data are log-transformed to eliminate scale effects.
16. Treatment effects are determined using contrasts that compare ratios obtained for opposite combinations. This test is most sensitive since a treatment that increases the ratio in one mixture should decrease the ratio in the opposite mixture.

3.3. Intrauterine Infusion of IFNτ to Study ISGs in the Ovine Uterus

1. Cyclic ewes are fitted with indwelling uterine catheters on day 5 post-estrus as originally described by Godkin et al. *(39)*.
2. Ewes are induced to a surgical plane of anethesia, and the uterus and ovaries are exteriorized through a midventral incision.
3. The V6 polyvinyl catheter is introduced into the lumen of the oviduct ipsilateral to the CL approx 1–2 cm above the tubo–uterine junction, and the tip of the catheter fed into the uterine lumen approx 2 cm below the tubo–uterine junction. The catheter has 3 cuffs (~0.5 cm wide) made of V8 polyvinyl catheter that are placed 4, 5, and 15 cm from the tip, which are used to secure it to the oviduct and the intercornual ligament.
4. Silk ligatures *(2)* are placed on either side of each cuff, securing the catheter to the exterior of the oviduct and to the uterine horn.
5. The catheter was exteriorized through the animal's flank.
6. The length of the exteriorized cannula (~20 cm) is stored in a sealable plastic bag, which is covered with surgical tape and sutured to the skin in each corner.
7. The ends of the exteriorized catheters are kept closed using dialysis tubing clips.
8. After recovery, the ewes are maintained in a large pen.
9. In order to infuse proteins into the uterus, the ewes are caught by hand and then briefly physically restrained as the proteins are infused into the uterus via the catheter. It is important to keep the bag securely affixed to the skin.
10. The uteri of ewes are infused daily with either ovine serum proteins as a control or roIFNτ (1×10^7 antiviral units) *(29)* at 0700 and 1900 h daily from days 11 to 16. Control and roIFNτ proteins are stored at –20°C and brought to room temperature before injection into the uterus via exteriorized catheters.

11. Protein treatments into the uterine horn via the exteriorized catheters are followed by 50 mg ampicillin in 0.1 mL sterile saline (0.9% w/v NaCl) and 1.0 mL sterile saline to clear the catheter.
12. The ewes are hysterectomized on day 17 to obtain the uterus (*see* **Notes 7** and **8**).

3.4. Human 2fTGH Cells to Discover IFNτ-Regulated Genes

The 2fTGH cell and its derivates (*see* **Table 1**) are excellent models for studying responses of endometrial stroma/GE and LE of the ovine uterus to IFNτ because they recapitulate cell type-specific responses of the ovine uterus to IFN(during pregnancy in terms of ISG expression *(7,24,25)*.

1. 2fTGH and U1-U6 cells are treated with roIFNτ (10^4 antiviral U/mL) for 6 to 24 h.
2. Untreated and treated cells are harvested for RNA and protein analysis (*see* **Note 9**).

4. Notes

1. When incubating endometrium with radiolabeled methionine, for example, the concentration of radioinert methionine is reduced to one-tenth that normally used to enhance incorporation of the radiolabeled amino acid into proteins that are synthesized and/or secreted by the endometrium in culture.
2. Most rabbit polyclonal and mouse monoclonal antibodies generated against human proteins and peptides are useful for the analysis of ISGs in ovine endometrium and endometrial cell lines as well as human cell lines.
3. This method uses radiolabeled leucine in supplemented MEM for detection of *de novo* synthesized and secreted proteins using 2D-PAGE and fluorography *(40,41)*. However, other radiolabeled amino acids may be used for the method.
4. The cultured endometrium can also be solubilized and analyzed by 2D-PAGE and fluorography to ascertain the molecular weight and pI of proteins synthesized *de novo*.
5. To increase incorporation of radiolabeled Met, no radioinert Met is included in the modified MEM.
6. Mixing media from the different cultures and measuring ratios of the two radioisotopes allows treatment comparisons independent of variation due to separate electrophoresis procedures (sample loading, efficiency of gel penetration, and so on).
7. At hysterectomy, the catheter should be checked to ensure it was maintained in the uterine lumen during the infusion period. In addition, the CL should be structurally intact in ewes infused with roIFNτ, but structurally regressed in control ewes. If necessary, daily blood samples can be taken for determination of circulating levels of progesterone, which is a sensitive indicator of CL function.
8. RNA can be extracted from the endometrium and analyzed by quantitative methods (Northern, slot blot, reverse-transcription polymerase chain reaction) to determine ISG mRNA levels. Protein can be extracted from the endometrium and analyzed by 1D- or 2D-PAGE followed by Western blot analysis to determine ISG protein levels. Endometrium can be fixed in 4% paraformaldehyde in PBS or frozen for sectioning and localization of ISG mRNAs and proteins by *in situ* hybridization or immunohistochemistry, respectively.

9. Comprehensive genome-wide gene profiling is possible in human tissues and cells, but not currently in tissues from domestic animals. Therefore, one can identify genes regulated by ovine IFNτ using commercially available human arrays *(7,42)*.

Acknowledgments

This work was supported by grants from the The National Institute of Child Health and Human Development (NICHD) (HD 32534) and United States Department of Agriculture (USDA) National Research Initiative Competitive Grants Program.

References

1. Spencer, T. E., Bazer, F. W. (2002) Biology of progesterone action during pregnancy recognition and maintenance of pregnancy. *Front. Biosci.* **7,** d1879–d1898.
2. Fleming, J. A., Choi, Y., Johnson, G. A., Spencer, T. E., and Bazer, F. W. (2001) Cloning of the ovine estrogen receptor-alpha promoter and functional regulation by ovine interferon-tau. *Endocrinology* **142,** 2879–2887.
3. Spencer, T. E., Johnson, G. A., Burghardt, R. C., and Bazer, F. W. (2004) Progesterone and placental hormone actions on the uterus: insights from domestic animals. *Biol. Reprod.* **71,** 2–10.
4. Hansen, T. R., Austin, K. J., Perry, D. J., Pru, J. K., Teixeira, M. G., and Johnson, G. A. (1999) Mechanism of action of interferon-tau in the uterus during early pregnancy. *J. Reprod. Fertil.* **54,** 329–339.
5. Nagaoka, K., Sakai, A., Nojima, H., et al. (2003) A chemokine, interferon (IFN)-gamma-inducible protein 10 kDa, is stimulated by IFN-tau and recruits immune cells in the ovine endometrium. *Biol. Reprod.* **68,** 1413–1421.
6. Nagaoka, K., Nojima, H., Watanabe, F., et al. (2003) Regulation of blastocyst migration, apposition, and initial adhesion by a chemokine, interferon gamma-inducible protein 10 kDa (IP-10), during early gestation. *J. Biol. Chem.* **278,** 29,048–29,056.
7. Kim, S., Choi, Y., Bazer, F. W., and Spencer, T. E. (2003) Identification of genes in the ovine endometrium regulated by interferon tau independent of signal transducer and activator of transcription 1. *Endocrinology* **144,** 5203–5214.
8. Austin, K. J., Bany, B. M., Belden, E. L., Rempel, L. A., Cross, J. C., and Hansen, T. R. (2003) Interferon-stimulated gene-15 (Isg15) expression is up-regulated in the mouse uterus in response to the implanting conceptus. *Endocrinology* **144,** 3107–3113.
9. Li, Q., Zhang, M., Kumar, S., et al. (2001) Identification and implantation stage-specific expression of an interferon-alpha-regulated gene in human and rat endometrium. *Endocrinology* **142,** 2390–2400.
10. Vallet, J. L., Gross, T. S., Fliss, M. F., and Bazer, F. W. (1989) Effects of pregnancy, oxytocin, ovine trophoblast protein-1 and their interactions on endometrial production of prostaglandin F2 alpha in vitro in perifusion chambers. *Prostaglandins* **38,** 113–124.

11. Johnson, G. A., Spencer, T. E., Burghardt, R. C., Joyce, M. M., Bazer, F. W. (2000) Interferon-tau and progesterone regulate ubiquitin cross-reactive protein expression in the ovine uterus. *Biol. Reprod.* **62,** 622–627.

12. Johnson, G. A., Spencer, T. E., Hansen, T. R., Austin, K. J., Burghardt, R. C., Bazer, F. W. (1999) Expression of the interferon tau inducible ubiquitin cross-reactive protein in the ovine uterus. *Biol. Reprod.* **61,** 312–318.

13. Johnson, G. A., Stewart, M. D., Gray, C. A., et al. (2001) Effects of the estrous cycle, pregnancy, and interferon tau on 2',5'- oligoadenylate synthetase expression in the ovine uterus. *Biol. Reprod.* **64,** 1392–1399.

14. Choi, Y., Johnson, G. A., Burghardt, R. C., et al. (2001) Interferon regulatory factor-two restricts expression of interferon-stimulated genes to the endometrial stroma and glandular epithelium of the ovine uterus. *Biol. Reprod.* **65,** 1038–1049.

15. Choi, Y., Johnson, G. A., Spencer, T. E., and Bazer, F. W. (2003) Pregnancy and interferon tau regulate MHC class I and beta-2-microglobulin expression in the ovine uterus. *Biol. Reprod.* **68,** 1703–1710

16. Pru, J. K., Austin, K. J., Perry, D. J., Nighswonger, A. M., Hansen, T. R. (2000) Production, purification, and carboxy-terminal sequencing of bioactive recombinant bovine interferon-stimulated gene product 17. *Biol. Reprod.* **63,** 619–628.

17. Pru, J. K., Austin, K. J., Haas, A. L. , and Hansen, T. R. (2001) Pregnancy and interferon-tau upregulate gene expression of members of the 1-8 family in the bovine uterus. *Biol. Reprod.* **65,** 1471–1480

18. Nagaoka, K., Sakai, A., Nojima, H., et al. (2003) A chemokine, interferon (IFN)-gamma-inducible protein 10 kDa, is stimulated by IFN-tau and recruits immune cells in the ovine endometrium. *Biol. Reprod.* **68,** 1413–1421.

19. Ott, T. L., Yin, J., Wiley, A. A., et al. (1998) Effects of the estrous cycle and early pregnancy on uterine expression of Mx protein in sheep (Ovis aries). *Biol. Reprod.* **59,** 784–794.

20. Rosenfeld, C. S., Han, C. S., Alexenko, A. P., Spencer, T. E., Roberts, R. M. (2002) Expression of interferon receptor subunits, IFNAR1 and IFNAR2, in the ovine uterus. *Biol. Reprod.* **67,** 847–853.

21. Stark, G. R., Kerr, I. M., Williams, B. R., Silverman, R. H., and Schreiber, R. D. (1998) How cells respond to interferons. *Annu. Rev. Biochem.* **67,** 227–264.

22. Sato, M., Taniguchi, T., and Tanaka, N. (2001) The interferon system and interferon regulatory factor transcription factors—studies from gene knockout mice. *Cytokine Growth Factor Rev.* **12,** 133–142.

23. Mamane, Y., Heylbroeck, C., Genin, P., et al. (1999) Interferon regulatory factors: the next generation. *Gene* **237,** 1–14.

24. Stewart, M. D., Choi, Y., Johnson, G. A., Yu-Lee, L. Y., Bazer, F. W., Spencer, T. E. (2002) Roles of Stat1, Stat2, and interferon regulatory factor-9 (IRF-9) in interferon tau regulation of IRF-1. *Biol. Reprod.* **66,** 393–400.

25. Stewart, M. D., Johnson, G. A., Bazer, F. W., and Spencer, T. E. (2001) Interferon-tau (IFNtau) regulation of IFN-stimulated gene expression in cell lines lacking specific IFN-signaling components. *Endocrinology* **142,** 1786–1794.

26. Stewart, D. M., Johnson, G. A., Vyhlidal, C. A., et al. (2001) Interferon-tau activates multiple signal transducer and activator of transcription proteins and has complex effects on interferon-responsive gene transcription in ovine endometrial epithelial cells. *Endocrinology* **142**, 98–107.

27. Johnson, G. A., Burghardt, R. C., Newton, G. R., Bazer, F. W., and Spencer, T. E. (1999) Development and characterization of immortalized ovine endometrial cell lines. *Biol. Reprod.* **61**, 1324–1330.

28. Mahaboob Basha, S. M., Bazer, F. W., and Roberts, R. M. (1979) The secretion of a uterine specific, purple phosphatase by cultured explants of porcine endometrium: dependency upon the state of pregnancy of the donor animal. *Biol. Reprod.* **20**, 431–441.

29. Van Heeke, G., Ott, T. L., Strauss, A., Ammaturo, D., and Bazer, F. W. (1996) High yield expression and secretion of the ovine pregnancy recognition hormone interferon-tau by Pichia pastoris. *J. Interferon Cytokine Res.* **16**, 119–126.

30. Pontzer, C. H., Torres, B. A., Vallet, J. L., Bazer, F. W., Johnson, H. M. (1988) Antiviral activity of the pregnancy recognition hormone ovine trophoblast protein-1. *Biochem. Biophys. Res. Commun.* **152**, 801–807.

31. Pellegrini, S., John, J., Shearer, M., Kerr, I. M., and Stark, G. R. (1989) Use of a selectable marker regulated by alpha interferon to obtain mutations in the signaling pathway. *Mol. Cell. Biol.* **9**, 4605–4612.

32. John, J., McKendry, R., Pellegrini, S., Flavell, D., Kerr, I. M., Stark, G. R. (1991) Isolation and characterization of a new mutant human cell line unresponsive to alpha and beta interferons. *Mol. Cell. Biol.* **11**, 4189–4195.

33. McKendry, R., John, J., Flavell, D., Muller, M., Kerr, I. M., Stark, G. R. (1991) High-frequency mutagenesis of human cells and characterization of a mutant unresponsive to both alpha and gamma interferons. *Proc. Natl. Acad. Sci. USA* **88**, 11,455–11,459.

34. McKendry, R., Pellegrini, S., Kerr, I. M., and Stark, G. R. (1994) Constitutive production of alpha and beta interferons in mutant human cell lines. *J. Virol.* **68**, 4057–4062.

35. Muller, M., Laxton, C., Briscoe, J., et al. (1993) Complementation of a mutant cell line: central role of the 91 kDa polypeptide of ISGF3 in the interferon-alpha and -gamma signal transduction pathways. *EMBO J.* **12**, 4221–4228.

36. Muller, M., Briscoe, J., Laxton, C., et al. (1993) The protein tyrosine kinase JAK1 complements defects in interferon-α/β and -γ signal transduction. *Nature* **366**, 129–135.

37. Velazquez, L., Fellous, M., Stark, G. R., and Pellegrini, S. (1992) A protein tyrosine kinase in the interferon alpha/beta signaling pathway. *Cell* **70**, 313–322.

38. Vallet, J. L., Bazer, F. W., and Roberts, R. M. (1987) The effect of ovine trophoblast protein-one on endometrial protein secretion and cyclic nucleotides. *Biol. Reprod.* **37**, 1307–1316.

39. Godkin, J. D., Bazer, F. W., Thatcher, W. W., and Roberts, R. M. (1984) Proteins released by cultured Day 15-16 conceptuses prolong luteal maintenance when introduced into the uterine lumen of cyclic ewes. *J. Reprod. Fertil.* **71**, 57–64.

40. Godkin, J. D., Bazer, F. W., and Roberts, R. M. (1985) Protein production by cultures established from Day-14-16 sheep and pig conceptuses. *J. Reprod. Fertil.* **74,** 377–382.

41. Godkin, J. D., Bazer, F. W., and Roberts, R. M. (1984) Ovine trophoblast protein 1, an early secreted blastocyst protein, binds specifically to uterine endometrium and affects protein synthesis. *Endocrinology* **114,** 120–130.

42. Der, S. D., Zhou, A., Williams, B. R., and Silverman, R. H. (1998) Identification of genes differentially regulated by interferon alpha, beta, or gamma using oligonucleotide arrays. *Proc. Natl. Acad. Sci. USA* **95,**15,623–15,628.

V

Analysis of Placenta Adaptation to Disease

24

Reduced Uterine Perfusion Pressure (RUPP) Model for Studying Cardiovascular–Renal Dysfunction in Response to Placental Ischemia

Joey P. Granger, B. Babbette D. LaMarca, Kathy Cockrell, Mona Sedeek, Charles Balzi, Derrick Chandler, and William Bennett

Summary

Despite being one of the leading causes of maternal death and a major contributor of maternal and perinatal morbidity, the mechanisms responsible for the pathogenesis of preeclampsia are unknown. The initiating event in preeclampsia has been postulated to be reduced uteroplacental perfusion. Placental ischemia/hypoxia is thought to lead to widespread activation/dysfunction of the maternal vascular endothelium, vasoconstriction and hypertension. Experimental induction of chronic uteroplacental ischemia appears to be the most promising animal model to study potential mechanisms of preeclampsia since reductions in uteroplacental blood flow in a variety of animal models lead to a hypertensive state that closely resembles preeclampsia in women. This chapter details the methods we use in our laboratory to produce the reduced uterine perfusion pressure (RUPP) model in the pregnant rat.

Key Words: Preeclampsia; placenta; arterial pressure; rat; ischemia; pregnancy

1. Introduction

Preeclampsia is estimated to affect 7–10% of all pregnancies in the United States *(1,2)*. Preeclampsia in women is typically characterized by hypertension, proteinuria, and edema *(1–5)*. Despite being one of the leading causes of maternal death and a major contributor of maternal and perinatal morbidity, the mechanisms responsible for the pathogenesis of preeclampsia have not yet been fully elucidated. Hypertension associated with preeclampsia develops during pregnancy and remits after delivery, implicating the placenta as a central culprit in the disease *(1–5)*. An initiating event in preeclampsia has been postulated to be reduced placental perfusion, which leads to widespread dysfunction of the maternal vascular endothelium by mechanisms that remain to be defined *(6)*.

From: *Methods in Molecular Medicine, Vol. 122: Placenta and Trophoblast: Methods and Protocols, Vol. 2*
Edited by: M. J. Soares and J. S. Hunt © Humana Press Inc., Totowa, NJ

Although the physiological mechanisms that mediate the alterations in vascular function have been extensively studied during normal pregnancy, information regarding the mediators of the alteration in endothelial and vascular function during preeclampsia has been limited because of the difficulty in performing mechanistic studies in pregnant women. The main focus of this chapter is on the procedures used to produce an animal model to study mechanisms that link placental ischemia/hypoxia with the vascular pathophysiology of preeclampsia. Experimental induction of chronic uteroplacental ischemia appears to be the most promising animal model to study potential mechanisms of preeclampsia since reductions in uteroplacental blood flow in a variety of animal models lead to a hypertensive state that closely resembles preeclampsia in women *(7)*. In early studies of the relationship between placental blood flow and preeclampsia, Ogden et al. found that partially occluding the infrarenal aorta of pregnant, but not nonpregnant, dogs resulted in hypertension *(8)*. In subsequent studies, the bilateral ligation of the utero-ovarian arteries and placement of nonconstrictive bands around the uterine arteries resulted in hypertension in dogs only after they achieved pregnancy *(9)*. These animals uniformly developed hypertension. This hypertensive state persisted until the postpartum period, at which time pressures returned to normal. These findings were confirmed by studies in dogs in which precise constriction of the aorta below the renal arteries resulted in hypertension and proteinuria *(10,11)*. These animals also displayed glomerular endothelial lesions (termed glomerular endotheliosis) similar to those classically found in preeclamptic women. Losonczy et al. conducted experiments in which aortic constriction was performed and measurements were obtained from conscious, chronically instrumented rabbits *(12)*. These studies demonstrated elevated arterial pressures accompanied by increased peripheral resistance, a feature commonly observed in preeclamptic women .

The relationship between reduced uteroplacental perfusion and hypertension during pregnancy has also been demonstrated in nonhuman primates. Cavanagh and co-workers *(13,14)* conducted studies in baboons using a system similar to that used by Hodari with the ligation of the utero-ovarian arteries and placement of bands around the uterine arteries. Females bred after the surgery exhibited higher blood pressures than nonpregnant or sham-operated control pregnant animals. These animals were also found to have glomerular endothelial swelling. An aortic constriction model has also been reported in Rhesus monkeys *(15)* to study the effects of reduced utero-placental perfusion from early pregnancy through delivery. In this model, the degree of aortic constriction was precisely controlled, and progressive hypertension, proteinuria, and glomerular endotheliosis developed.

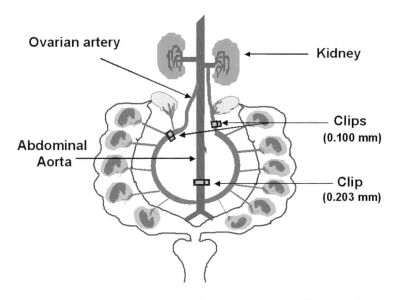

Fig. 1. Induction of reduced uterine perfusion pressure (RUPP) model in pregnant rats. Uterine perfusion pressure in the gravid rat is reduced by approx 40% by placing a silver clip (0.203 mm) around the aorta below the renal arteries. Because this procedure has been shown to cause an adaptive increase in uterine blood flow via branches of the ovarian artery, we also placed a silver clip (0.1mm) on both the right and left uterine arcade at the ovarian end just before the first segmental artery. RUPP results in significant and consistent elevations in arterial pressure of 20–30 mmHg at day 19 of gestation.

Hypertension in response to chronic reductions in uteroplacental perfusion pressure in gravid rats after day 14 of gestation has been reported by Eder and MacDonald *(16)*. Recently, we have modified and characterized this rat model in order to examine potential pathophysiological mechanisms that mediate the hypertension during chronic reductions in uteroplacental perfusion pressure *(17–23)*. We reduced uterine perfusion pressure in the gravid rat by approx 40% by placing a silver clip around the aorta below the renal arteries (*see* **Note 1**). Because this procedure has been shown to cause an adaptive increase in uterine blood flow via the ovarian artery, we also placed a silver clip on both the right and left uterine arcade at the ovarian end just before the first segmental artery *(24)* (**Fig. 1**). We found that reducing uteroplacental perfusion pressure (RUPP) results in significant and consistent elevations in arterial pressure of 20–30 mmHg as compared with control pregnant rats at day 19 of gestation *(17)*. We also reported that reducing uteroplacental perfusion pressure in nonpregnant rats had no effect on blood pressure *(17)*. Our data also indicate that the RUPP-induced hypertension is associated with proteinuria, reductions in renal plasma flow and glomerular filtration rate, and a hypertensive shift in the pressure natriuresis relationship *(17)*. Moreover, we found important evidence indicating that endothelial function is significantly impaired in the RUPP hypertensive rat *(20)*. We compared the relaxation responses to acetylcholine between aortic vessel strips of pregnant and RUPP hypertensive rats and found that endothelial-dependent vasodilatation was significantly attenuated in the RUPP hypertensive rats *(20)*. In addition, we reported that the production of nitric oxide is reduced in vascular tissue while the synthesis of thromboxane, endothelin, and 8-isoprostane (a marker of oxidative stress) are elevated in the RUPP hypertensive rat as compared to normal pregnant rats at day 19 of gestation *(17–23)*. Moreover, we have preliminary evidence that the inflammatory cytokine, tumor necrosis factor (TNF)-α is significantly elevated in the plasma of the RUPP hypertensive rat. Finally, we have found intrauterine growth restriction in the RUPP hypertensive rats because the average pup size in this group is smaller than in normal pregnant rats *(17)*. Thus, RUPP-induced hypertension in the pregnant rat has many of the features of preeclampsia in women.

2. Materials

The RUPP procedure is performed in female time pregnant Sprague-Dawley rats weighing approx 200–250 g. Pregnancy-induced hypertension has been produced in a variety of animals by mechanically reducing the uteroplacental perfusion pressure during pregnancy. We have chosen the rat model of reduced uterine perfusion pressure to study pregnancy-induced hypertension for several important reasons. Rats have the advantage of short gestation period of approx 21–22 d and are easy to maintain and less costly. Furthermore, the cardiovascular, renal, neural, and hormonal physiology of normal pregnancy has been extensively investigated in the conscious chronically instrumented rat model.

2.1. Silver Clips for Reducing Uterine Perfusion Pressure

1. Silver foil, AG000450, 0.25 mm thick (Goodfellow Cambridge, Devon, PA).
2. Feeler/thickness gage.
3. Fine metal file.

2.2. Materials for Surgical Procedure

1. Sprague-Dawley timed pregnant rats (Harlan, Indianapolis, IN).
2. Isofluorane anesthesia machine (Webster, Sterling, MA, Ohmeda Model No. BBTQ04288).
3. Oxygen 100% (E-tank).
4. Oxygen regulator set at 1 L.

5. Isofluorane anesthesia (Phoenix brand, Webster, Sterling, MA).
6. Anesthesia box for induction.
7. Sterile 0.9% sodium chloride (NaCl).
8. Gauze 4-in. × 4-in.
9. Cotton tipped applicators.
10. Forceps.
11. Scissors.
12. Needle holders.
13. Modified needle holders.
14. Hemostats.
15. Suture 3-0 Supramid Extra II (S. Jackson Inc., Alexandria, VA).
16. Suture three-eighths circle needle nylon, nonabsorbable. (S. Jackson Inc., Alexandria, VA).
17. Absorbable gelatin sponge (Gelfoam®).

3. Methods

3.1 Methods for Preparing Silver Vessel Constriction Clips

1. Uterine perfusion pressure in the gravid rat is reduced by placing a silver constriction clip around the aorta below the renal arteries. The clip is made from a sheet of silver with a thickness of 0.25 mm. Using a pair of surgical scissors, a small strip approx 1.25–1.75 mm in width is cut from the sheet. The strip will curl up as it is cut. Simply flatten and straighten the strip with the fingers and lay it on a hard flat surface, preferably a metal table. Hold the two ends down with one hand. Using the back of the scissors, rub along the edges of the strip to smooth out any sharp edges or burrs. This should be done on both edges of one side and for the full length of the strip.

2. Using a very fine metal file, file both edges of the strip to ensure that all burrs are removed. It may be difficult to hold the strip with enough support to file the edges. Holding the end of the strip between the thumb and side of the middle finger while supporting the bottom edge with the index finger works best.

3. Round off the end of the strip using the file. The edges and the end of the clip must be free from all burrs nicks or sharp edges. The rounded and smooth edges help the clip to slide on easily and prevent any damage to the vessel.

4. Place the strip of silver on the table so that the smoothed edges are on the top. This will be the inside of the clip, where the vessel will be sliding into place. Apply a feeler/thickness gage of 0.203 mm over the strip so that approx 3.5–4.5 mm of the strip is showing. Bend the strip over the feeler gage and press down firmly with the back of the scissors or the back of the file.

5. The spacing of the clip may be checked by removing the gage and holding the clip up to the light. If there are any deviations, simply replace the gage and press firmly with the scissors or file.

6. Remove the gage and cut the clip from the strip approx 4–5 mm behind the overlap, creating a tail to grab with forceps and leaving enough space to lay the vessel into the clip.

3.2. Method for Preparing Ovarian Clips

1. The ovarian clips are made from the same sheets of silver and the same strips are cut. The strips do not have to be rubbed and filed down unless there are any major burrs or nicks on them. These clips do not slide onto the vessel they are clamped on.
2. The silver strip is cut into 8- to 10-mm long pieces. These pieces are bent in half with the fingers to an approx 30–45° angle. The correct spacing of the clip is determined by the clamp, not the clip. The thickness of the silver is 0.25 mm, and the optimum space is 0.1 mm. The clamp is made from a pair of needle holders, which have been ground down so that, when they are closed, the space between the jaws is 0.6 mm.

3.3. Surgical Procedure for Reducing Uterine Perfusion Pressure

1. Surgical procedures are performed under aseptic conditions. Isoflorane is used to anesthetize the rats. After the rat is under anesthesia (2% isoflorane), shave the rat along the midline of the belly from the last pair of nipples to the rib cage. Wipe down the shaved area with alcohol and iodine prep solution.
2. Using a pair of surgical scissors (or surgical scalpel blade if you prefer), make a cut along the midline approx 2–2.5 inches in length. Then, make another cut through the muscle tissue of the abdominal wall. Be cautious not to cut or damage any organs.
3. Moisten some 4×4 gauze or sponge pads with saline. Then place them on each side of the cut.
4. Moisten a couple of cotton swabs and use them to pull out the uterus. The fingers may also be used, but in that case, ensure that too much pressure is not put on the uterus. If there is too much trauma to the pups, they will be reabsorbed.
5. Lay the uterus onto the wet gauze pads. Fold the pads over to cover the exposed uterus. This will prevent the uterus from drying while the procedure is being performed.
6. Next, use the moist cotton swabs to find the abdominal aorta. It is dorsal to the large intestine/colon. It may be necessary to pull apart some of the fatty tissue to expose the aorta. Keep at a minimum to prevent any excess bleeding.
7. The aortic clip must be placed directly anterior to the bifurcation of the aorta. Therefore, this is where the vessel must be isolated. For this portion of the procedure, it is best to use a pair of micro dissecting, serrated, slight (or full) curve forceps. A tip width of 0.8 mm is recommended, but a 0.5-mm tip may also be used (the smaller tip can tear or puncture a vessel much easier).
8. Be aware of a small feeder vessel, which cannot be seen, branching from the dorsal side of the aorta. It is often right around where the clip should be placed. When isolating the vessel, be extremely careful not to tear this feeder vessel. If it is ruptured, there will be excess bleeding and the rat is likely to die or at least reabsorb the pups. The bleeding can be stopped by placing a small piece of absorbable gelatin sponge (Gelfoam) into the area to induce clotting.
9. Using a pair of forceps in the right hand, go underneath the aorta from the left side of the rat. Place the closed tip of the forceps between the aorta and the vein.

Be sure the tip is between the two vessels; it is difficult to judge where the edge of the vein is. Lift to add slight pressure to the tip of the forceps. The vessels are very frail as a result of pregnancy so do not put too much pressure on them or they will tear.

10. Open and close forceps to help push through the connective tissue between the vessels. The tissue is tough and it may take a minute or two to do this (be patient and do not hurry). A cotton swab can also be used. Place the tip of the swab on the tip of the forceps with the tissue between the two and push slightly.

11. Once the tips of the forceps are through the connective tissue, open and close them to enlarge the opening between the two vessels. Do not force the opening any larger than the forceps themselves will make it, to prevent tearing the feeder vessel underneath.

12. Once the aorta has been isolated, pick it up with the forceps underneath (not too much lift) to hold the opening and to help flatten the artery. With a second pair of forceps in the left hand, hold the aortic clip by the end and slide it underneath the vessel from the right. If it will not go easily, do not force it. The small feeder vessel may be blocking it between the tips of the forceps holding the vessel. Remove the forceps from underneath the aorta and reposition them.

13. Once the clip is all the way under the aorta, lay the vessel on the tail end of the clip, which is being held by the forceps in the left hand. Lift the vessel to decrease blood flow and very gently slide the clip onto the vessel. It is a tight squeeze, but it will go on. The aortic clip will stay in place by itself once it is on the vessel.

14. Because clipping of the aorta above the uterine arteries has been reported to cause an adaptive increase in uterine blood flow via branches of the ovarian artery, we also place a silver clip on both the right and left uterine arcade at the ovarian end just before the first segmental artery. The silver ovarian clips are placed on the main artery between the ovarian branch and the first branch leading to the uterus and first pup.

15. The moist cotton swabs can be used to find the vessels. The fatty tissue is full of tiny blood vessels, which are very delicate. It may take a minute to figure out were to place the clip. Sometimes the fatty tissue gets in the way, but do not try to get through it or an unseen vessel may be torn.

16. Once you have determined where to place the clip, use the small forceps to isolate the vessel. Open and close the forceps to help push through the fat underneath and directly around the vessel. Do not try to clean the vessel excessively because it is too delicate. Next, place the clip around the vessel with the open end toward you. Also, place the vessel at the folded end of the clip.

17. Place the open end of the clip toward the inside of the clamp and the folded end away from the clamp. Be sure that the whole clip is inside the jaws of the clamp to ensure proper closure. Repeat these steps for the opposite uterine horn.

18. Once all the clips are in place, gently put the uterus back into the abdomen and pour some saline into the cavity.

19. Use an interlocking mattress stitch or a simple tie stitch to suture the abdominal muscle wall. A simple continuous stitch may be used to close the skin.

20. Clean all blood and fluids around the cut with hydrogen peroxide after closure.
21. All rats are allowed to recover for 4–5 d before physiological measurements are obtained (*see* **Note 2**).

4. Notes

1. Eder and McDonald *(16)* utilized silk ties to constrict the blood vessels leading to the uteroplacental unit. We utilize silver clips (the same material used to produce renovascular hypertension in rats). The silver clips are less tissue-reactive and provide more precise control of vessel constriction. Timing of the vessel constriction is another important issue. During a series of pilot studies to determine the appropriate clip size and the ideal gestational time for reducing uterine perfusion pressure, we found that placement of the clips prior to d 14 of gestation in the rat resulted in a significant increase in pup deaths. We have found that reducing perfusion pressure at day 14 of gestation produces a consistent blood pressure effect (measured at days 19–20 in conscious rats).

2. Blood pressure measurements are typically measured at d 19–20 of gestation. This time period allows the animals to fully recover from the effects of anesthesia and surgery. It is critical that blood pressure is measured in the conscious state because anesthesia markedly influences systemic hemodynamics in pregnant animals. Blood pressures are measured by chronic indwelling arterial catheters, which are placed in the animal at the time of the clipping procedure. A more detailed description of catheter placement can be obtained in **ref. *17***.

   Measurements of 24 h urinary protein excretion are performed on d 18–19 of gestation by placing the animals in metabolic cages. Although we have observed significant increases in protein excretion and consistent increases in blood pressure in response to reductions in uterine perfusion pressure, the proteinuria response has been somewhat variable in the pregnant rats. The reason for the variability is unknown, but it may be due to the short time frame of exposure to placental ischemia. Another possibility is that the variable proteinuric response is due to the preglomerular constriction and subsequent reduction in glomerular hydrostatic pressure may protect the glomerular membrane from further damage caused by placental ischemia.

References

1. August, P. and Lindheimer, M. D. (1995) Pathophysiology of preeclampsia, in *Hypertension*, 2nd Edition (Laragh, J. L. and Brenner, B. M., eds.). Raven, New York: pp. 2407–2426.
2. Roberts, J. M., Taylor, R. N., Musci, T. J., Rodgers, G. M., Hubel, C. A., and McLaughlin, M. K. (1989) Preeclampsia: an endothelial cell disorder. *Am. J. Obstet. Gynecol.* **161,** 1200–1204.
3. Alexander, B. T., Bennett, W. A., Khalil, R. A., and Granger, J. P. (2001) Pathophysiology of pregnancy-induced hypertension. *News Physiol. Sci.* **16,** 282–286.
4. Granger, J. P., Alexander, B. T., Bennett, W. A., and Khalil, R. A. (2001) Pathophysiology of pregnancy-induced hypertension. *Am. J. Hypertens.* **14,** 178–185.

5. Granger, J. P., Alexander, B. T., Llinas, M. T., Bennett, W. A., and Khalil, R. A. (2001) Pathophysiology of hypertension during preeclampsia: Linking placental ischemia with endothelial dysfunction. *Hypertension* **38,** 718–722.

6. Fisher, S. J. and Roberts, J. M. (1999) Defects in placentation and placental perfusion, in *Chesley's Hypertensive Disorders in Pregnancy*, 2nd Edition (Linhheimer, M. D., Roberts, J. M., and Cunningham, F. G., eds.). Appleton & Lange, Stanford, CT: pp. 377–394.

7. Conrad, K. P. (1990) Animal models of pre-eclampsia: do they exist? *Fetal Medicine Rev.* **2,** 67–88.

8. Ogden, E., Hildebrand, G. J., and Page, E. W. (1940) Rise in blood pressure during ischemia of the gravid uterus. *Proc. Soc. Exper. Biol. Med.* **43,** 49–51.

9. Hodari, A. A. (1967) Chronic uterine ischemia and reversible experimental "toxemia of pregnancy". *Am. J. Obstet. Gynecol.* **97,** 597–607.

10. Abitbol, M. M., Gallo, G. R., Pirani, C. L., and Ober, W. B. (1976) Production of experimental toxemia in the pregnant rabbit. *Am. J. Obstet. Gynecol.* **124,** 460–470.

11. Abitbol, M. M., Pirani, C. L., Ober, W. B., Driscoll, S. G., and Cohen, M. W. (1976) Production of experimental toxemia in the pregnant dog. *Obstet. Gynecol.* **48,** 537–548.

12. Losonczy, G., Brown, G., and Venuto, R. C. (1992) Increased peripheral resistance during reduced uterine perfusion pressure hypertension in pregnant rabbits. *Am. J. Med. Sci.* **303,** 233–240.

13. Cavanagh, D., Rao, P. S., Tung, K. S., and Gaston, L. (1974) Eclamptogenic toxemia: The development of an experimental model in the subhuman primate. *Am. J. Obstet. Gynecol.* **120,** 183–196.

14. Cavanagh, D., Rao, P. S., Tsai, C. C., and O'Connor, T. C. (1977) Experimental toxemia in the pregnant primate. *Am. J. Obstet. Gynecol.* **128,** 75–85.

15. Combs, C. A., Katz, M. A., Kitzmiller, J. L., and Brescia, R. J. (1993) Experimental preeclampsia produced by chronic constriction of the lower aorta: Validation with longitudinal blood pressure measurements in conscious rhesus monkeys. *Am. J. Obstet. Gynecol.* **169,** 215–223.

16. Eder, D. J. and McDonald, M. T. (1987-1988) A role for brain angiotensin II in experimental pregnancy-induced hypertension in laboratory rats. *Clin. Exp. Hyper. Preg.* **B6,** 431–451.

17. Alexander, B. T., Kassab, S. E., Miller, M. T., et al. (2001) Reduced uterine perfusion pressure during pregnancy in the rat is associated with increases in arterial pressure and changes in renal nitric oxide. *Hypertension* **37,** 1191–1195.

18. Alexander, B. T., Rinewalt, A. N., Cockrell, K. L., Bennett, W. A., and Granger, J. P. (2001) Endothelin-A receptor blockade attenuates the hypertension in response to chronic reductions in uterine perfusion pressure. *Hypertension* **37,** 485–489.

19. Alexander, B. T., Cockrell, K. L., Sedeek, M., and Granger, J. P. (2001) Role of the renin-angiotensin system in meditating the hypertension produced by chronic reductions in uterine perfusion pressure in the pregnant rat. *Hypertension* **38,** 742–745.

20. Crews, J. K., Herrington, J. N., Granger, J. P., and Khalil, R. A. (2000) Decreased endothelium-dependent vascular relaxation during reduction of uterine perfusion pressure in pregnant rats. *Hypertension* **35,** 367–372.

21. Llinas, M. T., Alexander, B. T., Abram, S. R., Sedeek, M., and Granger, J. P. (2002) Enhanced production of thromboxane A2 in response to chronic reductions in uterine perfusion pressure in pregnant rats. *Am. J. Hypertens.* **15,** 793–797.

22. Llinas, M. T., Alexander, B. T., Capparelli, M., Carroll, M. A., and Granger, J. P. (2004) Cytochrome P-450 inhibition attenuates hypertension induced by reductions in uterine perfusion pressure in pregnant rats. *Hypertension* **43,** 623–628.

23. Alexander, B. T., Llinas, M. T., Kruckeberg, W. C., and Granger, J. P. (2004) L-arginine attenuates hypertension in pregnant rats with reduced uterine perfusion pressure. *Hypertension* **43,** 832–836.

24. Nienartowicz, A., Link, S., and Moll, W. (1989) Adaptation of the uterine arcade in rats during pregnancy. *J. Develop. Physiol.* **21,** 101–108.

25

In Vivo Rat Model of Preeclampsia

S. Ananth Karumanchi and Isaac E. Stillman

Summary

Preeclampsia is characterized by the clinical triad of new hypertension, proteinuria, and edema after 20 wk of gestation. Recent evidence suggests that disturbances in angiogenic factors (such as vascular endothelial growth factor and placental growth factor) signaling and endothelial health may play a major role in the pathogenesis of preeclampsia. Exogenous administration of soluble fms-like tyrosine kinase-1 (sFlt-1; a circulating anti-angiogenic protein) results in a preeclampsia-like phenotype in rats. This chapter describes the methods we use in our laboratory to create the sFlt-1 induced-rat model of preeclampsia.

Key Words: Albuminuria; hypertension; angiogenesis; pregnancy; glomerular endotheliosis.

1. Introduction

Preeclampsia is one of the least well understood and most prevalent disorders of pregnancy and leads to significant morbidity and mortality to the mother and the baby. It is believed to be a two-stage disease, with an initial placental trigger with no maternal symptoms followed by a maternal syndrome characterized by hypertension, proteinuria, and endothelial dysfunction *(1–3)*. The clinical picture may be dominated by mild to severe microangiopathy in which the chief target organ may be the brain (eclampsia), the liver (Hemolysis, Elevated Liver, Low Platelet [HELLP] syndrome) or the kidney (glomerular endotheliosis and proteinuria) *(4)*. Preeclampsia occurs only in the presence of the placenta and can occur even when there is no fetus (as in hydatidiform mole) or in extrauterine pregnancy (where preeclampsia persists after the delivery of fetus but not the placenta). It remits dramatically in the postpartum after the delivery of the placenta *(5)*. All of the clinical manifestations of preeclampsia can be attributed to endothelial cell dysfunction leading to end-organ damage and hypoperfusion. Based on this observation, it has been suggested that there may be a circulating factor, likely placental in origin, which

From: *Methods in Molecular Medicine, Vol. 122: Placenta and Trophoblast: Methods and Protocols, Vol. 2*
Edited by: M. J. Soares and J. S. Hunt © Humana Press Inc., Totowa, NJ

affects systemic endothelial cell function and leads to the clinical syndrome of preeclampsia *(6,7)*.

Recently, gene expression profiling has been used to search for candidate factors produced by the placenta in preeclampsia. Using this approach, we found that placental soluble fms-like tyrosine kinase-1 (sFlt-1 or sVEGFR-1) mRNA is upregulated in preeclampsia *(8)*. sFlt-1, a splice variant of the vascular endothelial growth factor (VEGF) receptor, Flt-1, which lacks the transmembrane and cytoplasmic domains, is made in large amounts by the placenta and is released into the maternal circulation *(9,10)*. sFlt-1 acts as a potent VEGF and placental growth factor (PlGF) antagonist by binding these molecules in circulation. Circulating sFlt-1 concentrations are increased in women with established preeclampsia *(8,11)* and may begin to rise before the onset of clinical symptoms *(12)*. Consistent with the antagonistic effect of sFlt-1, free (or unbound) VEGF and free (or unbound) PlGF concentrations are decreased in preeclamptic women at disease presentation and even before the onset of clinical symptoms *(8,12–14)*. When administered to pregnant and nonpregnant rats, sFlt-1 produces a syndrome of hypertension, proteinuria, and glomerular endotheliosis that recapitulates the human syndrome of preeclampsia *(8)*. This chapter will highlight the generation of the rat model of preeclampsia with details on characterization of the systemic signs and symptoms of preeclampsia. The effects of sFlt1 on the fetus and the placenta are currently being characterized in our laboratory and will not be discussed here.

2. Materials

1. Adenoviruses expressing sFlt-1 or control Fc were obtained from Dr. Richard Mulligan at Children's Hospital, Boston, MA. The detailed construction of the adenoviral plasmid has been previously described *(15)*.
2. Adenovirus dialysis buffer: sterile 20 mM Tris pH 8.0, 25 mM NaCl, 2.5% glycerol.
3. Plaque dilution based titration assay kit (BD Biosciences Clontech, Palo Alto, CA, cat. no. K1653-1)
4. Day 5–6 pregnant Sprague-Dawley Rats (Harlan, Indianapolis, IN).
5. Nephrat II . Enzyme-linked immunosorbent assay (ELISA) for urinary albumin (Exocell, Philadelphia, PA, cat. no. NR002).
6. Mouse sVEGF receptor-1 (otherwise referred to as sFlt-1) ELISA kit (R&D Systems, Minneapolis, MN, cat. no. MVR100).
7. 3-Fr high fidelity microtip catheter connected to a pressure transducer (Millar Instruments, Houston, TX).
8. Metra urinary creatinine assay (Quidel Corp, San Diego, CA, cat. no. 8009).
9. Bouin's solution (Sigma-Aldrich, St. Louis, MO, cat. no. HT10-1-32) and glutaraldehyde fixative (Sigma-Aldrich, cat. no. G5882).
10. Anti-rat fluorescein isothiocyanate (FITC)-onjugated fibrinogen antibody (MP Biomedicals, Aurora, Ohio, cat. no. 55752).

11. Reagents for electron microscopy: 3% glutaraldehyde, 2% osmium, 2% uranyl acetate, Epon, and methylene blue.

3. Methods

Procedures described in this section include methods for (1) adenoviral preparation and injection, (2) blood pressure measurement, (3) blood and urine chemistry, and (4) renal histology and electron microscopy.

3.1. Adenovirus Preparation and Injection

1. Adenoviruses expressing Fc or sFlt1 (obtained from Dr. Mulligan) are amplified from a single plaque by serial infection of 293A cells and purified by two cycles of CsCl gradient and dialyzed. Adenovirus expressing murine Fc protein (a soluble protein) in equivalent doses is used as a control to rule out non-specific effects of adenoviruses.
2. The final products are titered by an optical absorbance method *(16)*. The titer is expressed as plaque forming units (pfu)/mL based on a formula derived from previous virus preps that were titered using the standard plaque dilution based titration assay kit and the optical absorbance method.
3. We typically amplify the adenovirus at the university core facility and store the final preparation at –70°C.
4. We inject per animal an adenoviral dose that is approx $1-2 \times 10^9$ pfu, which is dissolved in phosphate-buffered saline (PBS) to give a total volume of 400 µL.
5. The adenoviruses are injected through the tail vein of Sprague-Dawley rats at days 8–9 of pregnancy (early second trimester). We use a 31-gage, 0.5-cc tuberculin syringe for the tail vein injections.
6. Blood pressures are measured at day 16–17 (corresponds to early third trimester).

3.2. Blood Pressure Measurement

Blood pressures of the rats are measured through the carotid arterial catheter.

1. Rats are first anesthetized with sodium pentobarbital (60 mg/kg intraperitoneally).
2. Using standard dissection tools, the carotid artery of the rat is isolated and cannulated with a 3-Fr high fidelity microtip catheter connected to a pressure transducer.
3. Blood pressures are recorded and averaged over a 10-min period. Mean arterial pressure is then calculated using the formula as follows: MAP = diastolic pressure in mmHg + one-third (systolic pressure – diastolic pressure in mmHg).

3.3. Blood and Urine Chemistries

1. We collect blood from the rats in ethylenediamine tetraacetic acid (EDTA) tubes.
2. Plasma from the blood is separated by centrifugation at 500*g* for 5 min.
3. We also collect urine from the rats at the time of sacrifice by direct puncture of the urinary bladder using a 1-mL tuberculin syringe.

Table 1
Blood Pressure and Proteinuria in Rats

Treatments	N	MAP (mmHg)	U Alb:Cr ratio in µg/mg
Fc (P)	5	75 ± 11	62 ± 21
SFlt-1 (P)	4	109 ± 19*	6923 ± 658**
Fc (NP)	5	89 ± 6	138 ± 78
SFlt-1 (NP)	6	118 ± 13*	12947 ± 2776**

Pregnant (P) and nonpregnant (NP) rats were administered adenovirus expressing Fc (control) or sFlt-1. Mean arterial blood pressure (MAP = diastolic + one-third
pulse pressure in mmHg) ± S.E.M and mean urine–Alb:Cr ratio (µµg of albumin per
mg of creatinine) ± S.E.M were measured eight days after adenoviral administration
corresponding to the early third trimester in the pregnant rats. n = the number of
animals in each experimental group. Statistical significance is represented with *
for $p < 0.05$ and ** for $p < 0.01$ when compared with the control group (Fc). Mean
plasma sFlt-1 levels were 388 ng/mL (P) and 101 ng/mL (NP) in the sFlt-1 treated
rats. This table is reproduced from Maynard et al. *(8)* with permission.

4. If the plasma and urine specimens are not being processed immediately, we recommend storing these specimens at –70°C.
5. Plasma samples must be processed for the measurement of sFlt-1 protein using a
   commercially available ELISA for murine sFlt-1.
6. We also measure urinary albumin using commercial ELISA kit. To normalize the
   albumin excretion for varying urine outputs, we also measure urinary creatinine
   and report proteinuria as a ratio of urinary albumin over creatinine.
7. Blood pressure and urinary proteinuria data from previously published experiments *(8)* are shown in **Table 1**.

3.4. Renal Histology and Electron Microscopy

1. Kidneys are serially sectioned into three pieces, to allow for light and electron
   microscopy, as well as immunofluorescence.
2. The first slice, to be processed for light microscopy, is fixed in Bouin's solution
   for 6 h and stored in 70% ethanol at room temperature until processing.
3. Following paraffin embedding, sections are cut at 3 µm, and stained with hematoxylin and eosin (H&E), periodic acid–Schiff (PAS) and Masson Trichrome
   (MT) stains, using routine methods.
4. The second slice is embedded in optimum cutting temperature (OCT) compound
   and frozen in a standard type cryostat. Frozen sections for immunofluorescence
   studies are cut at 4 µm, and using standard techniques immunostained for fibrin
   (anti-rat fibrinogen).
5. The last slice, for electron microscopy, is fixed in 3% glutaraldehyde, and
   postfixed in 2% osmium. Blocks are stained with 2% uranyl acetate and embed-

PAS   **EM**

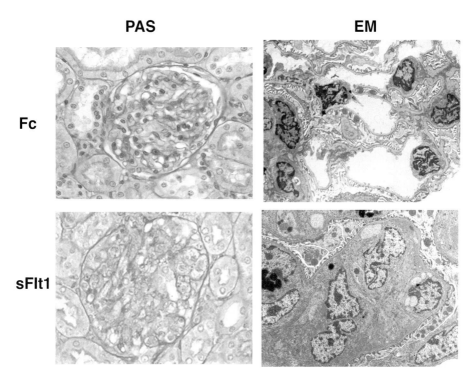

Fig. 1. Histology and electron microscopy (EM) of rat kidneys demonstrating glomerular endotheliosis. Histopathological analysis of renal tissue from one representative Fc pregnant (upper panel), one sFlt-1 treated pregnant (lower panel) treated pregnant rat (lower panel) is shown here. Periodic acid–Schiff (PAS) stain shows capillary occlusion in the sFlt-1 treated animal with enlarged glomeruli and swollen endocapillary cells compared to the Fc control animal. The sFlt-1 treated rat glomerulus also demonstrates the PAS negative swollen cytoplasm of the endocapillary cells (endotheliosis). These pathologic changes are absent in the Fc treated rat. EM was performed for the same rats shown in light microscopy. EM of glomeruli from a sFlt-1 treated rat (lower panel) confirmed cytoplasmic swelling of the endocapillary cells. There is relative preservation of the podocyte foot processes and the basement membranes. All light photomicrographs were taken at 60×, original magnification. The EM pictures were taken at 2400×, original magnification. All figures reproduced with permission from Maynard et al *(8)*.

ded in Epon. One micron sections are cut and stained with methylene blue for light microscopy. Thin sections are cut (at about 130 nm) and assessed by ultrastructural study. Representative light microscopy and EM pictures from a previously published study *(8)* are shown in **Fig. 1**.

4. Notes

1. We would recommend amplifying the adenoviruses at a university-based core facility (such as Harvard Gene Therapy Initiative, Boston, MA) or a commercial entity (such as Q-biogene, Montreal, Canada).
2. The glomerular lesion of endotheliosis does not involve an increase in cellularity, and can be subtle in mild cases, especially when assessed by light microscopy alone. Electron microscopy or even just the semi-thin plastic sections can be helpful in confirming minor changes. In more florid cases protein resorption droplets are often seen within glomerular epithelial cells. We strongly recommend that a pathologist with expertise in glomerular diseases evaluate the renal histology.
3. Because of tremendous variability with the various adenoviral preparations, we recommend that plasma levels of sFlt-1 be confirmed using ELISA and/or Western blotting. It is important to document the expression of sFlt-1 protein in the bloodstream prior to evaluating histology or urine/blood chemistries. We prefer the ELISA procedure, but if western blotting is used we recommend screening with an antibody directed against the extra-cellular domain of mouse Flt-1 (Sigma-Aldrich, cat. no. V1139).
4. One could also measure blood pressure noninvasively using a tail-cuff method (Visitech BP-2000 Systems, Cary, NC). However, we have found a lot of variability in blood pressures measured non-invasively and hence always resort to intra-carotid monitoring.
5. Similar results can also be obtained with adenoviral injection of sFlt1 into nonpregnant rats as previously described *(8)*. However, we recommend using pregnant rats to fully recapitulate the human situation.

Acknowledgments

The authors would like to thank Dr. Richard Mulligan for help with generation of adenoviruses, Dr. Jiang-Yong Min for help with blood pressure measurements in rats, and Cathy Grant at the Animal Care Facility for help with tail vein injections. S. A. K is funded by National Institutes of Health (NIH) grants (DK64255 and DK065997) and the American Society of Nephrology Carl W. Gottschalk Research Scholar Award.

References

1. Walker, J. J. (2000) Pre-eclampsia. *Lancet* **356,** 1260–1265.
2. Roberts, J. M. (2000) Preeclampsia: what we know and what we do not know. *Semin. Perinatol.* **24,** 24–28.
3. Roberts, J. M. and Cooper, D. W. (2001) Pathogenesis and genetics of pre-eclampsia. *Lancet* **357,** 53–56.
4. Karumanchi, S. A., Lim, K. H., Sukhatme, V. P., and August, P. (2004) Pathogenesis of Preeclampsia, in *Obstetrics—UpToDate* (Rose, B. D., ed.). UpToDate, Wellesley, MA.

5. Page, E. W. (1939) The relation between hydatid moles, relative ischemia of the gravid uterus and the placental origin of eclampsia. *Am. J. Obstet. Gynecol.* **37,** 291.

6. Roberts, J. M., Taylor, R. N., Musci, T. J., Rodgers, G. M., Hubel, C. A., and McLaughlin, M. K. (1989) Preeclampsia: an endothelial cell disorder. *Am. J. Obstet. Gynecol.* **161,** 1200–1204.

7. Ferris, T. F. (1991) Pregnancy, preeclampsia, and the endothelial cell. *New Engl. J. Med.* **325,** 1439–1440.

8. Maynard, S. E., Min, J. Y., Merchan, J., et al. (2003) Excess placental soluble fms-like tyrosine kinase 1 (sFlt1) may contribute to endothelial dysfunction, hypertension, and proteinuria in preeclampsia. *J. Clin. Invest.* **111,** 649–658.

9. Kendall, R. L. and Thomas, K. A. (1993) Inhibition of vascular endothelial cell growth factor activity by an endogenously encoded soluble receptor. *Proc. Natl. Acad. Sci. USA* **90,** 10,705–10,709.

10. Clark, D. E., Smith, S. K., He, Y., et al. (1998) A vascular endothelial growth factor antagonist is produced by the human placenta and released into the maternal circulation. *Biol. Reprod.* **59,** 1540–1548.

11. Koga, K., Osuga, Y., Yoshino, O., et al. (2003) Elevated serum soluble vascular endothelial growth factor receptor 1 (sVEGFR-1) levels in women with preeclampsia. *J. Clin. Endocrinol. Metab.* **88,** 2348–2351.

12. Levine, R. J., Maynard, S. E., Qian, C., et al. (2004) Circulating angiogenic factors and the risk of preeclampsia. *New Engl. J. Med.* **350,** 672–683.

13. Taylor, R. N., Grimwood, J., Taylor, R. S., McMaster, M. T., Fisher, S. J., and North, R. A. (2003) Longitudinal serum concentrations of placental growth factor: evidence for abnormal placental angiogenesis in pathologic pregnancies. *Am. J. Obstet. Gynecol.* **188,** 177–182.

14. Polliotti, B. M., Fry, A. G., Saller, D. N., Mooney, R. A., Cox, C., and Miller, R. K. (2003) Second-trimester maternal serum placental growth factor and vascular endothelial growth factor for predicting severe, early-onset preeclampsia. *Obstet. Gynecol.* **101,** 1266–1274.

15. Kuo, C. J., Farnebo, F., Yu, E. Y., et al. (2001) Comparative evaluation of the antitumor activity of antiangiogenic proteins delivered by gene transfer. *Proc. Natl. Acad. Sci. USA* **98,** 4605–4610.

16. Sweeney, J. A. and Hennessey, J. P., Jr. (2002) Evaluation of accuracy and precision of adenovirus absorptivity at 260 nm under conditions of complete DNA disruption. *Virology* **295,** 284–288.

26

A Novel Mouse Model for Preeclampsia by Transferring Activated Th1 Cells into Normal Pregnant Mice

Ana Claudia Zenclussen

Summary

Immunological imbalances have been hypothesized as a cause for the onset of preeclampsia, which is a very severe, pregnancy-related disease. We recently described a novel preeclampsia mouse model by adoptively transferring activated BALB/c Th1-like splenocytes into allogeneically pregnant BALB/c female mice during late gestation. This cell transfer provoked preeclampsia symptoms (increased blood pressure and glomerulonephritis accompanied by proteinuria). Interestingly, preeclampsia-like symptoms could not be detected in nonpregnant animals receiving activated Th1-like cells. Adoptive cell transfer further affected pregnancy outcome by increasing fetal rejection through an inflammatory profile of uterine immune cells. This chapter describes the methods employed to develop the model as well as additional experiments developed to analyze cellular and molecular mechanisms involved.

Key Words: Cell transfer; preeclampsia; murine pregnancy; Th1/Th2 balance; tolerance; blood pressure.

1. Introduction

Preeclampsia is a severe pregnancy complication associated with immunological imbalances. Preeclampsia affects about 10% of late-pregnancies (*1*). The clinical symptoms of preeclampsia include elevated maternal blood pressure, proteinuria, and abnormal fluid retention (*1*).

The etiology of preeclampsia remains controversial. Several hypotheses have been proposed, such as shallow trophoblast invasion during the second physiological wave of trophoblasts invasion (*2,3*), or the so-called "inflammatory theory" which proposes an excessive maternal inflammatory response as the stimulus leading to generalized endothelial cell dysfunction and finally resulting in preeclampsia (*4*). Several data indicate that the placenta itself as well as some of its secretory products, e.g., tumor necrosis factor (TNF)-α, are the stimuli leading to an immune activation and preeclampsia (*4–9*). A systemic response of activated maternal inflammatory cells (including elevated

From: *Methods in Molecular Medicine, Vol. 122: Placenta and Trophoblast: Methods and Protocols, Vol. 2*
Edited by: M. J. Soares and J. S. Hunt © Humana Press Inc., Totowa, NJ

numbers of granulocytes and monocytes) has been reported in patients suffering from preeclampsia (9–11), accompanied by increased levels of pro-inflammatory Th1-type cytokines, especially TNF-α (8,12,13).

Using an immunological approach, we have recently established an animal model for preeclampsia (14). The model was developed by adoptively transferring activated immune cells, mainly of a Th1 phenotype, into normal pregnant mice (BALB/c females mated with C57BL/6 males) during pregnancy. Using this model we were able to show that the transfer of activated Th1-like cells leads to preeclampsia-like symptoms (hypertension, proteinuria, and kidney pathology) exclusively in pregnant mice (14). We conclude that this animal model will be useful in analyzing immune pathways associated with preeclampsia and opens possibilities for the development of new therapeutic strategies. This chapter describes the methods used to establish the mouse preeclampsia model.

2. Materials

1. BALB/c and C57BL/6 female and male mice (BgVV, Berlin, Germany).
2. Phosphate-buffered saline (PBS) (PAA Laboratories GmbH, Linz, Austria).
3. Blood Pressure Detection System (TSE BP-Systems, Bad Homburg, Germany).
4. RPMI culture medium (Biochrom AG, Berlin, Germany) (store at 4°C).
5. Fetal calf serum (FCS) (Seromed, Berlin, Germany) (store at –20°C, inactivate before use).
6. 100 µm cell strainer (Becton Dickinson Labware, Franklin Lakes, NJ).
7. Lympholyte-M Solution (Cedarlane, Ontario, Canada) (store at room temperature in darkness).
8. anti-CD3 mAb (BD Biosciences, Heidelberg, Germany) (store at 4°C).
9. HEPES (25 mM) (Biochrom AG, Berlin, Germany).
10. Glutamine (2 mM) (Biochrom AG, Berlin, Germany).
11. Antibiotic mix (Gibco, Karlsruhe, Germany).
12. Recombinant mouse (rm) interleukin (IL)-2 (R&D Systems, Wiesbaden-Nordenstadt, Germany) (store at –20°C, make small aliquots, avoid cycles of freeze–thaw).
13. rm IL-12 (R&D Systems, Wiesbaden-Nordenstadt, Germany) (store at –20°C, make small aliquots, avoid cycles of freeze–thaw).
14. Hank's balanced salt solution (HBSS) without Ca^{2+} and Mg^{2+} (stable for up to 2 mo at 4°C).
15. Freezing medium (Jung, Nussloch, Germany).
16. Hematoxylin and eosin (H&E) (Roth, Germany).
17. Dithiothreitol (DTT) (Sigma, Germany). Please be aware of the toxicity of this chemical.
18. Brefeldin A (BD Pharmingen, Heidelberg, Germany) (Toxic).
19. Fix™ solution (Becton Dickinson, Erembodegem, Belgium).
20. FACS™ Permeabilizing Solution (Becton Dickinson, Heidelberg, Germany).

21. Bovine serum albumin (BSA) (Sigma, Germany) (store at 4°C).
22. 0.1 % Natrium azid (Merck, Germany).
23. FACS Calibur (Becton Dickinson)
24. Phycoeritrin (PE)-labeled antibodies against interferon (IFN)-γ, TNF-α, IL-12, IL-4, IL-10, and CD25 (BD Pharmingen, Heidelberg, Germany) (store at 4°C).
25. Fluorescein isothiocyanate (FITC)-conjugated antibodies against CD2 and CD8 (BD Pharmingen, Heidelberg, Germany) (store at 4°C).
26. PerCP-Biotin-labeled antibody against CCR5 (BD Pharmingen, Heidelberg, Germany) (store at 4°C).
27. Proteinuria test, Combur Test, Roche, Mannheim, Germany.
28. Carboxyfluorescein diacetate succinimidyl ester (CSFE) (Molecular Probes, Eugene, OR) (store at –20°C until use, make small aliquots).

3. Methods

3.1. Spleen Cell Harvest and Th1 Activation

1. BALB/c spleens are crushed in culture dishes with RPMI medium containing 10% FCS and filtered through a 100-μm cell strainer (*see* **Note 1**).
2. Mononuclear cells are isolated with a density gradient and polyclonally activated by incubation with anti-CD3 mAb for 20 min at 3 μg/mL *(16)*.
3. The cells (1.5×10^6 cells/mL) are placed in RPMI culture medium containing HEPES (25 mM), glutamine (2 mM), antibiotic mix, 1.022 ng/mL rm IL-2, and 4 ng/mL rm IL-12) and incubated for an additional 30 h in 5% CO_2 at 37°C in a humidified incubator (*see* **Notes 2** and **3**).
4. Cell viability and fold increase in cell number are determined by light microscopy using Trypan Blue.
5. After two washes with PBS, cells are adjusted to a concentration of 10^7 cells/100 μL with sterile PBS and are ready for injection into recipient mice.

3.2. Mice and Treatments

Animal care and experimental procedures need to meet institutional guidelines. We obtain female and male mice from BgVV and maintain them in a barrier animal facility.

1. Two-month-old BALB/c females are housed with 3-mo-old C57BL/6 males and checked for vaginal plugs every morning. The day of the plug is considered day 0 of pregnancy; pregnant females are removed from breeding cages and randomized (*see* **Note 4**).
2. Pregnant females are administered two doses of 10^7 Th1-activated splenocytes (100 μL) intravenously (IV) on gestation days 12 and 14, between 0900 and 1200 h. Nonpregnant controls can also be injected (*see* **Note 5**).
3. Additional pregnant or nonpregnant control females receive 100 μL of sterile PBS IV.
4. Mice can be sacrificed on day 14 of gestation or as determined by the experimental protocol (*see* **Note 6**).

3.3. Measurement of Blood Pressure

1. We condition BALB/c females in the tail-cuff blood pressure apparatus for about 20 min every other day between 09:00 and 11:00 h for 10 d (*see* **Note 7**).
2. Pregnant and nonpregnant mice are evaluated for blood pressure at d 1, 3, 5, 7, 9, 11, 13, and 14 of pregnancy, or as determined by the experimental protocol.
3. For measuring blood pressure, animals are placed onto a warm plate (temperature set at 37°C). A 17-mm tail cuff is applied to the tail base and a pulse transmitter is applied to the tail. The apparatus is calibrated to inflate from 90 mmHg to 300 mmHg. A rest period of 1 s is allowed between each measurement.
4. We record 10 tracings without movement artifacts. The tracings are averaged and considered as the systolic blood pressure value for each mouse (*see* **Notes 8** and **9**).

3.4. Sample Collection

1. On d 14 of pregnancy or as indicated by the experimental protocol, blood samples can be obtained by retroorbital puncture, collected in tubes containing heparin, and stored at 4°C.
2. Urine samples can be obtained by gently pressing the mouse abdominal region and stored at 4°C. The animals are then sacrificed and the uteri removed.
3. Fetal rejection sites are identified by their small size and hemorrhagic appearance.
4. Uterine decidua samples are cut into small pieces and stored in HBSS at 4°C until used (average time: 1 h) for flow cytometry studies.
5. Tissues (feto–maternal unit, kidney, and so on) can be dissected, embedded in freezing medium, snap-frozen in liquid nitrogen, and kept at –80°C. Alternatively the tissues can be fixed in 10% neutral buffered formalin, embedded in paraffin and cut at 5 μm. H&E-stained samples (uterus, kidneys, and so on) can be evaluated microscopically for histopathological characteristics (*see* **Note 10**).

3.5. Flow Cytometry Analysis

A method for isolating large numbers of uterine cells for flow cytometry has been previously developed (*17*).

1. Tubes containing pieces of uteri are filled with HBSS containing 1 mM DTT and incubated under agitation and rotation for 20 min at 37°C.
2. The cells (at the interface) are transferred to a new tube by filtration through a 100-μm mesh and washed with RPMI-10% FCS. Filtration through the mesh is repeated twice with HBSS without DTT. All supernatants are collected and washed with RPMI medium containing 10% FCS, counted, and used for flow cytometry (*see* **Notes 11** and **12**).
3. White blood cells are obtained from whole blood following erythrocyte lysis and collected in RPMI with 10% FCS.
4. Blood cells and uterine cells are incubated for 3 h with Brefeldin A (10^6 cells/mL medium containing 1 μL/mL of Golgi Plug(tm)) in 5% CO_2 at 37°C (*see* **Note 13**).
5. Cells are washed, incubated with surface antibodies for 20 min at room temperature in the dark, fixed (Fix solution), and incubated overnight at 4°C.

6. The cells are then washed, permeabilized (FACS Permeabilizing Solution), and incubated with the intracellular antibody for 30 min at room temperature in the dark.
7. All wash steps are performed using PBS containing 1% BSA and 0.1% sodium azide.
8. The labeled cells are read in a FACS Calibur cytometer. The lymphocyte population is gated based on size and granularity and used for further analysis.
9. We have used phycoeritrin-labeled antibodies against IFN-γ, TNF-α, IL-12, IL-4, or IL-10 and FITC-conjugated antibodies against CD2 and CD8 as well as the respective isotype controls. All antibody incubations are performed at 4°C for optimal results (*see* **Note 14**).

3.6. Proteinuria

Urine samples can be analyzed for proteinuria using a qualitative method. The test allows the differentiation of values between 0, 0.3, 1, and 5 g/L. Proteinuria is considered positive when urine samples are >1 g/L (*see* **Notes 15** and **16**).

3.7. Tracking Labeled Cells After Adoptive Transfer

1. C57BL/6-mated BALB/c and non-pregnant BALB/c female can be used as recipients for fluorescent Th1-like cells.
2. The Th1-like cells are obtained as previously described, washed three times in PBS, and re-suspended in 5 μM CSFE solution (10^7 cells/mL) for 3–4 min at room temperature (*see* **Note 17**).
3. The reaction is stopped by washing the cells four times with culture medium containing 10% FCS and three times with PBS.
4. Before cell transfer, cell viability and cell number are determined.
5. Thirty-five hours after the second cell transfer the animals (*18*) are sacrificed and tissues processed for flow cytometry studies (*see* **Notes 18** and **19**).
6. Immune cells are analyzed using flow cytometry for CFSE detection.
7. For histological analysis of CSFE-labeled cell distribution, organs are frozen in Tissue-Tek medium, cut in 5-μm sections, mounted on slides, and dried at room temperature.
8. For further analysis, we counterstain our slides with 4',6-diamidino-2-phenylindole (DAPI) and analyze them under a fluorescence microscope.

4. Notes

1. One mouse is usually required as a donor for cells to be transferred per recipient mouse.
2. The incubation of the cells with IL-12 and IL-2 leads to a Th1-like phenotype as demonstrated by the expression of Th1 markers such as CCR5 and the secretion of high quantities of Th1 cytokines and low levels of Th2 cytokines (*14*).
3. Check periodically the cells for their Th1 profile by flow cytometry, enzyme-linked immunosorbent assay, or reverse-transcription polymerase chain reaction (RT-PCR). Wash the cells carefully with PBS before injecting them to the animals.

4. When checking for vaginal plugs, it is convenient to do it twice a day, once early in the morning and once late in the afternoon. This minimizes the possibility of missing some plugs.

5. When injecting the mice intravenously, it is recommended to expose them to an infrared lamp about half an hour before injection, this helps visualization of the tail vein. Do not inject more than 200 μL.

6. The transfer of Th1-like activated cells transfer leads to an apparent increased fetal rejection rate. In some mice, preterm labor could be observed on gestation day 14 (preterm labor was diagnosed by the presence of blood at the vagina of the mice or in the cage bedding).

7. It is very important to "condition" the animals to the blood pressure apparatus in order to avoid aberrant results caused by stress. It is recommended to do this training every other day for at least 10 d before initiating the experimental measurements.

8. It is recommended to make 10 measurements because of the inherent variability due to stress. The measurements take about half an hour for each conditioned mouse. It is also very important to carry out the measurements at the same time each day. This will also help reduce variability. It is also recommended to limit the number of investigators handling the mice (maximum two).

9. The adoptive transfer of activated Th1 cells rapidly induces hypertension (from 124.13 (9.26 mmHg until 217.13 (12.54 mmHg, $p < 0.001$) exclusively in pregnant recipients (**Fig. 1A**). Before onset of pregnancy, the females display normal values of blood pressure, as well as during the early stages of pregnancy before cell transfer (**Fig. 1A**). Control pregnant mice injected with PBS show a mild decrease of blood pressure at the end of pregnancy, as expected (*15*). No significant changes in blood pressure values are seen in nonpregnant mice receiving activated Th1 cells (**Fig. 1B**), which confirms the pregnancy specificity of the treatment. **Figure 1C** depicts the blood pressure apparatus that we used throughout the entire experiment.

10. Interestingly, pregnant recipients of Th1-like activated cells show histopathological characteristics in their kidneys (enlarged glomeruli with increased glomerular cell density, presence of infiltrating immune cells). Kidneys derived from mice with preeclampsia-like symptoms show glomerular fibrosis, deposition of acidophilic material and increased vessel wall density. Placentas from pregnant mice treated with activated Th1 cells exhibit fibrosis associated with the spongiotrophoblast, extensive hemorrhagic sites in the labyrinth and spongiotrophoblast zones, and a massive immune cell infiltration (**Fig. 2A**) when compared with placentas from PBS-treated control pregnant mice (**Fig. 2B**). The decidua of mice with preeclampsia-like symptoms possesses blood vessels with much thicker vessel walls (**Fig. 2C**) than those observed in decidua from normal pregnant mice (**Fig. 2D**).

11. To obtain decidual immune cells, it is very important to incubate the cells no longer than 20 min with DTT, to work fast, and to always keep the cells on ice between steps in the procedure.

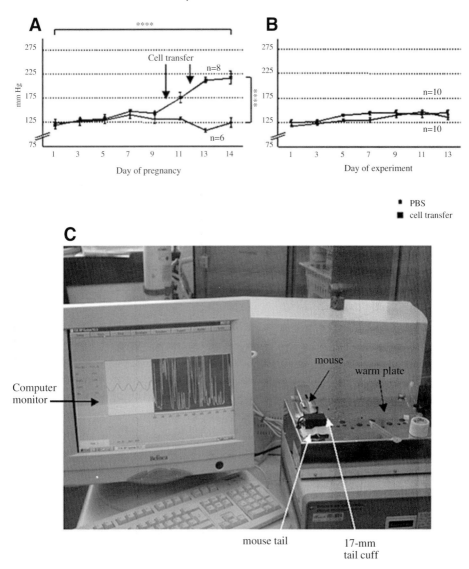

Fig. 1. Th1-activated cell transfer enhances blood pressure exclusively in pregnant recipients. **A** and **B** show blood pressure curves in mmHg (*x*-axis) and the gestational age or experiment day (*y*-axis) from pregnant (**A**) and nonpregnant mice (**B**) throughout the experiment. Mice received intravenous injections of phosphate-buffered saline (full circle) or activated Th1 cells (full square). **** means $p < 0.00001$, as analyzed by Mann Whitney or Friedman Test. **C** depicts the system that we use for measuring blood pressure. The arrows indicate the computer monitor, warming plate, mouse position, mouse tail, and tail cuff. **A** and **B** are reprinted from **ref. *14***, with permission of Wilry-VCH Verlag GmbH & Co. KGaA, Weinheim, Germany.

12. Using our DTT method to isolate decidual cells, the cell yield is about 1–4 million cells per animal. Additional cells can be retrieved by enzymatic digestion of the uterus; however, the potential for loss and/or damage of surface antigens (e.g., CD4) is increased.

13. Cytokine production can be evaluated with or without stimulation. Methods to stimulate the cells include treatment with 50 ng/mL phorbol myristate acetate (PMA) (Sigma) or 1 µg/mL Ionomycin (Sigma). This protocol stimulates mostly memory cells to produce cytokines. Alternatively, cells can be stimulated to produce cytokines with paternal antigens. For optimal results, both strategies require the addition of a Golgi blocker.

14. Uterine lymphocytes from pregnant mice produce significantly more Th1 cytokines (TNF-α and IL-12) (**Fig. 2E**) after Th1 cell transfer in comparison to PBS-treated pregnant mice. A modest increase in the percentage of IFN-γ^+ uterus cells could be observed in Th1 cell-treated mice (**Fig. 2E**). Th1-type cytokines are produced by $CD2^+$ lymphocytes, which are $CD4^+$ and $CD8^+$ cells. Additionally, the production of Th2 cytokines IL-10 and IL-4 by uterine lymphocytes is increased in mice with preeclampsia-like symptoms (**Fig. 2E**).

15. We measure protein in urine obtained at the time of autopsy. More accurate assessments can be obtained by assessing urine protein in 24-h urine collections.

16. Inoculation of activated Th1-like cells in pregnant mice results in proteinuria. PBS-treated pregnant mice or non-pregnant mice injected IV with PBS or activated Th1-like cells do not exhibit proteinuria, which again points towards the pregnancy restriction of the experimentally induced preeclampsia-like symptoms.

17. It is important to work fast with the CFSE reagent and always keep the cells on ice. The cell pellet should exhibit a yellow color if cells are correctly stained. Count the cells after staining, because many of them die during the staining process. If the number of dead cells is high, then use gradient separation (i.e., Lympholyte) to remove dead cells.

Fig. 2. (*opposite page*) Recipients of activated Th1-cells exhibit signs of inflammation at the feto–maternal interface. **A** and **C** show decidual histopathological signs in mice which previously received activated Th1-like cells intravenously. **A** is a representative field of placental samples from mice having preeclampsia-like symptoms showing fibrosis in the spongiotrophoblast area as well as a massive lymphocyte infiltration. **C** shows abnormally thick uterine blood vessel walls, as indicated by the arrows. **B** and **D** are placental and decidual samples from phosphate-buffered saline (PBS)-treated pregnant mice without pathological findings. **E** illustrates the percentage of uterine lymphocytes expressing tumor necrosis factor (TNF)-α, interleukin (IL)-12, interferon (IFN)-γ, IL-10, and IL-4 in pregnant mice that received PBS ($n = 6$) or activated Th1-like cells ($n = 8$), as analyzed by flow cytometry. * means $p < 0.05$ and *** is a $P < 0.001$, as analyzed by Mann Whitney nonparametric test. Reprinted from **ref. *14***, with permission of Wilry-VCH Verlag GmbH & Co. KGaA, Weinheim, Germany.

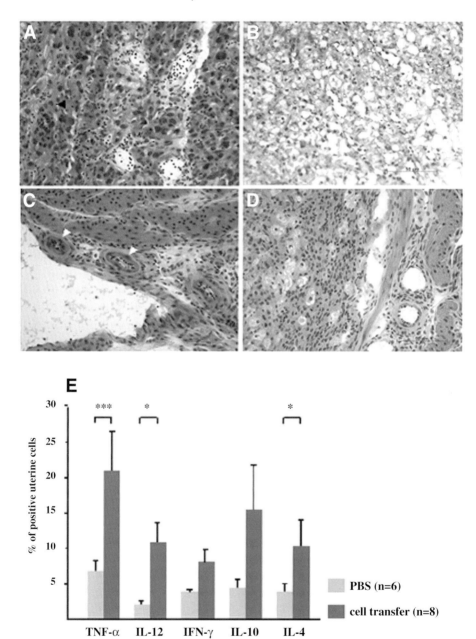

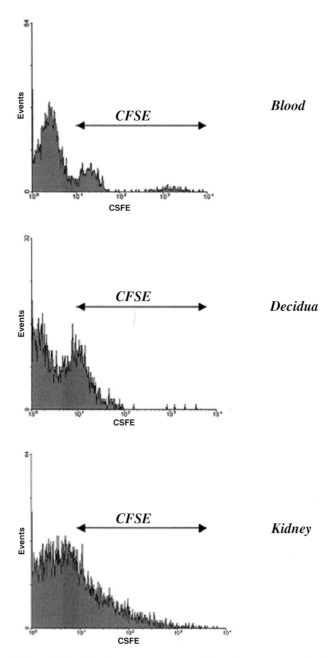

Fig. 3. Cell distribution in tissues, as analyzed by flow cytometric detection of carboxyfluorescein diacetate succinimidyl ester (CSFE)[+] cells. We confirmed the presence of the transferred CFSE[+] cells in blood (A), decidua (B), and kidneys (C) by flow cytometry. As a negative control, we used nonstained cells in culture as well as cells obtained from nontransferred animals. As positive controls, we included cultured cells, which were first stained with CFSE and maintained in vitro.

18. Tissue samples can also be processed for RT-PCR, Western blotting, or immuno-histochemistry.
19. By using flow cytometry, we have confirmed the presence of CFSE⁺ cells in organs from both nonpregnant and pregnant mice receiving the adoptive cell transfers (**Fig. 3**).

Acknowledgments

The preeclampsia model was developed with grants from the Charité. I developed this work while working as a guest scientist from the Alexander von Humboldt Foundation in Petra Arck´s laboratory, therefore I would like to especially thank Dr. Arck for this great opportunity and her support. I am grateful to Dr. Thomas Ritter for his excellent advice in performing the cell transfer experiments and for providing the CSFE reagents, to Dr. Stefan Fest and Dr. Ricarda Joachim for their contributions, to Dr. Eva Peters for assistance with the images, to Ruth Pliet for her excellent technical assistance measuring blood pressure, and to Petra Busse for her assistance in flow cytometry. Finally, I would like to thank Prof. Dr. Hans-Dieter Volk for his support.

References

1. Robillard, P. Y. (2002) Interest in preeclampsia for researchers in reproduction. *J. Reprod. Immunol.* **53,** 279–287.
2. Pijnenborg, R., Luyten, C., Vercruysse, L., and Van Assche, F.A. (1996) Attachment and differentiation in vitro of trophoblast from normal and preeclamptic human placentas. *Am. J. Obstet. Gynecol.* **175,** 30–36.
3. Zhou, Y., Damsky, C., and Fisher, S. (1999). Pre-eclampsia is associated with failure of human cytotrophoblasts to mimic a vascular adhesion phenotype. *J. Clin. Invest.* **99,** 2152–2164.
4. Redman, C. W. G., Sacks, G. P. and Sargent, I. L., Preeclampsia (1999) An excessive maternal inflammatory response to pregnancy. *Am. J. Obstet. Gynecol.* **180,** 499–506.
5. Roberts, J. M., Taylor, R. N. and Goldfien, A. (1991) Clinical and biochemical evidence of endothelial cell dysfunction in the pregnancy syndrome preeclampsia. *Am. J. Hypertens.* **8,** 700–708.
6. Faas, M. M., Schuiling, G., Baller, J. F. W., Visscher, C. A., and Bakker, W. W. (1994) A new animal model for human preeclampsia: ultralow dose endotoxin infusion in pregnant rats. *Am. J. Obstet. Gynecol.* **171,** 158–164.
7. Faas, M. M. and Schuiling, G. A (2001). Pre-eclampsia and the inflammatory response. *Eur. J. Obstet. Gynecol. Reprod. Biol.* **95,** 213–217.
8. Saito, S., Umekage, H., Sakamoto, Y., et al. (1999). Increased T-helper-1-type immunity and decreased T-helper-2-type immunity in patients with preeclampsia. *Am. J. Reprod. Immunol.* **5,** 297–306.
9. Sacks, G. P., Studena, K., Sargent, I. L., and Redman, C. W. (1997) CD11b expression on circulating neutrophils in pre-eclampsia. *Clin. Sci.* **93,** 187–189.

10. Oian, P., Omsjo, I., Maltau, J. M., and Osterud, B. (1985) Increased sensitivity to thromboplastin synthesis in blood monocytes from pre-eclamptic patients. *Br. J. Obstet. Gynaecol.* **92,** 511–517.

11. Greer, I. A., Haddad, N. G., Dawes, J., Johnstone, F. D., and Calder, A. A. (1989) Neutrophil activation in pregnancy-induced hypertension. *Br. J. Obstet. Gynaecol.* **96,** 978–982.

12. Darmochwal-Kolarz, D., Leszczynska-Gorzelak, B., Rolinski, I., and Oleszczuk, J. (1999) T helper 1- and T helper 2-type cytokine imbalance in pregnant women with pre-eclampsia. *Eur. J. Obstet. Gynecol. Reprod. Biol.* **86,** 165–170.

13. Stark, J. M. (1993) Pre-eclampsia and cytokine induced oxidative stress. *Br. J. Obstet. Gynaecol.* **100,** 105–109.

14. Zenclussen, A. C., Fest, S., Joachim, R., Klapp, B. F., and Arck, P. C. (2004) Introducing a mouse model for pre-eclampsia: adoptive transfer of activated Th1 cells leads to pre-eclampsia-like symptoms exclusively in pregnant mice. *Eur. J. Immunol.* **34,** 377–387.

15. Hefler, L. A., Tempfer, C. B., Moreno, R. M., O'Brien, W. E., and Gregg, A. R. (2001) Endothelial-derived nitric oxide and angiotensinogen: blood pressure and metabolism during mouse pregnancy. *Am. J. Physiol. Regul. Integr. Comp. Physiol.* **280,** 174–182.

16. Saxton, M. L., Longo, D. L., Wetzel, H. E., et al. (1997) Adoptive transfer of anti-CD3-activated CD4+ T cells plus cyclophosphamide and liposome-encapsulated interleukin-2 cure murine MC-38 and 3LL tumors and establish tumor-specific immunity. *Blood* **89,** 2529–2536.

17. Zenclussen, A. C., Blois, S., Stumpo, R., et al. (2003) Murine abortion is associated with enhanced Interleukin-6 levels at the feto-maternal interface. *Cytokine* **24,** 150–160.

18. Hammer, M. H., Zhai, Y., Katori, M., et al. (2001) Homing of in vitro-generated donor antigen-reactive CD4+ T lymphocytes to renal allografts is alpha 4 beta 1 but not alpha L beta 2 integrin dependent. *J. Immunol.* **166,** 596–601.

27

Working with Oxygen and Oxidative Stress In Vitro

Graham J. Burton, D. Stephen Charnock-Jones, and Eric Jauniaux

Summary

Oxygen has a profound influence on the behavior of many cell types, including trophoblast. The effects are mediated in part through the generation of oxygen free radicals, which act as signaling molecules. Because of their high reactivity, free radicals are, however, potentially damaging to a wide range of biomolecules, and if concentrations exceed homeostatic levels then cellular oxidative stress results. Responses of tissues to changes in oxygen concentration may therefore range from physiological adaptations to pathological insults. Placental development is heavily modulated by the prevailing oxygen concentration, and understanding the mechanisms involved is clearly important. Equally, trophoblastic oxidative stress plays a key role in the pathogenesis of pregnancy complications such as miscarriage and preeclampsia. This chapter describes techniques by which the effects of oxygen and oxidative stress on placental tissues can be systematically investigated in vitro.

Key Words: Oxygen; oxidative stress; placenta; trophoblast; free radicals.

1. Introduction

There is much evidence that oxygen has a powerful influence of placental development and function (1–3), although the molecular mechanisms underlying these effects are only beginning to be understood. Equally, oxidative stress of placental tissues is now recognized as a major component in the pathophysiology of many complications of pregnancy, such as preeclampsia and miscarriage (4–7). There is, therefore, considerable interest on the effects of oxygen and reactive oxygen species (ROS) on trophoblast behavior. This chapter outlines some of the opportunities offered by experimental manipulations of the prevailing oxygen tension in vitro, and some of the potential pitfalls in this approach.

Oxygen is both an essential and a toxic gas for mammalian tissues (8). It is required as the final electron recipient for the mitochondrial electron transport chain, enabling oxidative phosphorylation and the generation of large quanti-

From: *Methods in Molecular Medicine, Vol. 122: Placenta and Trophoblast: Methods and Protocols, Vol. 2*
Edited by: M. J. Soares and J. S. Hunt © Humana Press Inc., Totowa, NJ

ties of ATP to support energy-dependent cellular functions such as protein synthesis and ionic pumping. Oxygen can, however, participate in the formation of potentially harmful free radicals, chemical species that contain an unpaired electron. The commonest of these is the superoxide anion ($O_2^{\cdot-}$), and there are three principal intracellular sources. Under physiological conditions mitochondria are probably the principal source, with electrons leaking from Complexes I and III of the respiratory chain (9). The rate of production is paradoxically increased under both hypoxic and hyperoxic conditions, and in metabolic disorders, such as diabetes, in which the rate of oxidative phosphorylation is generally raised. In hypoxia the lack of oxygen causes electrons to accumulate on the enzymes of the transport chain, whereas in hyperoxia the activity of the transport chain is generally elevated (8,10). In both situations, the risk of electron leakage is increased. A second source of $O_2^{\cdot-}$ is the enzyme NAD(P)H oxidase located on the apical surface of the syncytiotrophoblast (11,12). This enzyme is capable of producing large quantities of $O_2^{\cdot-}$ in vitro, and is more active in first-trimester tissues than at term (13). The third potential source of $O_2^{\cdot-}$ is the xanthine dehydrogenase/oxidase system. Under normoxic conditions, this enzyme exists in the dehydrogenase form, converting hypoxanthine to xanthine, and xanthine to urea. In the process it donates electrons to NAD^+. During episodes of hypoxia, however, the enzyme is proteolytically cleaved to the oxidase form. This utilises the same substrates, but transfers the electrons released onto molecular oxygen rather than NAD^+, so generating $O_2^{\cdot-}$. Because of this transformation, the contribution of this enzyme to intracellular generation of ROS will be greatest under conditions of fluctuating oxygen concentrations, in particular in ischemia-reperfusion injury (14).

Under normal physiological conditions, 1–2 % of the oxygen we consume is converted to ROS, mainly within the mitochondria but in the trophoblast also potentially through NAD(P)H oxidase. These ROS play essential roles in cell signalling processes that maintain many homeostatic functions (15,16). Oxygen can also influence cell behavior through its availability as a substrate for various hydroxylases. In particular, the activity of the redox sensitive transcription factor hypoxia inducible factor (HIF)-1 is regulated principally at the posttranslational level through two hydroxylations that are oxygen-dependent (17,18). In addition, oxygen is also a substrate for the various isoforms of nitric oxide synthase, although the concentration at which it becomes rate-limiting under physiological conditions is not clear. Nonetheless, nitric oxide is a powerful signaling molecule, and there is strong evidence that it can modulate trophoblast behavior in vitro (19). The activities of the endothelial and inducible isoforms of nitric oxide synthase are stimulated at different phases of the ischemia-reperfusion cycle, and both can contribute to increased nitric oxide production in this situation (20).

Because of their high reactivity, ROS and other radical species are potentially damaging to biological systems. A complex series of antioxidant defences has evolved to scavenge and detoxify ROS so that under normal conditions a homeostatic balance is achieved *(8)*. These are both enzymatic, such as superoxide dismutase and catalase, and nonenzymatic, such as Vitamins C and E and low-molecular-weight thiol compounds. It is important that these defences act in concert as an imbalance in the concentrations of physiological ROS can lead to the formation of powerful prooxidants. For example, the highly toxic hydroxyl ion can be generated from hydrogen peroxide in the presence of ferrous ions in the O_2^--dependent Fenton reaction *(8)*. Equally, O_2^- and nitric oxide can react together to form peroxynitrite, and in the excess of O_2^- this reaction is favored energetically over that between O_2^- and the detoxifying enzyme superoxide dismutase *(21)*. Both hydroxyl ions and peroxynitrite are capable of reacting indiscriminately with all biological molecules, leading to oxidative stress. The consequences may vary from disruption of signaling mechanisms and cellular functions, through to damage to cell structure and even apoptosis *(8,22)*.

Thus the biggest challenge faced when performing experiments with oxygen is to be able to manipulate concentrations so as to elicit physiological effects while at the same time guarding against nonphysiological oxidative stress, which may confound results. There are a number of difficulties that must be overcome. First, there is the issue of delivering an adequate quantity of oxygen to the cells in vitro in the absence of an oxygen carrier. It is important here to distinguish between the oxygen tension, which is a measure of the force driving oxygen into a cell, and the oxygen content, which is a measure of the amount of oxygen available to a cell. The unique properties of hemoglobin ensure that it is capable of delivering large quantities of oxygen to tissues at relatively low tensions. This situation is impossible to reproduce in the laboratory for the amount of oxygen held in solution in plasma is very small compared with that carried by hemoglobin, yet only the former is available to cells in vitro. In attempts to increase the oxygen content of their medium, some investigators have increased the oxygen tension in the gas phase. Although this will increase the content, the effect is small, and there is the added danger that the higher tension will drive what oxygen is available into the mitochondria at too great a rate, increasing the risk of ROS formation. The best that can be achieved for tissues is to have the samples at the gas–medium interface so that the diffusion distance through the medium is minimal, and to constantly replenish the gas phase. Although this may provide sufficient for the trophoblast on the villous exterior, it should be recognized that the cells in the villous core are probably hypoxic. For cell cultures, the situation is easier because the oxygen requirements are less and the surface area for diffusion is greater.

The second major problem is ensuring that the tissues or cells are not stressed during delivery/collection and handling prior to culture. During normal vaginal delivery, the placenta is most likely subjected to repeated hypoxia/reoxygenation events as a result of intermittent restriction of intervillous blood flow during uterine contractions *(23)*. This is evidenced indirectly by the increased activity of xanthine oxidase in vaginally delivered placentas compared with those delivered by caesarean section *(24)*, and by the finding that maternal plasma Vitamin C levels are depleted during vaginal deliveries *(25)*. We are currently testing this hypothesis further, but in the meantime we routinely use nonlabored placentas obtained from elective caesarean sections for our work. Even with these placentas, however, one must ensure that a hypoxia/reoxygenation event is not induced during the period between placental separation and the tissues being placed in culture. For example, villous explants are by their nature ex vivo samples. The concentration of ATP falls rapidly in the term placenta after delivery *(26)*, and so it is important that samples are obtained as quickly as possible after separation and placed into oxygenated medium. Good relationships and liaison among scientists, clinicians, and nursing staff are essential here. For first-trimester samples, there is the additional problem of potential mixing with maternal blood during the termination procedure. It is now recognized that the maternal blood flow to the human placenta is not fully established until 10–12 wk of gestation. As a result, the early villi develop bathed in a clear fluid that probably arises as a plasma filtrate supplemented by secretion from the uterine glands *(27,28)*, at a low oxygen concentration *(29,30)*. Consequently, the tissues are susceptible to oxygen-mediated damage, in particular the syncytiotrophoblast which contains low concentrations of antioxidant enzymes such as superoxide dismutase and catalase *(31)*. Exposure to maternal blood during suction curettage constitutes both a hyperoxic insult and increases the risk of hydroxyl ion generation through the Fenton reaction catalyzed by iron released from hemolyzing maternal erythrocytes. We recently confirmed that high levels of oxidative stress can be induced in first-trimester tissues collected by chorionic villous sampling if they are exposed to maternal blood, and that this is associated with stabilization of the α subunit of HIF-1 *(32)*. The method of sample collection must therefore be considered when interpreting results. At present no data are available on the effects of medical termination procedures on placental tissues, but it is likely that these will also induce considerable stress through mixing with maternal blood.

Finally, there is the question of what is the most appropriate oxygen concentration to use. The oxygen concentration measured within the intervillous space prior to 10 wk is <20 mmHg, rising to >50 mmHg after 12 wk *(29,30)*. Onset of the maternal circulation is normally a periphery-center phenomenon, however, and so it is to be expected that regional differences in oxygenation and villous morphology will be present *(33)*. This is another reason why collection of samples using an ultrasound guided chorionic villous sampling technique is beneficial, because tissues can be obtained from a consistent location. From early in the second trimester to term there is then a progressive slow fall in the mean oxygen concentration in the intervillous space to approx 40 mmHg *(34)*. Again, because of the pattern of maternal blood flow, regional variations will occur. Although definite figures are not available, it is likely that the oxygen concentration in the center of a lobule will be approx 80 mmHg, as compared with 40 mmHg at the periphery *(35)*. Sampling from a consistent site may therefore again help to reduce experimental variability. Cell lines are routinely cultured under ambient conditions of 21% oxygen, and so will have enhanced antioxidant defences. The impact this has on subsequent exposure to variations in oxygenation within the physiological range has not been investigated.

In view of the difficulty in recreating physiological conditions of oxygenation in vitro, it has been suggested that investigators explore the effects of a range of oxygen concentrations in order to establish a dose–response effect rather than simply comparing, for example, 21% with 2.5% oxygen *(36)*. The latter will most likely generate a difference, but because 21% oxygen is clearly unphysiological, interpreting such data is problematic. We would also advise investigators to perform many repeats of experiments in order to overcome the inherent variability in placental oxygenation and levels of endogenous oxidative stress.

2. Materials

1. Culture medium: standard medium such as Medium-199 with 25 m*M* HEPES, Earle's salts, and L-gluatamine supplemented with 5% heat-inactivated fetal bovine serum, 100 U/mL penicillin, 100 µg/mL streptomycin, and 0.25 µg amphotericin B (all from Life Technologies, Paisley, UK).
2. Culture plastic ware and Costar Netwell inserts (24-mm diameter, 500 µm mesh, available from BDH Merck, Lutterworth, UK).
3. Gases (*see* **Note 5**).
   a. Special gas mixes can be purchased to order from most medical gas suppliers (for example, British Oxygen Corporation, Guildford, UK).
   b. The Pro-Ox and Pro-CO_2 oxygen and carbon dioxide gas controllers are available from Biospherix, Redfield, NY.
   c. Oxygen controlled incubators are available from most laboratory equipment suppliers.
   d. Dessicator chambers (21 × 18 × 13 cm; Scientific Laboratory Supplies Ltd., Nottingham, UK).
   e. Anaerocult IS is available from Merck KgaA, Darmstadt, Germany.
4. Oxygen-sensitive probes for measuring dissolved oxygen concentrations (World Precision Instruments, Sarasota, FL) (*see* **Note 6**).

a. 2',7'-dichlorofluorescein diacetate (DCFH-DA) and 3-(4,5-dimethyldiazol-2-yl)-2,5-diphenyl-tetrazolium bromide (MTT; Sigma Chemical Co., St Louis, MO).
b. Antibodies to hydroxynonenal and peroxynitrite (Upstate Biotechnology, Lake Placid or Chemicon, Nottingham, UK).

3. Methods

1. Placental samples should be obtained as rapidly as possible after delivery to avoid depletion of ATP and hypoxia-induced oxidative stress (*see* **Note 1**). It is advisable to take samples (each ~40 to 50 mg wet weight) from a consistent region of each of four to five lobules to account for regional variations. After a brief rinse in cold phosphate-buffered saline (pH 7.4), one sample should be snap-frozen in liquid nitrogen or fixed in paraformaldehyde as a baseline control of endogenous placental oxidative stress.

2. The remaining samples should be placed in culture medium (*see* **Note 2**) equilibrated with the appropriate gas mix (*see* **Note 3**) and transferred to the laboratory on ice.

3. On arrival, the samples are further dissected into pieces weighing approx 5–10 mg in ice-cold medium in an atmosphere of 5% O_2 (*see* **Note 4**). One or more samples should be snap-frozen and/or fixed as a time-zero control. The samples are then transferred to Costar Netwell supports in six-well flat-bottom culture plates with sufficient medium that the samples should be at the gas–liquid interface. These are then placed in a humidified incubator at the required oxygen concentration (*see* **Note 5**).

4. The dissolved oxygen concentration in the medium should be monitored at the start and end of experiments (*see* **Note 6**).

5. Length of culture and the oxygen concentrations used will depend on the question to be addressed. We routinely monitor the viability of the syncytiotrophoblast at the end of experiments as it notoriously difficult to maintain in culture *(37–40)* (*see* **Note 7**). This can be done in a variety of ways *(31,41)*:

   a. The quickest, and arguably the most physiological, is to monitor mitochondrial activity, for if this is lost, ATP levels will drop precipitously. The simplest test is using an adaptation of the MTT cleavage assay, in which tissues are incubated for 20 min at 37°C in a 0.5 mg/mL solution of MTT in culture medium *(41)*. After a brief rinse in culture medium, the tissues are frozen in an aqueous embedding medium for subsequent sectioning at 10 μm. The MTT is converted to stable formazan precipitates within active mitochondria, which therefore appear as blue dots on sections viewed by phase-contrast. Some crystallisation of the precipitates may subsequently occur, so if necessary sections are best photographed soon after preparation. Mitochondrial activity can also be monitored using Rhodamine 123, although this requires use of live tissue and confocal microscopy.

   b. Syncytiotrophoblast integrity can be checked using classical dye-exclusion methods such as trypan blue or dansyl lysine.

c. For morphological assessment, transmission electron microscopy remains the "gold standard." Although this is relatively time consuming and expensive for routine use, it can be very informative when initially validating a protocol.

6. Oxidative stress can be generated in placental tissues in a variety of ways:

a. Hypoxia-reoxygenation. Maintaining term tissues for a period of 20 min under hypoxic conditions followed by 2 h reoxygenation is a potent stimulus of oxidative stress within the syncytiotrophoblast and cytotrophoblast cells, and cells of the villous core *(42–44)*. Hypoxic conditions can be created using a glove box or a special incubation bag containing moistened Anaerocult IS. Medium is pre-equilibrated with 95% N_2/5% CO_2, and the bag is continuously flushed with the same mix, giving an oxygen concentration in the gas phase of <1%. The dissolved oxygen concentration is 12–16 mmHg. Reoxygenation with 5 or 21% oxygen is equally effective at generating oxidative stress and downstream consequences in terms of apoptosis or cytokine secretion. We have also used this technique with explants from the mouse labyrinth and found it to be similarly effective *(45)*.

b. Oxidative stress has also be generated in human and mouse placental tissues using the xanthine/xanthine oxidase system *(45,46)*. Samples are incubated in medium containing 2.3 mM xanthine and 15mU/mL xanthine oxidase for 2 h under 5% oxygen. Exposure to 500 µM hydrogen peroxide for 120 min also generates substantial oxidative stress in first-trimester tissues, as does exposure to 0.1 µg/mL tumor necrosis factor (TNF)-α *(32)*.

7. The oxidative stress generated in placental tissues can be monitored in a variety of ways:

a. Formation of free radicals. A simple method for detecting the formation of ROS is to incubate the tissues in 20 µM DCFH-DA. This is transformed into the fluorescent product DCF in the presence of ROS, which is excited at 780 nm *(42)* (*see* **Note 8**).

b. Immunological detection of lipid peroxidation using antibodies to hydroxynonenal, and of nitrosylated proteins using antibodies to peroxynitrite. These allow localization of the oxidative stress to particular cell types *(30,33,42)*. Quantification can be performed using a visual scoring system or by using a fluorescent secondary antibody and quantifying mean pixel intensity along lines drawn through the tissue of interest using the software on a confocal microscope *(30)* (*see* **Note 9**).

c. Increased concentrations of protein carbonyls and isoprostanes have been reported in oxidatively stressed placentas from cases of preeclampsia *(47,48)*, and so may have potential for in vitro work (*see* **Note 10**).

4. Notes

1. Levels of ATP within the term placenta fall steadily after delivery, and approach 25% of in vivo concentrations 20 min after separation. Evidence of ROS-medi-

ated lipid peroxidation is also first seen at this time point *(26)*, and so it would seem unwise to collect tissue from a placenta if more than 15–20 min have elapsed since delivery.

2. We routinely use Medium-199 supplemented with 5% serum. The concentration of serum (0–20%) has little effect on trophoblast viability. We add antibiotics to the medium as the original material is never sterile, although our cultures are usually only of short duration.

3. For samples from the peripheral regions of term placental lobules, we routinely collect material into medium equilibrated with 5% O_2/90% N_2/5% CO_2. Equilibration is achieved by bubbling the gas mix through the medium in a Dreschel bottle for 30 min, and should give a dissolved oxygen concentration of 45–62 mmHg. This can be monitored using a dissolved oxygen probe. The medium is transported to the Delivery Suite in a glass bottle filled to the top in order to reduce diffusion of oxygen into the medium.

4. We initially performed our dissections in a biological safety cabinet, but in order to prevent exposure to ambient concentrations of oxygen, we delivered an atmosphere of 5% O2/90% N2/5% CO_2 over the Petri dish from a large inverted funnel. We now use a glove box gassed with the same mix so that all dissection and handling is performed under a low-oxygen environment.

5. Incubators that allow control of oxygen as well as carbon dioxide are available commercially, but are relatively expensive. Other potential disadvantages are that many allow only one oxygen concentration to be set, and because of their volume, it can take some time for the final concentration to be achieved. We have devised our own system utilizing four dessicator chambers that are stacked on an orbital shaker. Initially, each chamber was continuously flushed with a different commercially purchased gas mix. Although a cheap option in terms of capital outlay, the range of concentrations is limited by the gas mixes held in store. We now have each chamber equipped with Pro-Ox and Pro-CO_2 probes enabling individual concentrations to be set by the researcher. This provides greater flexibility, and also a constant readout of the actual oxygen and carbon dioxide concentrations within each chamber. The relatively small size of the dessicator chambers ensures that the oxygen concentration is restored rapidly (1–2 min) after opening the door to add or remove samples.

6. The dissolved oxygen concentration as well as the oxygen concentration in the gas phase should be measured to check that equilibration has occurred. We routinely agitate our cultures using an orbital shaker at 70 rpm so that an oxygen gradient is not established within the medium.

7. Despite all efforts, we are not able to maintain mitochondrial activity within the syncytiotrophoblast of first-trimester or term placental explants for more than 10–12 h. Therefore, we currently restrict all experiments using primary tissues to 7 h or less. Mitochondrial activity is maintained within the cytotrophoblast cells and stromal cells for a number of days. Indeed, a new syncytiotrophoblast layer is generated over 48–72 h *(38,39)*, but the cells in the villous core ultimately undergo apoptosis or necrosis.

8. DCFH is a quick and easy technique that has the added advantage that is localizes generation of ROS to particular cell types within a tissue. It has been criticized on the basis that it is a self-propagating reaction, because the fluorescent signal itself generates ROS within cells. Nonetheless, it is widely used in other systems. Electron spin resonance remains the gold standard for the detection of ROS. Spectral analysis allows the species of ROS to be identified, although in tissues they cannot be localized to individual cell types. The technique has been used successfully to identify increased production of ROS in placentas from preeclampsia *(49)*.

9. The oxidative stress generated in different cell types will depend on their endogenous antioxidant defenses. One may therefore wish to quantify trophoblastic stress separately from that of stromal cells. Immunohistochemical staining is the only technique that allows one to do this. Visual scoring is at best semi-quantitative, but reliability can be enhanced using two observers blinded to the nature of the material. By contrast, measuring mean pixel intensity provides numerical data for statistical comparison *(7,30)*. The start points for lines drawn within the trophoblast layer can be identified with simple grids, using the intersection of a line with the villous surface as a start point. Western blotting can be used to back up the immunohistochemistry. For nitrotyrosine, we observe multiple bands of nitrosylated proteins, making quantification difficult, but hydroxynonenal produces only a few bands and so is preferred *(42)*. Problems can arise, however, if the stress is restricted to just the syncytiotrophoblast. Because this represents only a small fraction of the overall tissue mass of villous explants, significant stress in this compartment may not be reflected in the tissue homogenate. A combination of immunohistochemistry and Western blotting is therefore useful, for discrepancies can occur between the two techniques *(7)*.

10. Our own experience with measuring isoprostanes is that the assays are problematic when using tissues because they are compromised by the presence of hemoglobin. Because it is impossible to remove the fetal erythrocytes from the villous capillary network without perfusion, this limits use of the assays for tissue samples but not, of course, for supernatants or other fluid samples.

Acknowledgments

The authors would like to thank Drs. Tereza Cindrova-Davies, Joanne Hempstock, Tai-Ho Hung, Jeremy N. Skepper, Adrian L. Watson, and Billy Yung for their help in developing many of these techniques. The work has been supported by the Medical Research Council (MRC), Tommy's The Baby Charity, the Special Trustees of University College Hospital London, and The Wellcome Trust.

References

1. Genbacev, O., Zhou, Y., Ludlow, J. W., and Fisher S. J. (1997) Regulation of human placental development by oxygen tension. *Science* **277,** 1669–1672.

2. Burton, G. J., Jauniaux, E., and Watson, A. L. (1999) Influence of oxygen supply on placental structure, in *Fetal Programming: Influences on development and disease in later life* (O'Brien, P. M. S., Wheeler, T., and Barker, D. J. P., eds.). RCOG, London: pp. 326–341.

3. Caniggia, I. and Winter, J. L. (2002) Adriana and Luisa Castellucci Award Lecture 2001 Hypoxia Inducible Factor-1: Oxygen regulation of trophoblast differentiation in normal and pre-eclamptic pregnancies—a review. *Placenta* **23(Suppl A),** S47–S57.

4. Hubel, C. A. (1999) Oxidative stress in the pathogenesis of preeclampsia. *Proc. Soc. Exp. Biol. Med.* **222,** 222–235.

5. Redman, C. W. G. and Sargent, I. L. (2000) Placental debris, oxidative stress and pre-eclampsia. *Placenta* **21,** 597–602.

6. Burton, G. J., Hempstock, J., and Jauniaux, E. (2003) Oxygen, early embryonic metabolism and free radical-mediated embryopathies. *Reprod. BioMed. Online* **6,** 84–96.

7. Hempstock, J., Jauniaux, E., Greenwold, N., and Burton, G. J. (2003) The contribution of placental oxidative stress to early pregnancy failure. *Hum. Pathol.* **34,** 1265–1275.

8. Halliwell, B. and Gutteridge, J. M. C. (1999) *Free Radicals in Biology and Medicine.* Oxford Science, Oxford, UK.

9. Raha, S., McEachern, G. E., Myint, A. T., and Robinson, B. H. (2000) Superoxides from mitochondrial complex III: the role of manganese superoxide dismutase. *Free Radic. Biol. Med.* **29,** 170–180.

10. Freeman, B. A. and Crapo, J. D. (1981) Hyperoxia increases oxygen radical production in rat lungs and lung mitochondria. *J. Biol. Chem.* **256,** 10,986–10,992.

11. Matsubra, S. and Tamada, T. (1991) Ultracytochemical localisation of NAD(P)H oxidase activity in the human placenta. *Acta Obstet. Gynaecol. Jap.* **43,** 117–121.

12. Manes, C. (2001) Human placental NAD(P)H oxidase: solubilization and properties. *Placenta* **22,** 58–63.

13. Raijmakers, M. T. M., Burton, G. J., Jauniaux, E., Seed, P. T., Peters, W. H. M., Steegers, E. A. P., and Poston, L. (2005) Placental NAD(P)H oxidase mediated superoxide generation in early pregnancy. *Placenta*, in press.

14. Schachter, M. and Foulds, S. (1999) Free radicals and the xanthine oxidase pathway, in *Ischaemia-Reperfusion Injury* (Grace, P. A. and Mathie, R. T., eds.). Blackwell Science Ltd., Oxford: pp. 137–147.

15. Droge, W. (2002) Free radicals in the physiological control of cell function. *Physiol. Rev.* **82,** 47–95.

16. Chen, K., Thomas, S. R., and Keaney, J. F. (2003) Beyond LDL oxidation: ROS in vascular signal transduction. *Free Radic. Biol. Med.* **35,** 117–132.

17. Semenza, G. L. (1998) Hypoxia-inducible factor 1; master regulator of O_2 homeostasis. *Curr. Opin. Genet. Dev.* **8,** 588–594.

18. Lando, D., Peet, D. J., Whelan, D. A., Gorman, J. J., and Whitelaw, M. L. (2002) Asparagine hydroxylation of the HIF transactivation domain: a hypoxic switch. *Science* **295,** 858–861.

19. Graham, C. H., Postovit, L. M., Park, H., Canning, M. T., and Fitzpatrick, T. E. (2000) Adriana and Luisa Castellucci Award Lecture 1999: Role of oxygen in the regulation of trophoblast gene expression and invasion. *Placenta* **21,** 443–450.

20. Stewart, A. G., Barker, J. E., and Hickey, M. J. (1999) Nitric oxide in ischaemia-reperfusion injury, in *Ischaemia-Reperfusion Injury* (Grace, P. A. and Mathie, R. T., eds.). Blackwell Science Ltd., Oxford, UK: pp. 180–195.

21. Radi, R., Peluffo, G., Alvarez, M. N., Naviliat, M., and Cayota, A. (2001) Unravelling peroxynitrite formation in biological systems. *Free Radic. Biol. Med.* **30,** 463–488.

22. Hensley, K., Robinson, K. A., Gabbita, S. P., Salsman, S., and Floyd, R. A. (2000) Reactive oxygen species, cell signalling, and cell injury. *Free Radic. Biol. Med.* **28,** 1456–1462.

23. Burton, G. J. and Hung, T.-H. (2003) Hypoxia-reoxygenation; a potential source of placental oxidative stress in normal pregnancy and preeclampsia. *Fetal Mat. Med. Rev.* **14,** 97–117.

24. Many, A. and Robert, J. M. (1997) Increased xanthine oxidase during labour-implications for oxidative stress. *Placenta* **18,** 725–726.

25. Woods, J. R., Jr., Cavanaugh, J. L., Norkus, E. P., Plessinger, M. A., and Miller, R. K. (2002) The effect of labor on maternal and fetal vitamins C and E. *Am. J. Obstet. Gynecol.* **187,** 1179–1183.

26. Serkova, N., Bendrick-Peart, J., Alexander, B., and Tissot van Patot, M. C. (2003) Metabolite concentrations in human term placentae and their changes due to delayed collection after delivery. *Placenta* **24,** 227–235.

27. Schaaps, J. P. and Hustin, J. (1988) In vivo aspect of the maternal-trophoblastic border during the first trimester of gestation. *Troph. Res.* **3,** 39–48.

28. Burton, G. J., Watson, A. L., Hempstock, J., Skepper, J. N., and Jauniaux, E. (2002) Uterine glands provide histiotrophic nutrition for the human fetus during the first trimester of pregnancy. *J. Clin. Endocrinol. Metabol.* **87,** 2954–2959.

29. Rodesch, F., Simon, P., Donner, C., and Jauniaux, E. (1992) Oxygen measurements in endometrial and trophoblastic tissues during early pregnancy. *Obstet. Gynecol.* **80,** 283–285.

30. Jauniaux, E., Watson, A. L., Hempstock, J., Bao, Y.-P., Skepper, J. N., and Burton, G. J. (2000) Onset of maternal arterial bloodflow and placental oxidative stress; a possible factor in human early pregnancy failure. *Am. J. Pathol.* **157,** 2111–2122.

31. Watson, A. L., Skepper, J. N., Jauniaux, E., and Burton, G. J. (1998) Susceptibility of human placental syncytiotrophoblastic mitochondria to oxygen-mediated damage in relation to gestational age. *J. Clin. Endocrinol. Metabol.* **83,** 1697–1705.

32. Dyson, C. A. J., Hempstock, J., Jauniaux, E., Charnock-Jones, D. S., and Burton, G. J. (2003) Regulation of the level of immunoreactive HIF-1a by oxidative stress in the early human placenta. *Placenta* **24,** A6.

33. Jauniaux, E., Hempstock, J., Greenwold, N., and Burton, G. J. (2003) Trophoblastic oxidative stress in relation to temporal and regional differences in mater-

nal placental blood flow in normal and abnormal early pregnancies. *Am. J. Pathol.* **162,** 115–125.

34. Soothill, P. W., Nicolaides, K. H., Rodeck, C. H., and Campbell, S. (1986) Effect of gestational age on fetal and intervillous blood gas and acid-base values in human pregnancy. *Fetal Therapy* **1,** 168–175.

35. Hempstock, J., Bao, Y.-P., Bar-Issac, M., et al. (2003) Intralobular differences in antioxidant enzyme expression and activity reflect oxygen gradients within the human placenta. *Placenta* **24,** 517–523.

36. Burton, G. J. and Caniggia, I. (2001) Hypoxia: implications for implantation to delivery-a workshop report. *Placenta* **22(Suppl A),** S63–S65.

37. Burton, G. J., Mayhew, T. M., and Robertson, L. A. (1989) Stereological re-examination of the effects of varying oxygen tensions on human placental villi maintained in organ culture for up to 12 h. *Placenta* **10,** 263–273.

38. Palmer, M. E., Watson, A. L., and Burton, G. J. (1997) Morphological analysis of degeneration and regeneration of syncytiotrophoblast in first trimester villi during organ culture. *Hum. Reprod.* **12,** 379–382.

39. Siman, C. M., Sibley, C. P., Jones, C. J., Turner, M. A., and Greenwood, S. L. (2001) The functional regeneration of syncytiotrophoblast in cultured explants of term placenta. *Am. J. Physiol.* **280,** R1116–R1122.

40. Sooranna, S. R., Oteng-Ntim, E., Meah, R., Ryder, T. A., and Bajoria, R. (1999) Characterization of human placental explants: morphological, biochemical and physiological studies using first and third trimester placenta. *Hum. Reprod.* **14,** 536–541.

41. Watson, A. L., Palmer, M. E., Jauniaux, E., and Burton, G. J. (1998) Evidence for oxygen-derived free radical mediated damage to first trimester human trophoblast in vitro. *Troph. Res.* **11,** 259–276.

42. Hung, T.-H., Skepper, J. N., and Burton, G. J. (2001) In vitro ischemia-reperfusion injury in term human placenta as a model for oxidative stress in pathological pregnancies. *Am. J. Pathol.* **159,** 1031–1043.

43. Hung, T.-H., Skepper, J. N., Charnock-Jones, D. S., and Burton, G. J. (2002) Hypoxia/reoxygenation: a potent inducer of apoptotic changes in the human placenta and possible etiological factor in preeclampsia. *Circ. Res.* **90,** 1274–1281.

44. Hung, T.-H., Charnock-Jones, D. S., Skepper, J. N., and Burton, G. J. (2004) Secretion of tumour necrosis factor-α from human placental tissues induced by hypoxia-reoxygenation causes endothelial cell activation in vitro: a potential mediator of the inflammatory response in preeclampsia. *Am. J. Pathol.* **164,** 1049–1061.

45. Mann, C. A., Hempstock, J., Charnock-Jones, D. S., Ferguson-Smith, A. C., and Burton, G. J. (2003) Oxidative stress and apoptosis in the labyrinth of the normal mouse placenta increase with gestational age. *Placenta* **24,** A21.

46. Malek, A., Sager, R., and Schneider, H. (2001) Effect of hypoxia, oxidative stress and lipopolysaccharides on the release of prostaglandins and cytokines from human term placental explants. *Placenta* **22(Suppl A),** S45–S50.

47. Zusterzeel, P. L. M., Rutten, H., Roelofs, H. M. J., Peters, W. H. M., and Steegers, E. A. P. (2001) Protein carbonyls in decidua and placenta of pre-eclamptic women as markers of oxidative stress. *Placenta* **22,** 213–219.
48. Walsh, S. W., Vaughan, J. E., Wang, Y., and Roberts, L. J. (2000) Placental isoprostane is significantly increased in preeclampsia. *FASEB J.* **14,** 1289–1296.
49. Sikkema, J. M., van Rijn, B. B., Franx, A., et al. (2001) Placental superoxide is increased in pre-eclampsia. *Placenta* **22,** 304–308.

28

Hypobaric Hypoxia as a Tool to Study Pregnancy-Dependent Responses at the Maternal–Fetal Interface

Jennifer K. Ho-Chen, Rupasri Ain, Adam R. Alt, John G. Wood, Norberto C. Gonzalez, and Michael J. Soares

Summary

Establishment of proper oxygen and nutrient supply to the fetus is essential for a successful pregnancy. The maternal–fetal interface is the site of vascular modifications, providing a conduit for the delivery of essential nutrients to the developing fetus. Pregnancy-dependent adaptive vascular responses within the uteroplacental compartment can be exaggerated by exposure to a physiological stressor such as hypoxia. A simple procedure for exposing pregnant rats and mice to hypobaric hypoxia is presented.

Key Words: Hypoxia; pregnancy; rat; metrial gland; vascular remodeling; trophoblast.

1. Introduction

Oxygen is an essential component of life, and is especially important in pregnancy because oxygen tension has a regulatory role in placental development *(1)*. Vascular remodeling at the maternal–fetal interface is necessary in order to deliver an adequate oxygen and nutrient supply to the fetus *(2–4)*. Hypoxia has been implicated in pregnancy-associated diseases such as intrauterine growth restriction (IUGR) and preeclampsia, which elucidates the importance of oxygen regulation in pregnancy.

The rodent has been used as a model to study the role of oxygen in pregnancy. When rats and mice are exposed to hypoxia, gene expression is altered, impacting placental and fetal development *(5–7)*. The effect of low oxygen can vary—it can lead to IUGR and termination of pregnancy at one extreme or, alternatively, it can elicit maternal adaptations that allow a successful pregnancy to be achieved. The outcome of maternal hypoxia is dependent on the level of oxygen restriction, the duration of exposure, and the gestational period in which the insult is made.

From: *Methods in Molecular Medicine, Vol. 122: Placenta and Trophoblast: Methods and Protocols, Vol. 2*
Edited by: M. J. Soares and J. S. Hunt © Humana Press Inc., Totowa, NJ

During normal human and rat pregnancy, erythrocyte, hematocrit, and hemoglobin concentrations decrease as pregnancy progresses as a result of hemodilution *(8,9)*. There are also many reports of complications in pregnancies at high-altitudes in which chronic hypoxia has a role in the etiology of pregnancy-associated disease *(1)*. High altitude, defined as >2500 meters, has been shown to reduce uterine blood flow and increase the incidence of IUGR and preeclampsia *(1,10,11)*. Blood vessel development is stimulated by low oxygen tension from high altitude, which results in increased vascularity *(12,13)*.

In this chapter, we describe a simple in vivo model that allows induction of maternal adaptive responses to hypoxia, sparing the fetus from IUGR. In this model, pregnant rats or mice are exposed to hypobaric hypoxia, which activates maternal uterine vascular remodeling and hematological adaptations *(14,* Ho-Chen, J. K. and Soares, M. J., unpublished results). This profound maternal response largely protects the fetus from IUGR.

2. Materials

1. Animals: Holtzman rats are obtained from Harlan-Sprague Dawley (Indianapolis, IN) and CD-1 mice are obtained from Charles River Laboratories (Wilmington, MA).
2. The hypobaric chamber was designed and constructed by Alt Manufacturing (Kansas City, KS). A hypobaric chamber has four main components: a vacuum pump, a vacuum breaker valve, a differential vacuum gauge, and a chamber (*see* **Fig. 1**). The first three components are readily available and come from a manufacturer ready to be used. A one-fourth to one-half horsepower continuous duty, oil-less rotary vane vacuum pump that is capable of pumping down to at least 26 inches of Hg and moving at least 3 cfm of air, is required (McMaster-Carr, Elmhurst, IL, cat. no. 9901K64). The vacuum breaker valve is used to maintain a preset vacuum in the chamber. A heavy-duty bronze diaphragm valve with a breaking range of 2–30 in. of Hg is recommended (McMaster-Carr, cat. no. 4614K11). This type of valve ensures a highly controlled and reproducible vacuum. A digital differential vacuum gauge can be purchased from Cecomp Electronics, Inc. (Cecomp Electronics, Inc., Libertyville, IL, cat. no. DPG1000AD). The vacuum gauge can be programmed at the factory to display one of several different units. Construction of the chamber is considerably more involved because it usually requires custom fabrication and has several unique requirements. The chamber can be made to accommodate a wide range of space and weight requirements, as long the chamber can withstand a differential pressure equivalent to 10 psi. It is useful for the chamber to have at least one transparent side, so that animal light–dark cycles are not disrupted. The pump is connected to the chamber using one-half- inch (inner diameter) braid reinforced tubing (McMaster-Carr, cat. no. 55425K33) and generic brass barbed hose fittings. The vacuum breaker valve and vacuum gauge are connected to the chamber using standard copper pipe and various fittings (*see* **Notes 1** and **2**).

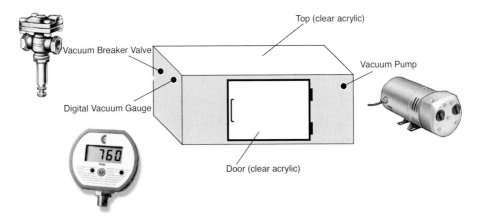

Fig. 1. Diagram of the hypobaric chamber, illustrating the essential components of the chamber.

3. Pediatric BD Vacutainer(tm) Tubes containing spray-dried K_2-ethylenediamine tetraacetic acid (EDTA) (Becton Dickinson, Franklin Lakes, NJ).
4. Act10 Hematological Analysis System (Beckman Coulter, Miami, FL).

3. Methods

3.1. Animal Preparations (see Note 3)

1. Male and female Holtzman rats are kept under controlled conditions of 14 h light and 10 h dark (14 h-L:10 h-D) or, alternatively, 12 h-L:12 h-D photoperiods with access to food and water *ad libitum*. To obtain timed pregnancies, female rats are caged overnight with fertile males. The presence of sperm in vaginal smear is designated as d 0 of pregnancy.
2. Male and female CD-1 mice are housed in 14 h-L:10 h-D photoperiod with access to food and water *ad libitum*. Timed mouse pregnancies are obtained by co-housing females with fertile males. The presence of a seminal plug in the vagina of females is designated as d 1 of pregnancy.

3.2. Chamber Calibration (see Table 1)

The barometric pressure adjustments are presented in **Table 1** and are based on the following equations:

$$P_{IO2} = (P_C - P_{H2O}) \times \%O_2 \text{ in air} = (P_B - P_{H2O}) \times \%O_2 \text{ inspired}$$

where:

P_{IO2} = Partial pressure of inspired oxygen
P_C = Pressure inside hypobaric chamber
P_B = Barometric pressure at experiment site
P_{H2O} = Partial pressure of water vapor = 47 Torr

Table 1
Calibration of the Hypobaric Chamber

Experimental conditions	Estimated O_2 concentrations at sea level	P_{IO2} (Torr)	P_B (Torr)	P_B (inches of Hg)	Differential Pressure (inches of Hg)	Simulated elevation (meters)
Sea level	21	149	760	29.9	–	0
Kansas City, KS	21	143	730	28.7	–	300
Chamber-10	10	71	385	15.2	14.7	5150
Chamber-11	11	78	418	16.5	13.4	4540
Chamber-12	12	86	454	17.9	12.0	3990
Chamber-13	13	93	490	19.3	10.6	3470
Chamber-14	14	100	523	20.6	9.3	2990
Chamber-15	15	107	556	21.9	8.0	2560

3.3. Exposure of Pregnant Rodents to Hypobaric Hypoxia

1. Prior to exposure, the rat or mouse is weighed and then placed in the hypobaric chamber. Food is measured and allocated. Each animal is caged separately to monitor food intake (*see* **Note 4**).
2. The chamber is sealed and the vacuum is activated. Different settings are used for the pregnant Holtzman rat vs the pregnant CD-1 mouse (*see* **Note 5**).
   a. For the Holtzman rat we routinely use conditions where air is circulated at a barometric pressure of approx 386 Torr, which results in an inspired PO_2 of approx 71 Torr, equivalent to breathing 10% O_2 at sea level (*see* **Table 1**).
   b. For the CD-1 mouse, we routinely use conditions in which air is circulated at a barometric pressure of approx 420 Torr, which results in an inspired PO_2 of approx 78 Torr, equivalent to breathing 11% O_2 at sea level (*see* **Table 1**).
3. On a daily basis, the vacuum is released and the chamber opened for 15–20 min in order that the cages may be cleaned, the animals and their food weighed, and food and water replenished (*see* **Note 6**).
4. At the termination of the experiment, the animals are removed from the chamber and analyzed, as dictated by the experimental design.
5. Two types of controls are used: (1) *ad libitum*-fed animals and (2) pair-fed animals. *Ad libitum*-fed controls are weighed and food intake monitored daily. Pair-fed controls are weighed daily and are fed the amount of food that the hypoxic animals ate on that day of gestation (*see* **Note 7**).

3.4. Phenotypic Assessment

1. Systemic assessment: blood samples are collected by cardiac puncture of anesthetized animals in Pediatric BD Vacutainer Tubes containing spray-dried K_2-EDTA and stored at 4°C until analyzed. Hematological parameters are measured using an Act10 Hematological Analysis System. This provides a complete hematological analysis, including: total leukocytes, total erythrocytes, hemoglobin, hematocrit, mean-corpuscular hemoglobin, mean cell hemoglobin concentration, total platelets, and mean platelet volume (*see* **Note 8**).
2. Strategies for assessing the maternal–fetal compartments of animals exposed to hypoxia and their respective controls have been presented in Chapters 20, 21, and 26 of Vol. 1 *(15–17)* (*see* **Note 9**).

4. Notes

1. Additional information about the hypobaric chamber design can be obtained by contacting Alt Manufacturing (Phone: 913-588-5690). The vacuum pump we have selected is relatively quiet, but optimally it should be housed in an adjoining room or utility closet, and the vacuum hose run through the wall thus minimizing the noise. If this is not possible, then it is essential that control animals be exposed to the same level of noise.
2. There are several alternatives to using a hypobaric chamber that can be used to create a hypoxic environment. Most utilize gas dilution. One approach is to use

an oxygen controller (e.g., Pro-Oxy Controller, Biospherix, Syracuse, NY). The controller monitors the oxygen concentration in a sealed box and regulates the rate of infusion of nitrogen gas. The oxygen controller releases nitrogen into the box, diluting the concentration of oxygen down to a set-point. The initial cost of such a controller is approximately twice that of fabricating a hypobaric chamber. Unlike the hypobaric system, the gas dilution system continues to require expenditures for nitrogen gas adding to the operational costs.

3. All animal experimentation should be approved by the institutional animal care and use committee.

4. Animals usually reduce their appetite the first few days and exhibit decreased physical activity. Overtime they adapt and regain some of their food intake; however, their physical activity remains limited during the course of exposure. The reduced food intake affects body weight and necessitates additional controls (see below).

5. Responses to maternal hypoxia are affected by species, strain, and gestational stage. In general, mice are more sensitive than rats and at least some inbred strains are more sensitive than outbred strains. Furthermore, the period of gestational exposure affects responses. Both rats and mice appear to be able to more effectively adapt to hypoxia during the interval immediately after implantation to midgestation. Adaptive responses to hypoxia during the last week of gestation are more variable, especially in the mouse. We have focused on two time intervals in the Holtzman rat: (1) d 6 to 12 of gestation and (2) d 13 to 20 of gestation. In the CD-1 mouse, we have focused on a time interval between d 6 and 12 of gestation.

6. A few issues are relevant regarding the opening of the chamber during the course of an experiment. First, the rate of pressure release from the chamber must be slow. We typically shut off the vacuum pump and let the chamber passively equilibrate with the ambient environment. Opening the chamber daily provides a convenient means for tracking responses of the animals during the course of an experiment and maintaining their food and water supply. This brief daily exposure to ambient pressure has also proved to be essential for maintaining viable pregnancies during the last week of gestation.

7. *Ad libitum* fed and pair-fed controls are required. These two control groups are important because hypobaric hypoxia influences food intake. Body weight gain in pregnant females exposed to hypobaric hypoxia is less than pregnant animals housed under ambient conditions. Restricting food intake of pregnant females housed under ambient conditions matches the maternal body weight changes in hypobaric hypoxia-exposed females. Pair-feeding is an essential control because maternal food restriction independently impacts placental and fetal growth.

8. Typical systemic responses to maternal hypoxia include increases in hemoglobin and hematocrit. The magnitude of the response appears to be more evident during the first half of gestation in comparison to responses observed during the last week of gestation (Ho-Chen, J. and Soares, M. J., unpublished results).

9. The most reproducible responses in pregnant rats or mice exposed to hypoxia are changes that occur in the uterine mesometrial compartment (also called the metrial gland). Maternal hypoxia increases vascularity and the diameter of uterine mesometrial blood vessels (*14*, Ho-Chen, J., Ain, R., and Soares, M. J., unpublished results). Additional responses are also noted in metrial gland gene expression profiles (Ain, R. and Soares, M. J., unpublished results). For the latter experiments, it is important to appreciate that some commonly used housekeeping genes are affected by hypoxia (e.g., glyceraldehyde-3-phosphate dehydrogenase).

Acknowledgments

This work is supported by National Institutes of Health (NIH) (F31HD45052, HD20676, HD39878) and the Hall Family Foundation.

References

1. Zamudio, S. (2003) The placenta at high altitude. *High Alt. Med. Biol.* **4,** 171–191.
2. Genbacev, O., Joslin, R., Damsky, C. H., Polliotti, B. M., and Fisher, S.J. (1996) Hypoxia alters early gestation human cytotrophoblast differentiation/invasion in vitro and models the placental defects that occur in preeclampsia. *J. Clin. Invest.* **97,** 540–550.
3. Caniggia, I., Mostachfi, H., Winter, J.,et al. (2000) Hypoxia-inducible factor-1 mediates the biological effects of oxygen on human trophoblast differentiation through TGFβ3. *J. Clin. Invest.* **105,** 577–587.
4. Burton, G. J. and Jaunaiux, E. (2001) Maternal vascularization of the human placenta: does the embryo develop in a hypoxic environment? *Gynecol. Obstet. Fertil.* **29,** 503–508.
5. De Grauw, T. J., Myers, R. E., and Scott, W. J. (1986) Fetal growth retardation in rats from different levels of hypoxia. *Biol. Neonate* **49,** 85–89.
6. Schwartz, J. E., Kovach, A., Meyer, J., McConnell, C., and Iwamoto, H. S. (1998) Brief, intermittent hypoxia restricts fetal growth in Sprague-Dawley rats. *Biol. Neonate* **73,** 313–319
7. Huang, S-T. J., Vo, K. C. T., Lyell, D. J., Fet al. (2004) Developmental response to hypoxia. *FASEB J.* **18,** 1348–1365.
8. Monga, M. (2004) Maternal cardiovascular and renal adaptation to pregnancy, in: *Maternal–Fetal Medicine: Principles and Practices, Fith Edition*(Creasy, R. K. and Resnik, R., eds.). Saunders, Philadelphia, PA, pp. 111–120.
9. De Rijk, E. P.C. T., Van Esch, E., and Flik, G. (2002) Pregnancy dating in the rat: placental morphology and maternal blood parameters. *Toxicol. Path.* **30,** 271–282
10. Moore, L. G. (2003) Fetal growth restriction and maternal oxygen transport during high altitude pregnancy. *High Alt. Med. Biol.* **4,** 141–156.
11. Moore, L. G., Shriver, M., Bemis, L., et al. (2004) Maternal adaptation to high-altitude pregnancy: an experiment of nature—a review. *Placenta* **25,** S60–S71.
12. Tissot van Patot, M., Grilli, P. A., Chapman, P., et al. (2003) Remodelling of uteroplacental arteries is decreased in high altitude placentae. *Placenta* **24,** 326–335.

13. Tissot van Patot, M. C., Bendrick-Peart, J., Beckey, V. E., Serkova, N., and Zwerdlinger, L. (2004) Greater vascularity, lowered HIF-1/DNA binding and elevated GSH as markers of adaptation to in vivo chronic hypoxia. *Am. J. Physiol. Lung Cell Mol. Physiol.* **287,** L525–L532.
14. Ain, R., Dai, G., Dunmore, J. H., Godwin, A. R., and Soares, M. J. (2004) A prolactin family paralog regulates reproductive adaptations to a physiological stressor. *Proc. Natl. Acad. Sci. USA* **101,** 16,543–16,548.
15. Natale, D. R. C., Starovic, M., and Cross, J. C. (2006) Phenotypic analysis of the placenta in the mouse, in: *Placenta and Trophoblast: Methods and Protocols, Vol. 1.* (Soares, M. J. and Hunt, J.S., eds.). Humana, Totowa, NJ.
16. Ain, R., Konno, T., Canham, L. N., and Soares, M. J. (2006) Phenotypic analysis of the placenta in the rat, in: *Placenta and Trophoblast: Methods and Protocols, Vol. 1.* (Soares, M. J. and Hunt, J. S., eds.). Humana, Totowa, NJ.
17. Whitely, K. J., Pfarrer, C. D., and Adamson, S. L. (2006) Vascular corrosion casting of the uteroplacental and feto-lacental vasculature in mice, in: *Placenta and Trophoblast: Methods and Protocols, Vol. 1.* (Soares, M. J. and Hunt, J. S., eds.). Humana, Totowa, NJ.

29

Infection With *Listeria monocytogenes* as a Probe for Placental Immunological Function

Ellen M. Barber, Indira Guleria, and Jeffrey W. Pollard

Summary

This chapter will describe the use of infection with *Listeria monocytogenes*, a Gram-positive intracellular bacterium, to study immunological responses in the placenta. This bacterium is chosen because it has a predilection for replication in the placenta. As such, it is a significant pathogen for pregnant women, being a major cause of fetal mortality and morbidity if appropriate public health precautions are not observed. Furthermore, this bacterium has been a major tool for studying innate immune responses and their transition to an acquired one, characterized by a Th1-type response. Details are given for the culture and maintenance of bacteria stocks, infection of mice, and analysis of the resultant infection. Such studies have revealed a unique pattern of immune responses in the placenta that, through the methods described, should reveal the strategies that the placenta uses to eradicate pathogens while not rejecting allogenic fetuses.

Key Words: Placenta; *Listeria monocytogenes*; pregnancy; uterus; cytokines; reproductive immunology.

1. Introduction

Viviparity in mammals causes a particular immunological challenge because the fetus, with the exception of that of some laboratory animals, is genetically disparate (allogeneic) and consequently should be perceived as foreign and rejected. Clearly, this is not the case and therefore, mammals must have developed strategies that inhibit immune responses to fetal alloantigens *(11)*. There have been many suggestions regarding the mechanisms of this lack of response ranging from the fetal tissue being nonallogenic (immunologically hidden), to the antigens not being accessible to the immune system, to active immunosuppression at the maternal–fetal interface *(10,11)*. Although the mechanism of avoiding rejection of the fetus is obviously multi-factorial, it is clear in the highly vascularized placental milieu that the maternal immune system has access to fetal antigens and that there is active regulation of maternal immune responses to fetal alloantigens *(11)*. Consistent with this, there appears to be an exclusion

From: *Methods in Molecular Medicine, Vol. 122: Placenta and Trophoblast: Methods and Protocols, Vol. 2*
Edited by: M. J. Soares and J. S. Hunt © Humana Press Inc., Totowa, NJ

of cytotoxic T-cells from the placenta and when this exclusion is broken, allogeneic, but not syngeneic, fetuses are rejected *(13)*.

This view of the maternal–fetal interface as an immunosuppressed environment however, raises a perplexing question: "How can the mother mount an effective defense against pathogens without rejecting the fetus?" This is especially a problem in the placenta, which, because of its abundant blood supply, makes it a rich environment for pathogens to prosper. Indeed, some pathogens such as *Listeria monocytogenes* and cytomegalovirus seem to preferentially replicate in this site, and both pathogens are a significant cause of fetal morbidity and/or mortality *(20)*. However, despite this fact, it is clear that in the majority of cases the mother and her fetus are not inundated by infections suggesting robust immune responses.

To explore this immunological paradox, we and others *(1,6,9,16–19)* have used infection of mice with the Gram-positive intracellular bacterium, *L. monocytogenes*. This bacterium was chosen not only because of its predilection for replication in the placental bed of mice and humans, but also because it has been an organism of choice to study the switch from innate to adaptive immunity during systemic infections *(5,7,12,21,22)*. Furthermore, the adaptive response is dominated by a Th1 type resulting in the generation of cytotoxic T-cells that recognize the newly presented Listerial antigens and are required for the sterile eradication of the bacterium *(7,22)*. Earlier studies showed that immunization of pregnant mice conferred protection against systemic but not placental infection, indicating that the placental immune response is different from the systemic one *(16)*. Thus, this bacterium is ideal for studying the ability of the immune system to develop a regional response in the placenta that is different from other sites in the body.

Our studies have indicated that the placental responses are biased towards innate immune responses principally involving neutrophils but also induction of an ancient defense mechanism that includes the upregulation of indoleamine 2,3-dioxygenase (IDO). We have suggested that IDO in turn, prevents the recruitment of cytotoxic T-cells to the placenta that could result in fetal rejection *(1,6,9)*. In this way, the immune system is modulated to eliminate, or at least constrain, the infection until the placenta and its residual bacterial load is discarded, without allowing the adaptive system to gain access to the fetus. In this chapter, we will describe the techniques for studying Listerial infections to allow further exploration of the placental immune response in the presence of an allogenic fetus.

2. Materials

1. *L. monocytogenes*, strain EGD (American Type Culture Collection [ATCC], Manassas, VA).

2. Tryptic soy (Difco; Detroit, MI).
3. Bacto agar (Difco; Detroit, MI).
4. Sterile polystyrene petri dishes, 100×150 mm (Fisher; Pittsburgh, PA).
5. Phoshpate-buffered saline (PBS) (Gibco/BRL; Bethesda, MD).
6. 20% Glycerol.
7. Gram stain kit (Sigma, St. Louis, MO).
8. 10% buffered formalin.
9. Periodate-lysine-2% parformaldehyde-0.5% glutaraldehyde (PLPG) fixative: to make 1 L of PLPG:

   a. add 20 g paraformaldehyde to 200 mL double distilled H_2O, microwave for 1 min. Add a few drops of 5 N NaOH to buffer the solution, and allow the paraformaldehyde to dissolve. Cool on ice.
   b. Add 13.7 g lysine monohydrochloride and 1.4 g Na_2HPO_4 in 500 mL double distilled H_2O.
   c. Add solutions made in **steps 1** and **2** and bring volume to almost 1000 mL with 0.1 M phosphate buffer.
   d. Add 2.2 g Na m-Periodate and adjust pH to 6.8 with NaOH.
   e. Make to 1 L, filter through filter paper, and add 1 mL 50% glutaraldehyde (EM grade, Fluka, Sigma).

10. Freezing tubes.
11. Mouse restraining device.
12. 16- and 26-gage needles and compatible 1-mL syringes.
13. Heating lamp.
14. Tissue Tearor (Biospec Products, Bartlesville, OK).

3. Methods

The methods described below outline: (1) the growth, harvesting and titer calculation of *L. monocytogenes*; (2) infection of mice with *L. monocytogenes*; (3) detection and quantification of bacteria from infected mice; and (4) preservation of infected tissues and their histological analysis.

3.1. Growth of L. monocytogenes

3.1.1. Preparation of Bacterial Cultures

Liquid cultures are grown in sterile broth made with 30 g of Tryptic Soy in 1 liter of milliQ H_2O. For solid cultures, 15 g Bacto agar is added to the above liquid broth prior to autoclaving and then distributed in 10-cm disposable Petri dishes. Similarly to *Escherichia coli*, the optimum temperature for *L. monocytogenes* growth is 37°C. However, unlike laboratory *E. coli* strains, the EGD strain of *L. monocytogenes* does not have an antibiotic resistance gene. Therefore, when grown in tryptic soy broth, it grows more quickly than antibiotic selected bacteria and there is a greater chance of contamination with other bacteria. This makes sterile technique even more important. For added protection from both contamination of *L. monocytogenes* solid cultures and the environment with the bacterium, the agar plates are wrapped with aluminum foil prior to incubation (*see* **Note 1**).

1. Using standard microbiology procedures, a small amount (less than 50 µL) of *L. monocytogenes* from a frozen aliquot or single colony from an agar plate is used to inoculate a 2-mL starter culture.
2. This is grown to saturation and then used to inoculate a larger culture. Using a ratio of 1 µL saturated culture to 1 mL broth the log phase is reached after approx 6 h.
3. The bacteria are collected by centrifugation at approx 300*g* for 20 min at 4°C.
4. For storage, the bacterial pellet is resuspended in a sterile 20% glycerol solution, distributed in 300 µL aliquots into appropriate freezing tubes, and snap-frozen in an ethanol/dry ice bath prior to storage at −80°C. The virulence of the strain is also maintained by routine passage in mice (discussed later).

3.1.2. Calculation of L. monocytogenes Titer

1. To calculate the titer of a given batch of *L. monocytogenes*, serial dilutions in sterile PBS (the usual range is 10^{-5} to 10^{-7}) of 3–4 aliquots are plated in duplicate.
2. After growth for 24 h, the colonies are enumerated and the titer calculated accordingly. This titer is then used to calculate the dilution needed for mouse injections.
3. Prior to use in experiments, it should be confirmed that the bacteria is *L. monocytogenes* by performing a Gram stain of a film of a single colony sample from an agar plate. This is a quick and simple procedure that uses a standard bacteriological kit (see below) and should confirm the presence of Gram-positive rods (*see* **Note 2**).

3.2. Infection of Mice With L. monocytogenes

3.2.1. Intervenous Injection

In humans, infection with *L. monocytogenes* occurs through the ingestion of contaminated foods and subsequent traversement of the bacterium across the mucosa is mediated by its binding to E-cadherin. However, the mouse E-cadherin differs from human one by one amino acid in the binding domain for *L. monocytogenes* (*8*) and therefore, the oral route of infection provides a very sub-optimal murine model for *L. monocytogenes* infection. Therefore, for mice the preferred method is intravenous (IV) infection, a technique that also allows tight control of infectious bacterial titer.

1. Mice should be maintained in a category 2 biosafety area with appropriate approval of animal protocols and with a knowledgeable curatorial staff that is trained in the husbandry of mice infected with a human pathogen.
2. To establish infection of mice, the best inoculum volume is 200 µL. For most of our experiments, we use an inoculum titer of 10^4 colony-forming units (CFU) (*see* **Note 3**). The inoculum should be prepared to the proper dilution in sterile

PBS and kept on ice immediately prior to injection. If this procedure is not followed, the infectivity is variable and therefore not reliable.

3. The mice to be injected are warmed under a heating lamp for approx 2–5 min.
   This will vary with the age and size of the mice. Younger mice are more susceptible to overheating.
4. The warmed mouse is placed in the restraining device in such a way that the tail
   is accessible.
5. 70% ethanol is sprayed on the tail to further dilate the vein.
6. The bacterium is then injected into the lateral tail vein through a 26-gage needle.
7. In many of our studies we have used pregnant mice. In this case, the day of pregnancy is established by the detection of the vaginal plug, which we designate d 1
   of pregnancy. The placenta is formed by d 9 and therefore, according to the
   experimental plan, mice should be infected either around d 6 to study decidual
   immune responses or d 10–14 for placental ones.

3.2.2. Analysis of Infected Mice

L. monocytogenes is an intracellular bacterium that replicates principally in
macrophages. Thus, within a few hours all the bacteria are cleared from the
circulation *(4)* and are located in the macrophage-rich target organs—spleen
and liver—where they replicate. In pregnant mice, infection is also established
in the decidualized regions of the uterus, an area that is devoid of macrophages
(14,17,19).

The infected mice are processed according to the experimental design. If,
for example, comparisons are to be made between two genetically distinct
strains of mice or following an experimental therapy, then the progress of the
infection must be monitored.

1. Monitoring the progress of infection usually involves killing the mice according
   to a locally approved animal protocol and then dissecting out the liver, spleen,
   decidual areas, or placenta (including the uterine areas above the decidua basalis
   and trophoblastic layers).
2. We usually process each decidual unit or placenta individually.
3. Each decidual unit or placenta is weighed and homogenized in a Tissue Tearor in
   sterile PBS, and the resultant supernatant plated in serial dilutions onto tryptose
   phosphate agar in duplicate.
4. The plates are incubated overnight at 37°C and colonies counted to obtain the
   bacterial titer as described under **Subheading 3.1.2.** (*see* **Note 4**).
5. Occasionally, colonies will be selected to re-grow bacterial stocks to maintain
   virulence.
6. Tissue homogenates may also be analyzed for cytokine production by homogenizing in PBS containing 1% Triton-X100 (*see* **Note 5**).
7. Tissues may also be fixed in 10% buffered formalin overnight (*see* **Note 6**) and stained
   with Gram stain kit according to the manufacturers instruction (*see* **Note 2**). After

processing and sectioning at 5 μm, the hydrated sections are covered with crystal violet for 1 min, rinsed with tap water, and covered with Gram iodine solution for 5 min to mordant the crystal violet. Excess crystal violet is removed by adding a few drops of decolorizing solution (75% isopropyl alcohol, 25% acetone). Tissues are counterstained with Safarin O solution for 30–60 s, rinsed, and dipped in Tartrazine solution for 5–10 s. These are rinsed with distilled water for 5 min, dehydrated through graded alcohols, and mounted and coverslipped. This will indicate which cell types are infected and where the bacterium is replicating (*see* **Note 7**).

4. Notes

1. Because *L. monocytogenes* is a significant human pathogen for susceptible persons such as the very young, the very old, immunocompromised individuals, and pregnant women, all work with this bacterium must be performed while wearing gloves and in a category 2 biosafety hood. Liquid cultures and cultures on agar can be grown in a shared warm room facility, but the containers must be clearly labeled and any spilled contents immediately cleaned with an antibacterial agent such as Lysol® and/or 10% bleach. In addition, all nondisposable items such as flasks must be disinfected with Lysol and all waste must be autoclaved prior to disposal. Similarly, mouse bedding should be autoclaved and carcasses properly disposed of by incineration. These procedures may seem overly precautious because *L. monocytogenes* can be found ubiquitously in the environment, but is necessary when working with such concentrated quantities of bacteria.

2. Gram staining can be performed on a film of cells from a liquid culture or solid medium colony, or on tissue slices for a histological context. Sigma offers a package of all of the needed solutions and detailed instructions for both methods. Of note, the most variable step is "decolorizing" or removing alcohol soluble crystal violet that did not mordant with the iodine incubation. The best solution for this step for both films and tissue sections is a mixture of 75% isopropanol/25% acetone. Care should be taken to apply the solution slowly and follow it with a water rinse when the purple color begins to leach out.

3. The ideal inoculum titer varies based on the background strain of the mice because there are dominant resistance factors rendering some strains, such as C57BL/6, more resistant to *L. monocytogenes* infection (*3*). We used 10^4 CFU, a titer that tends to minimize strain differences but that may not be appropriate for all experimental designs.

4. It is necessary to determine the sensitivity of this plating assay because tissues can contain inhibitors of bacterial replication. This is estimated by spiking an uninfected homogenate with a known titer of bacteria. In our case, approx 40 CFU/mL could be detected in the placenta, giving this as the limit of sensitivity.

5. There is an infinite variety of ways to analyze the immune response and the tissue preparation should be adjusted accordingly. Often, the cytokine responses must be measured. This can be done in tissue homogenates, although caution must be exercised with tissue inhibitory factors that can influence enzyme-linked

immunosorbent assays (ELISAs) or radioimmunoassays (RIAs). Many companies provide appropriate cytokine assays and their instructions should be followed. Examples of the use of some of these assays are given in references from our laboratory *(5,6)*.

6. Fixation can be changed according to purpose. Formalin is often not the best fixative for immunohistochemistry (IHC). A very good fixation method is the use of PLPG fixation *(2)*, which allows both IHC and *in situ* hybridization. Use cold and fix overnight. Stocks can be made in advance, but the final solution must be made up on the day of use. Once fixed, tissue preparation is compatible for histology, although in some cases the use of low melting temperature wax is useful.

7. Recently, green fluorescent protein (GFP)-tagged *L. monocytogenese* has been engineered. This gives a sophisticated way of following infection *(15)*.

References

1. Barber, E. M. and Pollard, J. W. (2003) The uterine NK cell population requires IL-15 but these cells are not required for pregnancy nor the resolution of a *Listeria monocytogenes* infection. *J. Immunol.* **171,** 37–46.

2. Cecchini, M. G., Dominguez, M. G., Mocci, S., et al. (1994) Role of colony stimulating factor-1 in the establishment and regulation of tissue macrophages during postnatal development of the mouse. *Development* **120,** 1357–1372.

3. Cheers, C. and McKenzie, I. (1978) Resistance and susceptibility of mice to bacterial infection: genetics of listeriosis. *Infect. Immun.* **19,** 755–762.

4. Gregory, S. H., Sagnimeni, A. J., and Wing, E. J. (1996) Bacteria in the bloodstream are trapped in the liver and killed by immigrating neutrophils. *J. Immunol.* **157,** 2514–2520.

5. Guleria, I. and Pollard, J. W. (2001) Aberrant macrophage and neutrophil population dynamics and impaired Th1 response to *Listeria monocytogenes* in colony-stimulating factor 1- deficient mice. *Infect. Immun.* **69,** 1795–1807.

6. Guleria, I. and Pollard, J. W. (2000) The trophoblast is a component of the innate immune system during pregnancy. *Nat. Med.* **6,** 589–593.

7. Kaufmann, S. H. E. (1993) Immunity to intracellular bacteria. *Annu. Rev. Immunol.* **11,** 129–163.

8. Luo, Y., Lee, A., Shen, H., and Radice, G. L. (2003) Altering tissue tropism of *Listeria monocytogenes* by ectopically expressing human E-cadherin in transgenic mice. *Microb. Pathog.* **35,** 57–62.

9. Mackler, A. M., Barber, E. M., Takikawa, O., and Pollard, J. W. (2003) Indoleamine 2,3-dioxygenase is regulated by IFN-gamma in the mouse placenta during *Listeria monocytogenes* infection. *J. Immunol.* **170,** 823–830.

10. Medawar, P. B. (1953) Some Immunological and Endocrine Problems raised by evolution of viviparity in vertebrates. *Symp. Soc. Exp. Biol.* **7,** 320–328.

11. Mellor, A. L. and Munn, D. H. (2000) Immunology at the maternal-fetal interface: lessons for T cell tolerance and suppression. *Annu. Rev. Immunol.* **18,** 367–391.

12. Milon, G. (1997) *Listeria monocytogenes* in laboratory mice: a model of short-term infectious and pathogenic processes controllable by regulated protective immune responses. *Immunol. Rev.* **158,** 37–46.
13. Munn, D. H., Zhou, M., Attwood, J. T., et al. (1998) Prevention of allogeneic fetal rejection by tryptophan catabolism. *Science* **281,** 1191–1193.
14. Pollard, J. W., Hunt, J. S., Wiktor-Jedrzejczak, W., and Stanley, E. R. (1991) A pregnancy defect in the osteopetrotic (*op/op*) mouse demonstrates the requirement for CSF-1 in female fertility. *Dev. Biol.* **148,** 273–283.
15. Qazi, S. N., Rees, C. E., Mellits, K. H., and Hill, P. J. (2001) Development of gfp vectors for expression in *Listeria monocytogenes* and other low g+c Gram positive bacteria. *Microb. Ecol.* **41,** 301–309.
16. Redline, R. W. and Lu, C. Y. (1987) Role of local immunosuppression in murine fetoplacental listeriosis. *J. Clin. Invest.* **79,** 1234–1241.
17. Redline, R. W. and Lu, C. Y. (1988) Specific defects in the anti-listerial immune response in discrete regions of the murine uterus and placenta account for susceptibility to infection. *J. Immunol.* **140,** 3947–3955.
18. Redline, R. W., McKay, D. B., Vazquez, M. A., Papaioannou, V. E., and Lu, C. Y. (1990) Macrophage functions are regulated by the substratum of murine decidual stromal cells. *J. Clin. Invest.* **85,** 1951–1958.
19. Redline, R. W., Shea, C. M., Papaioannou, V. E., and Lu, C. Y. (1988) Defective anti-listerial responses in deciduoma of pseudopregnant mice. *Am. J. Pathol.* **133,** 485–497.
20. Silver, H. M. (1998) Listeriosis during pregnancy. *Obstet. Gynecol. Surv.* **53,** 737–740.
21. Unanue, E. R. (1997) Inter-relationship among macrophages, natural killer cells and neutrophils in early stages of Listeria resistance. *Curr. Opin. Immunol.* **9,** 35–43.
22. Unanue, E. R. (1996) Macrophages, NK cells and neutrophils in the cytokine loop of Listeria resistance. *Res. Immunol.* **147,** 499–505.

Index